D1189356

Practical Guide to Epilepsy

WITHDRAWN

Practical Guide to Epilepsy

Mark Manford, MD, FRCP

Consultant Neurologist, Addenbrooke's Hospital, Cambridge and
Bedford Hospital, Bedford
Associate Lecturer, University of Cambridge, United Kingdom

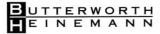

An Imprint of Elsevier Science

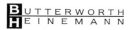

BUTTERWORTH
HEINEMANN

An imprint of Elsevier Science

200 Wheeler Road
Burlington, MA 01803

PRACTICAL GUIDE TO EPILEPSY   ISBN 0-7506-4621-7

Copyright © 2003, Elsevier Science, Inc. All rights reserved.

No part of this publication may be reproduced or transmitted in any form or by any means, electronic or mechanical, including photocopy, recording, or any information storage and retrieval system, without permission in writing from the publisher (Butterworth-Heinemann, 200 Wheeler Road, Burlington, MA 01803).

Notice

Medicine is an ever-changing field. Standard safety precautions must be followed but as new research and clinical experience broaden our knowledge, changes in treatment and drug therapy may become necessary or appropriate. Readers are advised to check the most current product information provided by the manufacturer of each drug to be administered to verify the recommended dose, the method and duration of administration, and contraindications. It is the responsibility of the treating physician, relying on experience and knowledge of the patient, to determine dosages and the best treatment for each individual patient. Neither the Publisher nor the author assumes any liability for any injury and/or damage to persons or property arising from this publication.

The Publisher

Library of Congress Cataloging-in-Publication Data
Manford, Mark.
  Practical guide to epilepsy / Mark Manford.
    p. ; cm.
  Includes bibliographical references.
  ISBN 0-7506-4621-7
   1. Epilepsy. I. Title.
  [DNLM: 1. Epilepsy. WL 385 M276p 2003]
  RC372 .M266 2003
  616.8'53–dc21
                                    2002038241

University of Nottingham
at Derby Library

Acquisitions Editor: Susan Pioli

CE/MVY

Printed in the United States of America.

Last digit is the print number: 9 8 7 6 5 4 3 2 1

100318 1948T

To Ruth and John, who made it all possible and to Catherine, Thomas, Evie, Anuska and Helena, who have to put up with the consequences.

Contents

SECTION 4   SPECIAL SITUATIONS

SECTION 5   PSYCHOSOCIAL ISSUES

Preface

Why buy this book rather than the other epilepsy texts on the shelves next to it. Is it the cheapest? Well, if true, that would be one good reason. Is it better than they are? As the author, I don't think my opinion is entirely impartial. You'll have to decide for yourself, but let me explain what I am trying to do. The aim of this book is to set out the rationales in the decision-making processes involved in looking after patients with seizures and epilepsy. How do you approach diagnosis in patients who present in different ways and how much reliance can you put on investigations in different situations? How do you navigate your way through the increasing maze of anti-epileptic drugs, with a near absence of good quality comparative trials? What are the special issues affecting different groups of patients and how do you deal with them? In this book I have tried to use the text to discuss these issues supported by many illustrative (true) case histories. The result is, I hope, a concise but readable text with the fine details kept in tables for reference. The style is hopefully not too didactic, except where I try to explode some medical myths. The text is also liberally sprinkled with flow charts and illustrations to summarise the points made in the text. I use the opening section to describe some of the basic science underpinning epileptology, highlighting the links between science and clinical practice. I hope you will find the result innovative, stimulating and most importantly, clinically useful. I would be interested to hear if you have any comments about the book. You never know, there might be a second edition!

Mark Manford

Acknowledgments

I wish to thank the following for their invaluable help and advice concerning various aspects of this book: Nagui Antoun; Simon Boniface; Alasdair Coles; Anne-Marie Laing; Belinda Lennox; Alasdair Parker and Steve Sawcer. Nagui, Simon, Justin Cross, Julia Bradford and Alasdair Parker also helped with some of the illustrations. Of course I would like to thank my family who were made into a computer widow and computer orphans – again!

Abbreviations

AD:	Alzheimer's disease
ADNFLE:	Autosomal dominant nocturnal frontal lobe epilepsy
ADRESD:	Autosomal dominant epilepsy with speech dyspraxia
AED:	Anti-epileptic drug
AMPA:	Alpha-amino-3-hydroxy-5-methyl-4-isoxazole propionate
AP:	Action potential
ASS:	Acute symptomatic seizure
AVM:	Arteriovenous malformations
BCOE:	Benign childhood occipital epilepsy
BECTS:	Benign epilepsy with centrotemporal spikes
BZ:	Benzodiazepine
CAE:	Childhood absence epilepsy
CPS:	Complex partial seizure
CSE:	Convulsive status epilepticus
CT:	Computerized tomography (scan)
DCD:	Disorder of cortical development
DNET:	Dysembryoplastic neuroepithelial tumor
ECSWS:	Epilepsy with continuous slow waves in sleep
EEG:	Electroencephalography
EMA:	Epilepsy with myoclonic absences
EOBCOE:	Early onset benign childhood occipital epilepsy
EPSP:	Excitatory postsynaptic potential
ETCSA:	Epilepsy with tonic–clonic seizures on awakening
FC:	Febrile convulsions
FDG:	2-[^{18}F]fluoro-2-deoxyglucose
FLAIR:	Fluid attenuated inversion recovery (scan)
FLE:	Frontal lobe epilepsy
FMSE:	Focal motor status epilepticus
FNI:	Functional neuroimaging
FS:	Febrile seizures
GABA:	Gamma amino butyric acid
GBP:	Gabapentin
GEFS+:	Generalized epilepsy with febrile seizures plus
GFR:	Glomerular filtration rate

GLU:	Glutamate
HLA:	Human lymphocytic antigen
HONC:	Hyperglycemic non-ketotic coma
HONH:	Hyperosmolar non-ketotic hyperglycemia
HVS:	Hyperventilation syndrome
IGE:	Idiopathic generalized epilepsy
IPSP:	Inhibitory postsynaptic potential
JAE:	Juvenile absence epilepsy
JME:	Juvenile myoclonic epilepsy
LGS:	Lennox-Gastaut syndrome
LKS:	Landau-Kleffner syndrome
LOBCOE:	Late onset benign childhood occipital epilepsy
LTP:	Long term potentiation
MAE:	Myoclonic astatic epilepsy
MAOI:	Monoamine oxidase inhibitor
MEG:	Magnetoencephalography
MELAS:	Mitochondrial encephalopathy, lactic acidosis and stroke-like episodes
MRC:	Medical Research Council
MRI:	Magnetic resonance imaging
MRS:	Magnetic resonance spectroscopy (scan)
MS:	Myoclonic seizures
MSE:	Myoclonic status epilepticus
MTS:	Mesial temporal sclerosis
NAA:	N-acetyl aspartate
NCS:	Neurocardiogenic syncope
NGPSE:	National general practice study of epilepsy
NMDA:	N-methyl-D-aspartate
NO:	Nitrous oxide
NREM:	Non rapid eye movement (sleep)
NTD:	Neural tube defects
OCD:	Obsessive compulsive disorder
OCP:	Oral contraceptive pill
PCO:	Polycystic ovaries
PDS:	Paroxysmal depolarizing shift
PET:	Positron emission tomography (scan)
PME	Progressive myoclonus epilepsy
PNES:	Psychogenic non-epileptic seizures
POSTS :	Positive sharp transients of sleep
PPR :	Photoparoxysmal response
QOL:	Quality of life
REM:	Rapid eye movement (sleep)
SECC:	Status epilepticus causing confusion
SK:	Saiko-Keishi-To
SLE:	Systemic lupus erythematosis
SMA:	Supplementary motor area
SMR:	Standardized mortality ratio
SPECT:	Single photon emission computerized tomography (scan)
SPM:	Statistical parametric mapping
SPS:	Simple partial seizure

SPSE:	Sensory partial status epilepticus
SSRI:	Selective serotonin reuptake inhibitor
SSW:	Slow spike and wave
S+W:	Spike and wave
SUDEP:	Sudden unexplained death in epilepsy
TCS:	Tonic–clonic seizure
TGA:	Transient global amnesia
TIA:	Transient ischemic attack
TLE:	Temporal lobe epilepsy
TRN:	Thalamic reticular nucleus
TS:	Tuberose sclerosis
UTI:	Urinary tract infection

SECTION 1
Clinical Science

1

Pathophysiology of Epilepsy

- Electroconvulsive therapy for depression shows that any brain has the circuits required for generating a convulsive seizure. We need to understand how this property becomes spontaneously activated in different forms of epilepsy and also how other types of seizure are generated.
- Epileptic seizures are due to abnormal, repeated, synchronous discharge of large groups of neurons. A gross simplification is that there is abnormal neuronal excitation and a lack of normal neuronal inhibition. Most efforts at treatment have been blunt attempts to redress this balance, but the subtleties of the problem remain elusive.
- There are numerous unanswered questions. How does abnormal synchronization come about in different situations and in different epilepsies? What are the structural, neurophysiological and chemical bases of different epilepsies? How do seizures start and stop? Why do seizures sometimes lead into status

epilepticus and why do they usually stop on their own? Why is epilepsy sometimes mild and sometimes severe? Why does epilepsy usually eventually go away and why does it sometimes persist? How do antiepileptic drugs work and how can we design ones that work better? How are EEG abnormalities generated, both ictal and interictal and how do they relate to the seizures themselves?

- Hypotheses must take account of the diversity of the epilepsies: focal epilepsies, generalized epilepsies and acute symptomatic seizures. The spectrum of aetiologies includes pathological foreign tissue lesions, developmental lesions and inherited disorders, where there may be no identifiable structural change at all.
- Evidence for the pathophysiology of epilepsy comes from a variety of experimental and clinical sources. These reflect the experimental models that it is possible to evaluate with current techniques. The challenge is to integrate these into a model of disturbances in the living human brain that has predictive value.

ANATOMY OF THE NEURON

- Neurons come in all sorts of shapes and sizes but they share three essential components.
- The cell body houses the nucleus and most of the metabolic processes of the cell. From the cell body there are two types of membrane-enclosed processes.
- The axon is the output process of the neuron. It may just reach to adjacent cells or may be very long, for example reaching from the cerebral motor cortex to the lower motor neurons of the anterior horn of the spinal cord. The axon branches and at the end of each branch is a synaptic terminal. The synaptic terminal releases packets of a neurotransmitter into a very narrow space, the synaptic cleft. On the other side of the cleft is the postsynaptic membrane. In the CNS, this membrane is usually the membrane on the electrical input side of another neuron.
- The input region of the neuron comprises a complex tree of processes called dendrites and the cell body itself. One axon will synapse onto many different target neurons and one dendritic tree will receive inputs from many neurons, generating a many-to-many relationship between neurons.
- When a neurotransmitter binds to its receptor on the postsynaptic membrane, it may induce a local change in the electrical properties of the neuron. This may either increase (excitatory postsynaptic potential, EPSP) or decrease (inhibitory postsynaptic potential, IPSP) the chance of the target cell's membrane reaching a critical electrical potential that causes an electrical impulse (action potential) to fire down its own axon.

NORMAL NEURONAL MEMBRANE FUNCTIONS

The Resting Potential

- In the intracellular fluid, sodium (Na^+) concentration is low and potassium (K^+) concentration is high under resting conditions.
- In the extracellular fluid the opposite is true, potassium concentration is low and sodium concentration is high.
- An ATP-dependent transporter creates and maintains these concentration gradients. It pumps three sodium ions out of the cell for every two potassium

Derby Hospital NHS
Foundation Trust

Think you and see you soon

np creates a negative membrane potential for the neuron.
l by changes in the intracellular sodium concentration. As
:ion increases, the sodium–potassium pump is activated
Jnder a chemical concentration gradient, some ions leak
mbrane, resulting in an equilibrium with a resting
f −90 millivolts for many neurons.
; from patients with epilepsy show a reduced activity
exchange and an inability to accumulate extracellular
rs to be due to reduced activity of the sodium–potassium
glia.

itatory synapses are stimulated, the excitatory post-
nmate to reach the threshold for an action potential (AP).
channels open briefly and sodium rapidly enters the cell,
hbrane and generating the AP. The AP is an electrical
own the axon to its synaptic terminals where it triggers
hitter, activating the next neuron in the chain.
tial reaches a certain level, potassium channels open and
potassium leaves the cell, reversing the depolarization. The cell becomes hyper-
polarized and there follows a brief refractory period when the cell cannot be
depolarized again.

- In some models of epilepsy, for example the kainate model of hippocampal
epilepsy in rats, this refractory period is missing, allowing higher frequencies of
action potentials and facilitating abnormal neuronal synchronization.

Secondary Ion Channels

- Some ion channels use the energy generated by the resting potential electrical
gradient across the membrane to drive ions in or out of the cell. For example the
sodium–calcium exchanger exchanges three sodium ions into the cell for every
calcium ion taken out.
- When the membrane potential becomes more positive than −30 millivolts, this
exchanger swaps direction, pushing calcium into the cell. This is important both
in physiological situations and in pathological situations where the cell is unable
to maintain the normal action potential.
- Abnormal fluxes of calcium in human cortical slices appear to correlate with the
initiation or termination of seizures.

The Control of Ion Channels

There are two main ways that ion channels may be activated:

- Voltage-gated channels open and close when the membrane potential reaches
specific voltages. These channels are usually selective for a specific ion, such as
sodium, potassium, calcium or chloride. The voltage dependence of these

channels means they may combine in individual neurons to produce voltage-dependent fluxes of ions back and forth across the membrane. This may result in spontaneous voltage oscillations that may form the basis of some of the rhythmical activity of neurons.
- Ligand-gated channels are opened by the binding of a specific substance, often a neurotransmitter.

The Effects of Ligand Binding

The binding of a ligand to its receptor may have two main types of action.

- Ionic receptors cause a fast response with ionic fluxes across the membrane.
- Metabotropic receptors cause a slow response with intracellular changes mediated via a second messenger such as cyclic adenosine monophosphate.

Ion Channel Disorders

- Numerous inherited ion channel disorders have been identified in recent years that may affect many levels of the nervous system. They often cause a paroxysmal disorder, for example, periodic paralyses. Many of the conditions respond to anticonvulsant drugs that alter sodium/potassium channel function, such as phenytoin or carbamazepine or the carbonic anhydrase inhibitor acetazolamide that affects pH so influencing ion fluxes.
- Epilepsy shares some of these characteristics pointing to the possible importance of ion channel disorders in inherited epilepsies. Recently, abnormalities of the sodium channel have been found in a syndrome that is probably relatively common: generalized epilepsy with febrile seizures plus (GEFS+). Two different potassium channel mutations have been described in the rare syndrome benign familial neonatal convulsions (Chapter 3). Abnormalities of the calcium channel have also been identified in an animal model of idiopathic absence epilepsy.

Neurotransmitters

- Excitatory neurotransmitters trigger depolarization of the postsynaptic membrane increasing the chance that the postsynaptic cell will produce an action potential. The main excitatory neurotransmitter is glutamate, which acts at three groups of receptors: AMPA, kainate and NMDA. Other excitatory neurotransmitters are serotonergic, puringergic and some nicotinic receptors.

  1. AMPA receptors are distributed widely throughout the brain. They open ion channels that tend to move the resting potential to 0 millivolts, resulting in depolarization. Four receptor subtypes have been identified: GluR1 to GluR4. In the kindling model of epilepsy, AMPA receptors are implicated in the expression of kindled seizures, but not in the development of kindling, which seems more related to NMDA receptors. Antibodies to the GluR3 receptor have been identified in Rasmussen's encephalitis

(Chapter 14, case 5) and immunization of rabbits with the Glu3 receptor protein produces a syndrome akin to Rasmussen's encephalitis. The antibodies activate the Glu receptor, triggering calcium-mediated cytotoxicity. Genetically modified mice without GluR2 also have a predisposition to seizures.

2. Kainate receptors are also divided into subgroups: low affinity GluR5 to GluR7 and high affinity KA1 and KA2. GluR5 and GluR6 are found in the hippocampus and have ionotropic effects. GluR7 is found widely but not in the hippocampus and may be important in regulating neurotransmitter release.

3. NMDA receptors act much more slowly than the other glutamate receptors, over hundreds of milliseconds rather than 5 to 10 milliseconds. They induce calcium entry, causing a biochemical cascade within the neuron, which alters the sensitivity of the neuron to further excitation, an event that may be crucial in epileptogenesis (long-term potentiation, below). NMDA receptors are voltage-dependent. They are unusual in that they require the binding of a co-agonist, glycine and the channel is blocked by magnesium. Hypomagnesemia is associated with recurrent seizures and magnesium sulfate may be used to treat seizures, especially those complicating eclampsia. A variety of other NMDA antagonists are effective anticonvulsants but their toxicity has precluded their clinical use.

• Inhibitory neurotransmitters trigger hyperpolarization of the postsynaptic membrane decreasing the chance of a postsynaptic action potential. The main inhibitory neurotransmitter is gamma-aminobutyric acid (GABA), which acts at two main kinds of receptor. Glycine is also an inhibitory neurotransmitter and nicotinic receptors may also be inhibitory at some synapses.

1. $GABA_A$ receptors are widespread in the CNS. They are ligand-gated chloride channels that mediate rapid inhibition. A number of animal models of epilepsy are associated with alterations of GABA activity. Angelman's syndrome is a condition characterized by severe epilepsy and mental retardation. It is due to a deletion on chromosome 15, which includes $GABA_A$ receptor subunits.

2. Many effective antiepileptic drugs act on the GABAergic system (below). GABA antagonists such as bicuculline or picrotoxin are potent proconvulsant agents, used in animal models.

3. Some but not all resections of human epileptic tissue show reduced $GABA_A$ receptor binding. Positron emission tomography (PET) studies of flumazenil (a $GABA_A$ receptor antagonist) in human temporal lobe epilepsy also show reduced binding *in vivo*. Qualitative studies of human epileptic tissue suggest that even where numbers of receptors are unchanged, the binding properties of the receptors may be altered and this varies depending on the type of pathology underlying the epilepsy.

• Other neurotransmitters are also implicated in epilepsy. Autosomal dominant nocturnal frontal lobe epilepsy (Chapter 3) is often due to defects of the alpha subunit of the nicotinic acetylcholine receptor. Acetylcholine is important in cortical arousal and influences a wide variety of other neurotransmitters including GABA, glutamate, serotonin and noradrenaline but how it is associated with seizures is unclear.

Paroxysmal Depolarizing Shift

- Animal models of focal epilepsy can be created by applying substances locally to the cerebral cortex such as penicillin, bicuculline or picrotoxin. One property is simultaneous electrographic discharges very similar to those seen in the inter-ictal EEG of patients with epilepsy. The neurophysiological basis of this is thought to be the paroxysmal depolarizing shift (PDS).
- PDS comprises a large EPSP generated by the synchronous activation of surrounding neurons converging on the cell being recorded. The PDS is thought to be dependent on sodium and calcium fluxes, which increase the excitability of the neuron for 50 to 200 milliseconds. During this period, any afferent impulses are much more likely to generate an action potential. This is followed by a GABA-mediated hyperpolarization of the neuron for 500 to 2000 ms that reduces excitability. This pattern occurring simultaneously in a large number of neurons leads to synchronous discharges, manifesting as the interictal spike on EEG.

Long-Term Potentiation (LTP)

- High frequency stimulation of the hippocampus in animals causes a poten-tiation of synaptic responses lasting many hours, which is called LTP. Repeating the process may cause potentiation that lasts months. In other words, certain kinds of stimuli lower the threshold of neurons to further stim-ulation. The positive feedback of LTP is a form of synaptic plasticity that is likely to play a key role in memory formation, but if LTP goes wrong, it may be an important substrate of pathological neuronal synchronization and epilepsy.
- *N*-methyl-D-aspartate (NMDA) receptors and protein kinases appear to be important in the first 3 hours of LTP. Protein kinases may act by modulating the effect of magnesium on NMDA receptors and facilitating further activation.
- The later phases of long-term potentiation are blocked by inhibiting platelet activating factor that mediates enhanced glutamate release.

Mechanisms of Neuronal Synchronization

- Blockade of GABA inhibition results in the PDS and unmasks recurrent excitatory circuits within the hippocampus.
- Non-synaptic mechanisms may be important. For example action potentials could spread between neurons via gap junctions. Alterations in electric fields generated by action potentials may also result in firing of adjacent neurons. Repeated firing of neurons probably enhances these field effects. As neurons fire, sodium moves into cells and with it goes extracellular water, bringing axons closer together. In addition, seizures increase extracellular potassium concentration in area CA3 of the hippocampus, and potassium enhances inter-ictal spikes.

Mechanisms of Action of Anti-Epileptic Drugs

Most drugs currently available have multiple effects. Nevertheless there are broad categories of actions that are common to many drugs and provide a basis for understanding drug actions on neuronal hyperexcitability (Figure 1.1).

- Sodium channel blockade is a major mode of action of phenytoin, carbamazepine and oxcarbazepine. The action is use-dependent so a normal axon firing at low frequencies is relatively unaffected but pathological firing at higher frequencies is reduced, so preventing seizures. These drugs are effective for focal epilepsy and are sometimes used to treat the tonic–clonic seizures of idiopathic generalized epilepsy (IGE) but may exacerbate absence and myoclonic seizures. Lamotrigine and topiramate also significantly block sodium channels but have additional actions on other sites, probably accounting for their broader spectrum of action.
- GABA augmentation is an effect of many drugs, achieved in different ways. Vigabatrin irreversibly blocks GABA breakdown by GABA transaminase and tiagabine blocks a GABA reuptake site. Benzodiazepines bind to a benzodiazepine receptor that is linked to the GABA$_A$ receptor. They augment inhibition by increasing the open time of the chloride channel. Barbiturates bind to the GABA$_A$ receptor and increase the duration of the chloride flux, augmenting hyperpolarization. Gabapentin appears to augment the action of a pump that pumps GABA out of cells into the extracellular space, increasing the concentration available to bind inhibitory receptors. Topiramate also enhances GABA currents.

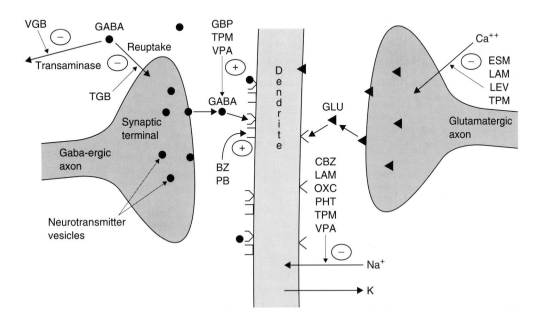

Figure 1.1. Excitatory glutamatergic and inhibitory GABAergic synapses showing major ion channels and sites of action of some antiepileptic drugs. BZ, benzodiazepines; Ca^{++}, calcium ions; CBZ, carbamazepine; ESM, ethosuximide; GBP, gabapentin; GLU, glutamate; K$^+$, potassium ions, LAM, lamotrigine; LEV, levetiracetam; OXC, oxcarbazepine; PB, phenobarbitone; PHT, phenytoin; Na$^+$, sodium ions; TGB, tiagabine; TPM, topiramate; VGB, vigabatrin; VPA, valproate.

- Different calcium channels occur at various sites in the CNS. Ethosuximide binds to calcium channels in the thalamus, reducing calcium influx and preventing the thalamocortical excitatory coupling that is characteristic of IGE absence epilepsy. It has virtually no effect on any other seizure type. Lamotrigine also acts on calcium channels reducing glutamate release, perhaps contributing to its actions in generalized epilepsies.
- Blocking excitation at glutamate receptors is another potential mechanism of action. Topiramate has been found to inhibit alpha-amino-3-hydroxy-5-methyl-4-isoxazole propionate (AMPA) but not NMDA receptors, which may decrease neuronal excitability. Other drugs with predominant effects on glutamate have been developed but have failed in clinical trials because of excessive neurotoxicity and sedation.

PATHOPHYSIOLOGY OF IDIOPATHIC EPILEPSIES

- The absence seizures of IGE have distinct electroclinical features. In childhood absence epilepsy (CAE) the EEG shows a very typical generalized spike and wave discharge at 3 hertz (Chapter 11, Figure 11.4). Between these discharges the EEG and the patient are normal. Almost as soon as the abnormal discharge starts, patients "switch off" and as soon as it is over they "switch on" with no sequelae apart from amnesia for the duration of the discharge. Stimulation of the midline and intralaminar nuclei in cats produces a similar bilateral cortical discharge. Abnormal thalamocortical circuits are implicated in animal models but the emphasis varies between species, as to whether cortex or thalamus is the most crucial in generating the abnormalities. PET studies show selectively increased thalamic blood flow in human absence epilepsy, supporting its role.
- The normal thalamus can switch between two modes: waking and sleeping. In waking mode, thalamic neurons fire at high frequency and low amplitude. In sleeping mode, thalamic neurons fire at low frequency and high amplitude. Switching between modes is achieved via the thalamic reticular nucleus (TRN). This structure forms a shell around the thalamus and projects an inhibitory (GABAergic) output to the thalamic relay nuclei and receives inputs both from collaterals of thalamocortical relay fibers and from corticothalamic fibers.
- A key membrane property controlling the ability of the TRN to switch modes is the low threshold calcium spike. $GABA_B$ inhibitory postsynaptic potentials give rise to a rebound burst of high frequency action potentials, mediated by the low-threshold calcium spike. This combination results in oscillations seen in slow wave sleep. Ethosuximide has a specific action on thalamic T-type calcium channels, suggesting that this mechanism is also central to the generation of absence seizures and supporting the role for an abnormality of this normal switching mechanism in IGE absences.
- NMDA antagonists reduce spike-wave discharges in animal models, probably influencing glutamatergic inputs from the thalamus and cerebral cortex. Lamotrigine is an effective anticonvulsant for IGE absences. It reduces glutamate release and may have some effect on calcium channels in addition to its other major effect on sodium channels. Pure sodium channel blockers tend to make absence seizures worse.

- GABA-mediated inhibition promotes neuronal synchronization and anticonvulsants that work through GABA, such as vigabatrin and tiagabine often make absence epilepsy worse, both in animal models and in people. Although benzodiazepines also augment GABAergic function in the TRN, their indirect effect seems to be to suppress $GABA_B$ receptors in the thalamic relay nuclei, reducing slow calcium spikes and leading to a reduction in spike-wave discharges. In one form of GEFS+ there is a mutation of the GABA receptor, reducing its sensitivity to benzodiazepines.

HOW SEIZURES START

Any model of the mechanisms of epilepsy must try to explain why seizures start at particular times, under particular circumstances and equally why they stop after a relatively consistent period of time.

- The common interictal spike is characterized by a depolarization followed by a hyperpolarization that protects against another immediate depolarization. Intracranial recordings undertaken preoperatively in patients with focal epilepsy tend to show high amplitude sharp waves at the onset of the seizure. As a tonic–clonic seizure develops, normal hyperpolarization is lost and the EEG shows an evolution of fast rhythmical activity – the recruiting rhythm – culminating in a seizure. Propagation from the site of onset of the seizure is usually associated with generation of a recruiting rhythm.
- In IGE absence seizures, the mechanism is different. The seizure is characterized by spike-wave discharges, in which the hyperpolarization is preserved and indeed, inhibitory mechanisms are likely to be important in enhancing synchronization of populations of neurons and in seizure development.

WHAT TRIGGERS SEIZURES?

- Some patients recognize a non-specific activation of their epilepsy such that seizures are more likely to occur under certain circumstances. These include sleep deprivation, emotional stress, alcohol withdrawal and phases of the menstrual cycle.
- Other patients recognize specific triggers for their seizures. These are stimuli that will reliably, though not necessarily invariably, lead to a seizure within seconds.

Non-Specific Activation

Careful study reveals that the timing of seizures is rarely totally random. In some cases specific factors can be identified that substantially increase the risk of seizures.

Fever

Febrile seizures are a specific entity of seizures occurring in young children without any other seizure precipitant. Febrile seizures may occur outside these age limits in GEFS+ (Chapter 3). Some older patients may have well controlled

epilepsy that only emerges with intercurrent infection and fever. Carers of handicapped children and young adults often notice a propensity to seizures at times
of infection. Early treatment with antipyretics such as paracetamol may help this
complication.

Case History 1

A 28-year-old woman suffered multiple sclerosis with a mild paraparesis and bladder disturbance. She was admitted to hospital with repeated convulsive seizures. She
was found to have a high fever secondary to urinary tract infection (UTI) that settled
with antibiotics and the seizures were controlled with benzodiazepines and phenytoin. She was discharged home and remained well until nine months later she was
readmitted with further seizures and another UTI.

Sleep Deprivation

Sleep deprivation activates epileptiform interictal EEG abnormalities. It can also
trigger seizures, especially in IGE. Avoiding the trigger factor may be all that is
required to prevent seizures. Antiepileptic drugs are not always effective, if the
individual continues to be sleep-deprived.

Case History 2

An 18-year-old woman suffered a tonic–clonic seizure the day after arriving on
holiday at a distant destination. She had taken an overnight flight and had had little
sleep during the night. She had an EEG that showed generalized epileptiform abnormalities. She remained well without treatment for a year until she had a further
seizure, the morning after a "stopover" birthday party with friends, where she had
consumed only one glass of wine.

Alcohol

Alcohol is strongly associated with epilepsy in many ways (Chapter 13). The most
immediate effect is alcohol withdrawal seizures, which commonly affect patients
with IGE but may occur in individuals after an alcoholic binge, even if they do not
suffer habitual seizures.

Specific Activation

Visual Stimuli

- Stroboscopic stimulation is a well-known trigger for seizures but is relevant
  in less than 5 percent of epilepsy. The prevalence of photosensitivity is about
  0.03 percent of the non-epileptic population but it is seen much more commonly
  in the relatives of those with photosensitive epilepsy (Figure 1.2).
- The definition of stroboscopic photosensitivity is based on EEG criteria
  (Chapter 7). Only the most abnormal photoparoxysmal response to photic
  stimulation is strongly associated with epilepsy. Usually, maximal sensitivity is
  at 15 to 20 hertz flicker and it is rare for individuals to be sensitive below 6 hertz
  or above 60 hertz. Over 95 percent of individuals who exhibit this response will
  develop epilepsy.

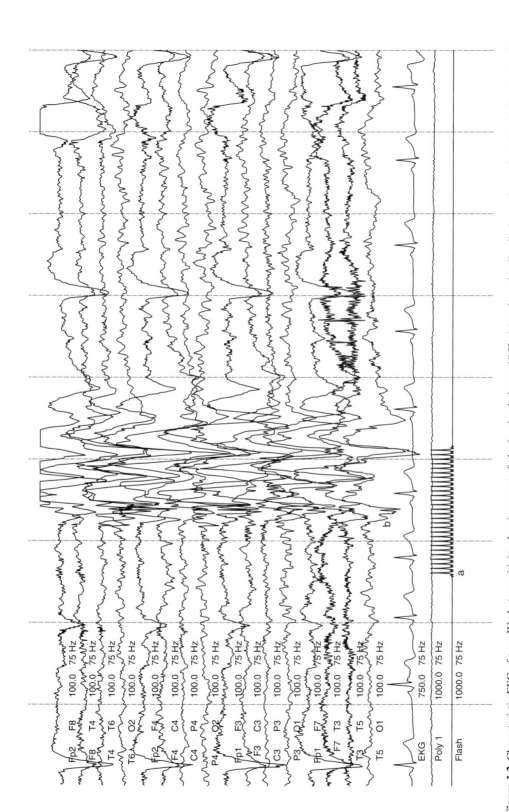

Figure 1.2. Characteristic EEG of type IV photosensitivity showing onset of photic stimulation at 18 Hz (a) and a polyspike discharge that outlasts the photic stimulus (b).

- Photosensitivity may trigger absences, myoclonus or tonic–clonic seizures and is nearly always part of an IGE syndrome. Occasionally photosensitivity is associated with focal occipital epilepsy.
- Most patients also have seizures that are not triggered by photic stimuli and for many patients the epilepsy will remit but photosensitivity commonly persists into adult life. Treatment may abolish seizures, without preventing EEG evidence of photosensitivity.
- A variety of other visual stimuli may trigger seizures (Table 1.1). In general a stimulus is more likely to cause a seizure if it occupies a large part of the visual field and it is viewed with both eyes. This provides potential strategies for treatment, including sitting back from the television and using a remote control, and covering one eye.
- Autoinduction of seizures may occur in up to a third of patients who suffer photosensitive seizures. Some individuals enjoy the sensation of an impending seizure. Others use the ability to induce seizures to deal with stressful situations. They may wave their hands in front of their eyes, sit close to the television or use video games.

Case History 3

A 37-year-old woman described tonic–clonic seizures that had occurred in adolescence. She also recalled that her father drove her along a tree-lined avenue to school and that often on this journey she felt disorientated if the sunlight flickered through the trees. After she married, she noticed she also felt uncomfortable when she ironed her husband's striped shirts but she had no further seizures until one day in a shopping centre, she collapsed after glancing down at a metallic escalator. Her EEG showed profound photosensitivity and she was treated with sodium valproate with a good response. High-contrast lines may trigger seizures.

Other Sensory Seizures

- Seizures have been reported to occur in response to all sensory modalities (Table 1.2), but these are much rarer than photosensitive seizures. For example some patients with focal motor seizures may experience seizures if there is contact with the body part involved in the seizure.

Table 1.1. Additional Forms of Photosensitivity

Seizure Stimulus	Characteristics
Patterns	High contrast vertical lines such as striped paper or runners on escalator steps
Specific wavelengths	May vary between individuals. EEG abnormality builds up more slowly over the posterior cortex than in stroboscopic sensitivity. Tinted spectacles may help
Television epilepsy	May be due to mains alternating current flicker at 50 Hz. This is less common in USA where mains is at 60 Hz. May also be due to stroboscopic images on screen and in video games
Fixation-off sensitivity	Seen when the patient is not fixating, usually in benign occipital epilepsies
Fixation-on sensitivity	Seen when the patient is actively fixating. Usually in occipital epilepsies

Table 1.2. Some Rarer Sensory Triggers for Seizures

Sensory Seizure Triggers
Somatosensory
Muscle stretch
Tapping
Hot water immersion (in India)
Vibration
Smell
Taste
Vestibular

- Rarely, somatosensory stimuli generate giant cortical somatosensory evoked potentials that provide additional evidence of abnormal cortical activation.
- If an external stimulus mimics a habitual aura, seizures may occasionally be triggered. For example a smell of onions may trigger a seizure in patients whose aura is a smell of onions. The external stimulus perhaps activates a well-trodden neuronal pathway that can also be activated endogenously to generate a seizure.

Startle Epilepsy

- Startle epilepsy is a moderately common form of reflex epilepsy. This form of epilepsy often occurs in children or adolescents with a developmental abnormality such as cortical dysplasia or birth injury. The attacks are most commonly tonic seizures, although patients with Down syndrome may develop absences. Seizures are triggered by a stimulus that is both sudden and unexpected. The same stimulus will not cause a seizure when the patient can anticipate it. Effective stimuli are usually loud noises, or sometimes sudden somatosensory stimuli. More than one modality may be effective in the same patient and most patients also suffer spontaneous seizures. The condition may be difficult to differentiate from idiopathic startle disease or psychogenic disturbances, especially as the EEG is often normal, even during the ictus.

Complex Reflex Epilepsies

- A higher cortical function is the trigger in these cases (Table 1.3). The more complex the task, the more likely that a seizure will be triggered in sensitive patients. This may be analogous to the effect in photosensitive seizures, reflecting recruitment of a larger volume of cerebral cortex.
- Treatments are usually valproate, clobazam or clonazepam, which may be very effective.

HOW SEIZURES STOP

- The duration of seizures varies between individuals and between syndromes. IGE absences often last only seconds and supplementary motor area focal seizures are usually less than a minute long. Tonic–clonic seizures usually last

Table 1.3. Complex Seizure Triggers

Seizure Trigger	Characteristics
Reading	After reading for some time. Jaw starts to click and myoclonus of face then tonic–clonic seizures. May be triggered by other language functions e.g. writing or speaking and may have a family history of seizures. EEG shows 3–6 Hz discharges in the temporo-parietal region. Possibly a variant of juvenile myoclonic epilepsy (JME)
Thinking	Intense mental concentration e.g. with card games, problem solving or chess, triggers a tonic–clonic seizure. EEG shows generalized spike and wave. Possibly a variant of JME
Music	May be highly specific, even just one tune. Usually manifests as temporal lobe seizures
Eating	Rare, mainly in Sri Lanka. Trigger is usually soon after eating but may be the sight of food, swallowing or abdominal distension. Usually partial seizures

2 to 3 minutes and it is rare for any seizure to last more than 5 minutes unless it is evolving into status epilepticus.

- The EEG at the end of the seizure and post-ictally also varies between different seizure types. It is likely that different mechanisms are at play in terminating each of these seizure types at different times.
- After focal seizures there is often focal slowing of the EEG in the region of seizure onset, associated with a focal disturbance of cerebral function, such as dysphasia after a temporal lobe seizure or Todd's paresis after a motor cortex seizure. Depression of the EEG and loss of clinical function after a seizure are associated with reduced cerebral blood flow. These effects appear to be partly mediated by opiates, as postictal effects are enhanced by pretreatment with opiates and reduced by the opiate antagonist, naloxone.
- After IGE absences the EEG returns immediately to normal and the patient has no postictal effect. With these seizures there appears to be no postictal alteration of blood flow.
- Why some seizures evolve into status epilepticus is unclear, but a failure of GABAergic inhibitory processes is possible. Persistent metabolic activity and high cerebral perfusion characterize status epilepticus, causing an eventual collapse of a number of homeostatic mechanisms. It evolves through a number of definable stages (Chapter 14) that become less coordinated, with a breakdown of neuronal synchronization and a decline in the clinical correlate of status epilepticus. When untreated status epilepticus seems to evolve to a state of "neuronal exhaustion" where the brain is unable to sustain the high rates of metabolic activity and ion fluxes necessary for continued seizure activity. Ultimately calcium influx may trigger apoptosis.

BIBLIOGRAPHY

Berkovic SF. Paroxysmal movement disorders and epilepsy: links across the channel. Neurology 2000;55:165–170.

Bliss TV, Lomo T. Long-lasting potentiation of synaptic transmission in the dentate area of the anaesthetized rabbit following stimulation of the perforant path. J Physiol 1973;23:331–336.

Delgado-Escueta AV, Wilson WA, Olsen RW, Porter RJ (eds). Jaspers basic mechanisms of the epilepsies. Section IV-A neuronal channels, receptors, and transporters: molecular structure, gating and pharmacology. Adv Neurol 1999;79:433–560.

Dichter M, Wilcox KS. Excitatory synaptic transmission. In Engel J Jr, Pedley TA (eds). Epilepsy: A Comprehensive Textbook. Lippincott Raven: Philadelphia, 1997;251–263.

Frucht MM, Quig M, Scwaner C, Fountain NB. Distribution of seizure precipitants among epilepsy syndromes. Epilepsia 2000;41:1534–1539.

Huguenard JR. Neuronal circuitry of thalamocortical epilepsy and mechanisms of antiabsence drug action. Adv Neurol 1999;79:991–1000.

Nayak A, Browning. Presynaptic and postsynaptic mechanisms of long term potentiation. Adv Neurol 1999;79:645–658.

Ritaccio AL. Reflex seizures. Neurologic Clinics 1994;12:57–83.

Sherman SM. A wake-up call from the thalamus. Nature Neuroscience 2001;4:344–345.

Takahashi Y, Fujiwara T, Yagi K, Seino M. Photosensitive epilepsies and mechanisms of the photoparoxysmal response. Neurology 1999;53:926–932.

2

Anatomy of Epilepsy

Abnormalities affecting neuronal excitability at a single cell level need to be expanded to explain abnormal, synchronous activation of large groups of neurons. In many of the focal epilepsies there are alterations in the anatomical relationships between cells and tissues and in their neurochemical properties. Magnetic resonance imaging (MRI) has also shown the high prevalence of different disorders of cortical development (DCD) and contributed substantially to our understanding. Animal models and resected human tissue have pieced together some of the changes at play in different forms of epilepsy.

MESIAL TEMPORAL LOBE EPILEPSY

- The mesial temporal structures include the amygdala, entorhinal cortex, and hippocampal formation. The normal hippocampal formation is divided into fields CA1 to CA4 and the dentate gyrus (Figure 2.1).
- Mesial temporal sclerosis (MTS) is the commonest cause of focal epilepsy. Commonly, the amygdala, hippocampus, and entorhinal cortex are all affected by MTS and there are highly specific alterations within these structures. In the entorhinal cortex there is severe loss of cells from layer III. These cells provide excitatory input to the CA1 region of the hippocampus. In most cases of MTS, there is marked reduction in cell numbers in the hippocampus, affecting CA1, CA3 and the hilar region of the dentate gyrus, with relative preservation of CA2. The hilum of the dentate gyrus appears to be the most consistently

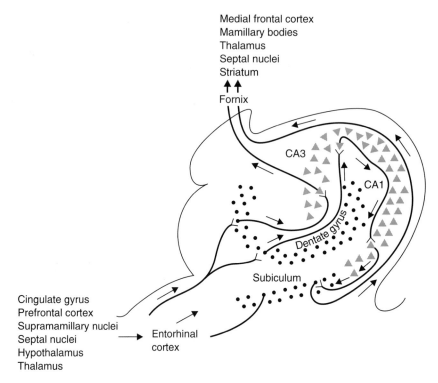

Figure 2.1. The structure of the hippocampus showing major internal circuits and inputs and outputs. Most inputs to the hippocampal formation are from the entorhinal cortex. The flow of information is then to the dentate gyrus, to CA3, CA1 and the subiculum. Most of the output of the hippocampus comes from the subiculum, through a pathway called the fornix. The targets are the mamillary bodies, ventral striatum and some cortical areas including the cingulate and orbitofrontal cortices.

affected in all the patterns of MTS. GABAergic cells are particularly prone to damage: up to 40 percent of these cells are lost from the dentate gyrus and smaller numbers from CA1 and elsewhere. These inhibitory cells are critical in regulating excitability in the hippocampus, especially in controlling the excitatory activity of mossy fibers. Their loss is likely to be an important factor in the failure of inhibition, predisposing to seizures.

- Major structural reorganization of the remaining elements within the mesial temporal structures follows this damage. Mossy fibers are the axons of the granule cells of the dentate gyrus and synapse mostly in the polymorph region of the dentate hilum. They represent the first stage of excitation in the hippocampus. When the hilum suffers seizure-induced cell loss, mossy fibers reorganize into the inner molecular layer. Here they appear to make a monosynaptic excitatory feedback circuit that may be a short-cut, upregulating excitation.
- The reorganized mossy fiber synapses exhibit long-term potentiation (Chapter 1) and neurophysiological studies of granule cells in slice preparations from patients with MTS, show markedly increased spiking that may be blocked by GABA. Prolonged stimulation of the perforant pathway creates the kindling model of hippocampal epilepsy. Cellular recordings of the dentate gyrus show this is followed by a long-lasting loss of $GABA_A$ inhibition in the dentate gyrus,

which at first is nearly complete, then becomes more patchy. Although the total numbers of GABAergic terminals are not altered, they may predispose to seizures because they originate from a smaller group of cells, promoting neuronal synchronization. The response of GABA to induced seizures is also much less in chronically epileptic hippocampi than in control contralateral hippocampi, implying a much reduced ability to control or terminate abnormal excitation.

• Several neurophysiological changes may be observed in abnormal hippocampal tissue. These include evoked bursts of activity, loss of polysynaptic inhibition, prolonged excitatory postsynaptic potentials, spontaneous depolarizing activity and commonly paroxysmal depolarizing shift (Chapter 1).

The Relationship between Febrile Convulsions and Temporal Lobe Epilepsy

• Febrile convulsions (FC) affect as many as 5 percent of children and are the commonest cause of seizures in children aged 3 months to 5 years. About 7 percent of affected children go on to develop epilepsy and these usually have had complex febrile convulsions. Temporal lobe epilepsy (TLE) with MTS is the commonest sequel to febrile convulsions.

• There is a strong genetic component to the risk of febrile seizures, depending on gender and relationship to the proband. For example, mother to son transmission of the trait is as high as 33 percent. Some of these may have generalized epilepsy with febrile seizures plus (GEFS+; Chapter 3).

• There are three hypotheses to explain the link between FC and TLE.

1. MTS underlies both febrile convulsions and TLE. In support of this hypothesis, MRI soon after the acute phase of complex FC has shown pre-existing hippocampal atrophy in some cases. However, it is rare to recognize an insult predisposing to MTS, prior to developing febrile convulsions.

2. Prolonged FC causes MTS. Status epilepticus is known to cause MTS in animal models. It is much more difficult to establish this relationship in humans but MRI in the acute phase of complex FC shows acute edema in the hippocampus in some cases and this progresses to MTS after 1 year.

3. A two stage process underlies MTS. By this hypothesis febrile seizures act on an already abnormal hippocampus to generate MTS. Careful assessment of human temporal tissue resected for refractory epilepsy reveals focal cortical dysgenesis in 35 percent. This finding must predate the development of FC. Dysgenesis in animal studies predisposes to febrile seizures. This hypothesis is clinically attractive since it could explain why the febrile seizure itself is more complex in most of those who go on to develop epilepsy.

CORTICAL DEVELOPMENT AND ABNORMALITIES OF DEVELOPMENT

• Developmental abnormalities of the nervous system are a very common cause of epilepsy, sometimes in association with other neurological problems.

Significant numbers of cases have only come to light since the advent of high resolution MRI.

- The severity of the clinical abnormality depends on the extent of the histological abnormality. Those with very extensive disease tend to suffer mental retardation with other neurological deficits and severe epilepsy. An intermediate histological picture may be associated with milder learning disability. The most subtle pathological findings may cause no deficits or may cause just epilepsy that is relatively easy to control. The pattern of developmental abnormality depends on the timing of the pathological changes in relation to the stages of normal cortical development (Figure 2.2).

Neural Tube Formation

- The central nervous system is formed from the ectoderm in the third to fourth week of gestation. The cells form the neural plate that folds and elongates to make the neural tube stretching the length of the fetus. This process is complete by 28 days of gestation.
- Failure of rostral closure causes anencephaly and failure of caudal closure causes spina bifida. Folic acid deficiency is important in sporadic neural tube defects (NTD) and folic acid supplementation can reduce NTD by 75 percent. Antiepileptic drugs also cause failure of neural tube closure, but whether folic acid has any impact on this form of spina bifida is not clear. Defects of the *Pax1* and *Pdgfra* genes are implicated in NTD in mice but their role in humans is not known.

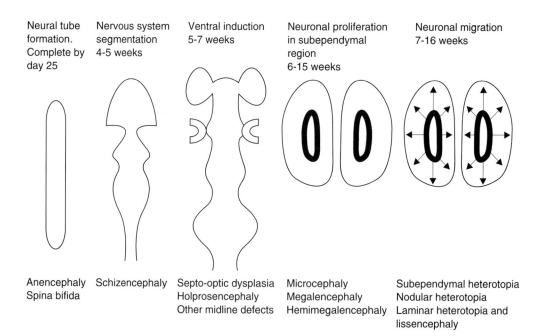

Neural tube formation. Complete by day 25

Nervous system segmentation 4-5 weeks

Ventral induction 5-7 weeks

Neuronal proliferation in subependymal region 6-15 weeks

Neuronal migration 7-16 weeks

Anencephaly
Spina bifida

Schizencephaly

Septo-optic dysplasia
Holprosencephaly
Other midline defects

Microcephaly
Megalencephaly
Hemimegalencephaly

Subependymal heterotopia
Nodular heterotopia
Laminar heterotopia and lissencephaly

Figure 2.2. Important stages of neural development and consequences of maldevelopment.

Nervous System Segmentation

- After closure the neural tube elongates, folds and starts to differentiate in a rostrocaudal direction into forebrain, midbrain, hindbrain and spinal cord. These structures further differentiate into the major regions of the CNS and then into the multiple smaller regions, nuclei and pathways of the brain and spinal cord over the ensuing weeks of gestation. Homeobox genes encode transcriptional factors that include sequences involved in DNA binding. There are a number of different genes expressed in different brain regions and they are important in local development.
- Deletions of the *Otx1* gene in the mouse cause abnormalities of cortical lamination and small hippocampi, resulting in epilepsy. A homologous defect has not been found in humans. Schizencephaly (Figure 2.3) describes clefts in the brain running from the pia to the ventricle and lined by gray matter that is abnormally laminated (polymicrogyria). The severity varies from a localized abnormality giving no symptoms to a severe, diffuse disturbance with microcephaly, mental retardation and severe epilepsy. Severe familial forms are seen in association with defects of the homeobox gene *EMX2*.

Ventral Induction

- Initially, the forebrain contains a single fluid-filled chamber. This then splits to form the two hemispheres connected by the corpus callosum, with lateral ventricles separated by the septum pellucidum.
- Failure of this split is often associated with other midline defects. In holoprosencephaly there are abnormalities of the anterior portions of the lateral

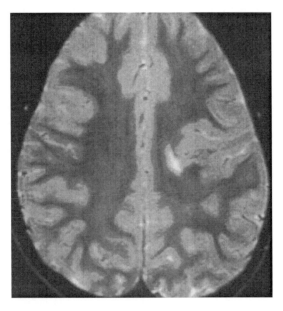

Figure 2.3. T_2 weighted MRI of schizencephaly showing a deep cleft extending into the white matter. These clefts are often lined by abnormally small gyri (polymicrogyria).

ventricles, the corpus callosum and the septum pellucidum. Some patients have a single midline "cyclops" eye, cleft lip and other facial abnormalities. This abnormality may be due to several gene defects and acquired causes include maternal diabetes, retinoic acid exposure, cytomegalovirus and rubella. Septo-optic dysplasia is characterized by absence of the septum pellucidum, optic nerve hypoplasia and hypothalamic dysfunction. Suggested acquired causes include maternal ingestion of antiepileptic drugs, alcohol and cocaine.

Neuronal Proliferation and Differentiation

- Neuroepithelial cells proliferate in units that later populate specific regions of the cerebral cortex. Proteins called cyclins and tumor-suppressor genes (including retinoblastoma protein and *p53* gene) are important in regulating the movement of cells between stages of the cell cycle. The number of cells produced is initially much larger than the number of cells in the final cerebral cortex. A proportion of the cells undergoes programmed cell death (apoptosis). Cysteine aspartate specific proteases (caspases) are probably important in this process.
- Animals without caspase 3 have abnormally big brains. Megalencephaly (big brain) is associated with a big head, mental retardation and epilepsy. There is an excess of brain cells and the cells themselves are also abnormally large. Hemimegalencephaly may be part of a neurocutaneous syndrome: hypomelanosis of Ito or linear sebaceous naevus syndrome. Microcephaly is associated with a variety of inherited diseases of the nervous system and may be due to numerous *in utero* insults, including alcohol, cocaine or infections by toxoplasmosis, cytomegalovirus, or human immunodeficiency virus. These severe structural abnormalities cause severe mental retardation and epilepsy.

Neuronal Migration

- The first cells to populate the cerebral cortex are Cajal-Retzius cells that inhabit layer one, the most superficial of the six layers. Billions of neurons are produced at the ventricular surface which then migrate to the future cortex. They move along glial processes that radiate from the ventricle to the cortex. This process involves molecules such as reelin, laminin, astrotactin, and fibronectin that enable the neuron to adhere to the glial process. The movement itself is probably mediated by the cycling of microtubules. The first cells to arrive populate the deepest layer (layer six of the cerebral cortex) and subsequent arrivals move through these cells to inhabit the more superficial layers. The cortex is formed from the inside-out. At the ventricle, the neurons are divided into populations that receive input from cells designated to become different thalamic nuclei. These groupings probably help to define different cortical regions by their thalamic connectivity.
- As well as arriving at the right place, cells have to make appropriate functional connections. Cytoskeletal elements cause processes to grow out from the cell body. These are guided by a variety of chemical cues including adhesion molecules such as the neural cell adhesion molecule (NCAM) family,

chemoattractants, and chemorepellants, such as collapsin and platelet activating factor, that guide growth to the target. There is an initial excess production of neurons and connections that are subsequently pruned. This pruning partly depends on functional use of the pathway by the animal as it matures. Hubel and Wiesel classically showed how geniculocortical connections can be disrupted by covering one eye of a kitten from birth. This suggests a mechanism whereby abnormal brain activity may be self-reinforcing by modification of connectivity.

Disorders of Cortical Development

Disorders of cortical development (DCD) are characterized by abnormalities of neuronal number, gyral pattern, cortical thickness, and location of neurons in the deep white matter. The classification of DCD is evolving but several types are recognized (Table 2.1). The commonest disorders are heterotopias, which are ectopic collections of normal-appearing neurons that failed to migrate to the cortical mantle. They may be focal or widespread. Their position may vary from band heterotopias subjacent to the cortex to subependymal heterotopias adjacent to the ventricular surface. They may be associated with metabolic disturbances such as leukodystrophy or gangliosidoses, neurocutaneous syndromes, chromosomal abnormalities, or exposure to teratogenic infections or drugs *in utero*. Focal heterotopias are amongst the commonest substrates underlying refractory partial epilepsy, accounting for 15 percent of patients in one study (Figures 2.4–2.6).

- The pathophysiological basis of seizure generation in cortical developmental abnormalities is not clear. There have been very limited cytoarchitectural or immunohistochemical studies of human dysplastic cortex. One small study recently suggested that there are shared common features. As well as break-up of cortical lamination, there is an alteration of the balance of cell types with a relative increase of excitatory neurons.
- The abnormal cortex appears to be highly epileptogenic. Intracranial EEG recordings of the abnormal cortex show almost continuous epileptic activity in as many as two thirds of patients. This is much higher than in other causes of cortical epilepsy. The finding of continuous spiking over one region of the cortex in the extracranial EEG may be more common in DCD than in other causes of epilepsy.
- Magnetoencephalography and *in vitro* studies have suggested that the seizures are generated in the dysplastic tissue itself, rather than from surrounding brain. These findings support the inherent epileptogenicity of the cortex in focal dysplasia, although the precise mechanisms remain unclear.

Neurocutaneous Syndromes

- A variety of neurocutaneous syndromes may be associated with abnormalities of cortical development. Some of these are associated with histological appearances that include features of abnormal cortical development. One of the commonest is tuberose sclerosis (TS, incidence 1/6000 births) which often causes very severe epilepsy in children, including West syndrome and Lennox-Gastaut

Table 2.1. Some Disorders of Cortical Development

Syndrome and Genetic Basis	Pathophysiology	Clinical Features
Lissencephaly (smooth brain) *LIS 1* gene chromosome 17	Abnormality of a microtubule-associated protein involved in neurite outgrowth. Arrest of cortical development at weeks 15–17. Causes a four-layered cortex with the worst abnormalities posteriorly. The same gene may cause band heterotopia in females (Figure 2.4)	Most commonly in Miller-Dieker syndrome with facial cardiac and sacral abnormalities. Other genes may also produce this phenotype. Most patients have severe retardation and epilepsy from the first year of life. Infantile spasms in 80%
X-linked lissencephaly and band heterotopia syndrome. *Doublecortin* gene	Abnormality of microtubule-associated protein involved in neurite outgrowth. Males have lissencephaly. Females have band heterotopia. Abnormalities are worst anteriorly	Males have severe mental retardation and epilepsy. Females have epilepsy. Lennox-Gastaut syndrome is common. Focal epilepsy with focal motor status and infantile spasms also occur
Type 2 (cobblestone) lissencephaly	Pachygyria (few gyri) or polymicrogyria (many small gyri). Whorls of cells project into subarachnoid space giving cobblestone appearance	Other tissues often affected, especially muscle. Polymicrogyria in Fukuyama muscular dystrophy (muscle merosin deficiency), muscle-eye-brain disease Walker-Warburg syndrome and Zellweger syndrome (peroxisomal disorder)
Polymicrogyria	Four-layered cortex or a single thick layer. Causes include peroxisomal disorders and leukodystrophies. Focal cortical ischemia at 24–26 weeks may cause local polymicrogyria	Focal, tonic or tonic clonic seizures. Bilateral perisylvian polymicrogyria causes learning disability, epilepsy and a characteristic pseudobulbar syndrome
Subependymal heterotopias *Filamin 1* gene	X-linked dominant mutation. MRI shows typical irregular pattern on ventricular surface (Figure 2.5)	Usually causes lethal abortion in males or severe handicap. Females have normal IQ and have epilepsy of variable severity
Focal heteroptopias	Abnormal rests of ectopic neurons in the subcortical white matter. Present in up to 15% of refractory epilepsy. May result from a variety of prenatal insults (Figure 2.6)	Epilepsy varies from mild to severe. IQ usually normal
Microdysgenesis	Small rests of abnormal neurons visible only on microscopic examination or subtle changes in neuronal density. May be associated with abnormal synapse formation	Microdysgenesis may be implicated in idiopathic generalized epilepsies and in Down, Fragile X and Rett syndromes

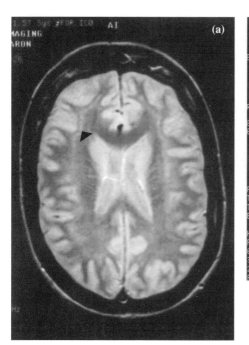
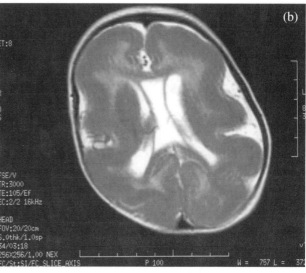

Figure 2.4. (a) T_2 weighted MRI of anteriorly predominant band heterotopia typical of that seen in doublecortin mutations. (b) T_2 weighted MRI of lissencephaly, which may be related genetically to band heterotopia (see Table 2.2).

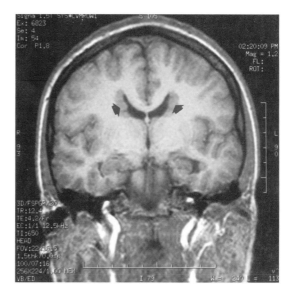

Figure 2.5. T1 weighted MRI of subependymal heterotopia in a woman with well-controlled epilepsy.

syndrome (Chapter 11). TS is due to mutations on chromosome 9q (hamartin) or 16p (tuberin). The pathological findings are cortical tubers composed of disorganized cortex, regions of loss of gray/white matter demarcation and subependymal nodules, reflecting a disorder of cortical development (see Figure 3.2 on p. 34).

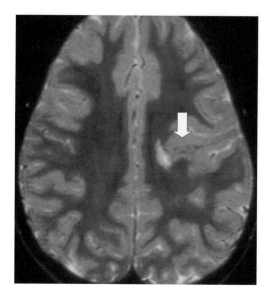

Figure 2.6. T_1 weighted MRI of focal nodular heterotopia adjacent to the occipital horn of the lateral ventricle.

Dysembryoplastic Neuro-Epithelial Tumors (DNET)

- DNET represent 2.5 to 25 percent of foreign tissue lesions removed in the treatment of refractory epilepsy. They occur most commonly in the temporal lobes. They are primarily intracortical accounting for the high risk of epilepsy and on neuroimaging may appear to expand the cerebral cortex (see Figure 8.1 on p. 129). They include both glial and neuronal cell types. The neurons may be mature and dysmorphic and the lesions are usually associated with dysplasia elsewhere in the cerebral cortex, implying a congenital origin, linked to cortical dysplasia. They are usually very slow growing and may not manifest with epilepsy until adulthood. Although the epilepsy is often refractory to medical treatment, the prognosis is very good after surgical resection.

BIBLIOGRAPHY

Andermann F. Cortical dysplasias and epilepsy: a review of the architectonic, clinical and seizure patterns. Adv Neurol 2000;84:479–496.

Clark GD, Swann JW, Miller G. From molecule to tissue: normal and abnormal brain development. In Miller G, Clark GD. The Cerebral Palsies. Causes, Consequences and Management. Boston: Butterworth-Heinemann, 1998;37–82.

Guerrini R, Andermann F, Canapicchi R, Roger J, Zifkin BG, Pfanner P (eds). Dysplasias of cerebral cortex and epilepsy. Philadelphia: Lippincott Raven, 1996.

Hubel DH, Wiesel TN. Ferrier Lecture: functional anatomy of macaque monkey visual cortex. Proc R Soc Lond B 1977;198:1–59.

Lewis D.V. Febrile convulsions and mesial temporal sclerosis. Curr Opin Neurol 1999;12:197–201.

Mathern GW, Babb TL, Armstrong DL. Hippocampal sclerosis. In Engel J Jr, TA Pedley TA (eds). Epilepsy: a Comprehensive Textbook. Philadelphia: Lippincott Raven, 1997;133–156.

Meencke H, Janz D. The significance of microdysgenesis in primary generalised epilepsy: an answer to the considerations of Lyon and Gastaut. Epilepsia 1985;26:368–371.

Morioka T, Nishio S, Ishibashi H, Muraishi M, Hisada K, Shigeto H, Yamamoto T, Fukui M. Intrinsic epileptogenicity of focal cortical dysplasia as revealed by magnetoencephalography and electrocorticography. Epilepsy Res 1999;33:177–187.

Parent A. Carpenter's Human Neuroanatomy. Chapter 18: The Limbic System. Baltimore: Williams & Wilkins, 1996.

Spreafico R, Battaglia G, Arcelli P, Andermann F, Dubeau F, Palmini A, Olivier A, Villemure JG, Tampieri D, Avanzini G, Avoli M. Cortical dysplasia. An immunocytochemical study of three patients. Neurology 1998;50:27–36.

Weissman, Z, Michowitz S, Shuper A, Kornreich L, Amir J. Dysembryoplastic neuroepithelial tumor: a curable cause of seizures. Pediatr Hematol Oncol 1996;13:463–468.

3

Genetics of Epilepsy

GENETIC RESEARCH IN EPILEPSY

- Assessing epilepsy pedigrees is difficult. There is no definitive test for epilepsy and inheritance of EEG abnormalities is not synonymous with inheritance of epilepsy. Epilepsy is expressed at different ages in different individuals and the investigator taking a cross-sectional view may miss some potentially positive cases. These factors mean separating epilepsy sufferers from unaffected relatives is problematic.
- Phenocopies are individuals who suffer from seizures that are not due to the genetic cause shared by the rest of the family but are due to some coincidental factor such as head injury, who complicate genetic analysis.
- Where single gene disorders cause epilepsy, the easiest to characterize have been autosomal dominant conditions as pedigrees contain large numbers of affected individuals.

TYPES OF GENETIC CONTRIBUTION TO EPILEPSY

A genetic contribution to epilepsy is common in many patients but the magnitude of this contribution is very variable, depending on the epilepsy syndrome. There are four main types of genetic input into epilepsy disorders:

1. Single gene inherited disorders whose only manifestation is epilepsy.
2. Inherited neurological disorders whose manifestations include epilepsy. There are over a hundred and some are listed in Table 3.1.
3. Epilepsy with complex inheritance. These are families where the incidence within the family is greater than would be predicted by chance. They are thought to be multifactorial, probably involving several genes. The idiopathic generalized epilepsies (IGE) and benign focal epilepsies of childhood are the most common in this category.
4. Epilepsy which is primarily due to environmental factors but in which genetic factors may play a smaller role for example the risk of epilepsy after head injury.

Table 3.1. Some Inherited Neurological Disorders Causing Epilepsy

Genetic Condition	Clinical Features
Chromosomal Abnormalities	
Down Syndrome (trisomy 21) usually sporadic	Short stature, typical face with large tongue. Epilepsy in 10% Absence seizures, startle-provoked seizures, tonic–clonic seizure (TCS)
Wolf-Hirschhorn syndrome Chromosome 4 deletion	Myoclonic seizures, atypical absences. Craniofacial anomalies, high voltage spike and wave on the EEG
Trisomy 13, usually sporadic	Developmental retardation, microcephaly and craniofacial dysgenesis. Seizures and apnoeic attacks both common
Trisomy 18	Failed somatic growth and hypoplasia of organs. Severe cerebral malformation and epilepsy. Death in early infancy
Contiguous Gene Disorders	
Angelman syndrome, maternal chromosome 15 $GABA_A$ abnormality in 70%.	Affects only females, mental retardation, epilepsy, inappropriate laughter and jerky movements with absent speech "Happy puppet syndrome." Severe epilepsy with absences, myoclonus and TCS and a typical EEG with high voltage spike and wave from infancy
Prader-Willi syndrome, paternal chromosome 15 abnormality in 70%	Obesity, short stature, hypotonia, small hands and feet and mental retardation. Epilepsy in 10–15% is less severe than in Angelman syndrome
Rett Syndrome	X-linked. Stereotypic motor behaviors, breathing disorders, seizures and cognitive decline from age 6–18 months. *MECP2* gene (DNA methylation protein)
Neurodevelopmental Disorders	See Chapter 2
Neurodegenerative Disorders	
Alzheimer's disease (AD)	Seizures occur most commonly in the inherited forms of AD. They are usually tonic–clonic seizures and relatively well controlled
Huntington's disease (Huntington gene triplet repeats)	Seizures are rare in adult onset cases but are more a feature in rarer juvenile onset cases
Progressive myoclonus epilepsies	See Table 3.3
Neurocutaneous Disorders	
Tuberose sclerosis (Figure 3.1), autosomal dominant prevalence 1/6 000 Due to defects of two genes: hamartin and tuberin, which interact *in vivo*	Skin: facial angiofibroma, subungual fibromas, Shagreen patches and ash leaf hypomelanotic lesions. Other: retinal hamartomas, cardiac rhabdomyoma, bone and renal cysts, renal angiomyolipoma. Seizures in 80% may be focal or malignant, including West syndrome and Lennox-Gastaut syndrome. Mental retardation (30%) and autism common. Subependymal nodules and calcification on neuroimaging
Hereditary hemorrhagic telangiectasia	Telangiectases on face and hands. Arteriovenous malformations (AVM) of brain causing hemorrhage and partial epilepsy. Pulmonary AVM causing right heart failure and paradoxical embolism

Table 3.1. *Continued*

Genetic Condition	Clinical Features
Sturge-Weber syndrome (usually sporadic, Figure 3.2)	Facial cutaneous angioma and leptomeningeal and brain angioma. Refractory partial epilepsy in 70–90%, West syndrome, hemiparesis mental retardation
Menkes syndrome, X-linked disorder of ATPase using copper transport.	Kinky fragile hair, neonatal jaundice, mental retardation, seizures, ataxia and numerous skeletal and soft tissue abnormalities.
Epidermal nevus syndrome, sporadic disorder	Epidermal nevus, usually on head or neck, seizures, including infantile spasms, hemimeganencephaly, hemiparesis, cranial nerve palsies
Hypomelanosis of Ito, sporadic disorder	Hypopigmented whorls, streaks and patches over the trunk, café-au-lait spots, dystrophic nails. Seizures and mental retardation, macrocephaly, microcephaly, polymicrogyria and heterotopias
Metabolic disorders	
Pyridoxine-dependent epilepsy. Recessive defect of glutamic acid decarboxylase	Presents with refractory seizures in neonatal period. Bilateral asynchronous 1–4 Hz waves. Responds rapidly to pridoxine
Peroxisomal disorders (autosomal recessive, 17 disorders described)	Neonatal seizures of all types including flexor spasms. Dysmorphic features: high palate, high forehead, shallow orbital ridges. EEG hypsarrhythmia or multifocal spikes. Elevated serum very long chain fatty acids. Cortical dysplasia on imaging
Urea cycle disorders. Autosomal recessive except ornithine transcarbamaylase deficiency (OTC, X-linked dominant)	Lethargy, vomiting and hyperventilation within 72 hours of birth. Hyperammonaemia, and alkalosis. OTC deficiency presents later with seizures and relapsing encephalopathy secondary to minor infection or drugs, especially valproate
Lysosomal disorders (autosomal recessive hexosaminidase and galactocerebrosidase deficiency)	Progressive encephalopathy, developmental regression, myoclonic jerks, exaggerated startle response. Peripheral neuropathy in galactocerebrosidase deficiency. Cherry red spot in ocular fundus of hexosaminidase deficiency
Pyruvate dehydrogenase or pyruvate carboxylase deficiency	Neonatal lactic acidosis with seizures or progressive neurological disturbance including malformations e.g. agenesis of the corpus callosum.
Leigh's syndrome (recessive or maternal inheritance)	Seizures and acute encephalopathy with thalamic infarction. Commonest in childhood but may be at any age. May be a maternally inherited disorder with pigmentary retinopathy
Mitochondrial disorders (MERRF see also Table 3.3)	MELAS (mitochondrial encephalopathy, lactic acidosis and stroke-like episodes). Short stature, cognitive decline, acute encephalopathic episodes and deficits with stroke-like onset. Tonic–clonic seizures and myoclonus
Methylene tetrahydrofolate reductase deficiency	Regression from infancy, myoclonus, partial, atonic seizures, infantile spasms. Later onset form: motor deterioration, psychosis, stroke-like episodes and homocystinuria
Organic acidurias (autosomal recessive)	Seizures in infancy: tonic–clonic seizures and infantile spasms. Encephalopathy, developmental delay and regression
Aminoacidurias (autosomal recessive)	Commonest is phenylketonuria, see Table 3.3. Others are tetrahydrobiopterin deficiency, tyrosinaemia and histidinaemia
Leukodystrophies (autosomal dominant, recessive and X-linked forms)	Seizures ataxia and cognitive decline. Some forms with myelopathy, peripheral neuropathy and adrenal failure. Marked white matter abnormalities on MRI. X-linked tends to present in adults with dementia
Acute intermittent porphyria, autosomal dominant	Crises of acute encephalopathy, seizures and abdominal pain. Presents in early adulthood. Triggered by illness and drugs that induce liver enzymes, including antiepileptic drugs

SINGLE GENE DISORDERS CAUSING EPILEPSY

Single gene disorders causing epilepsy are uncommon. Genetic disorders may provide insights into the pathophysiological mechanisms of commoner epilepsies

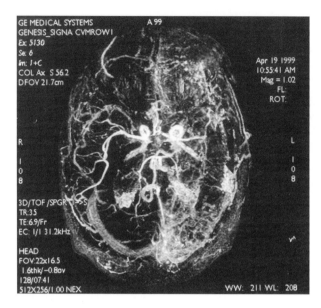

Figure 3.1. MR angiogram showing the unilateral, diffusely abnormal vascular pattern typical of epidermal naevus (Sturge-Weber) syndrome.

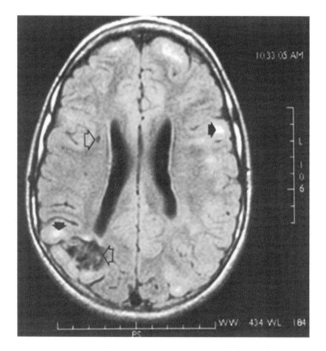

Figure 3.2. T_1 weighted MRI in tuberose sclerosis showing cortical tubers (closed arrows) and calcified lesions (open arrows).

but this remains to be clarified. To date only a few single gene causes of epilepsy have been identified (Table 3.2).

Progressive myoclonus epilepsies (PME) are a group of uncommon conditions, characterized by myoclonus, tonic-clonic seizures and cognitive decline (Table 3.3).

Table 3.2. Single Gene Disorders Causing Epilepsy

Diagnosis	Genetics and Pathophysiology	Clinical Features
Benign familial neonatal convulsions	Autosomal dominant mutations of voltage-gated potassium channels on chromosome 8 or 20 may slow membrane repolarization	Seizures typically start around the fifth day of life and remit within 3 months
Benign familial infantile convulsions	Cases linked to chromosome 16 and chromosome 19	Onset age 4–8 months. Focal attacks originate in parieto-occipital regions on EEG. Attacks easily controlled and usually remit by one year of age
Autosomal dominant nocturnal frontal lobe epilepsy (ADNFLE)	Abnormalities of the alpha 4 subunit of the nicotinic acetyl choline receptor. This is concentrated in the thalamus and may be involved in regulating sleep–waking cycles	Typical frontal lobe seizures are nocturnal and occasionally diurnal. Severity is very variable within the same family. Some patients have only a few seizures, others have many each night. Interictal EEG is often normal and ictal EEG is non-diagnostic in up to half. MRI is normal
Generalized epilepsy with febrile seizures plus (GEFS+)	GEFS+ may be quite common. Probably many mutations. Those identified involve alpha and beta subunits of voltage-gated sodium channels and GABA receptor, reducing benzodiazepine sensitivity	Febrile seizures start before age 3 months and continue after age 6 years. Afebrile seizures: myoclonic, absences, tonic atonic or tonic–clonic. EEG is often photosensitive with slightly irregular generalized abnormalities
Familial temporal lobe epilepsy	Autosomal dominant. Unrelated to febrile seizures and MRI scan is normal. Genetic basis is unknown	Focal seizures with or without loss of consciousness and tonic-clonic seizures. Symptoms include déjà vu, sensory and autonomic features
Autosomal dominant epilepsy with auditory features	Rare. Linked to chromosome 10q	Seizure onset age 9–18 years. Usually with spontaneous remission. Auditory hallucinations with simple sounds, music or speech
Familial partial epilepsy with variable foci	Rare. Autosomal dominant. Linked to chromosome 22q	Median onset age 13 years. Focal seizures with a consistent region of onset for each individual but differing between affected relatives and arising from any lobe
Autosmal dominant epilepsy with speech dyspraxia (ADRESD)	Rare. Genetic basis unknown but pedigrees may exhibit anticipation suggesting a triplet repeat syndrome	Features intermediate between benign epilepsy with centrotemporal spikes and Landau-Kleffner syndrome (see Chapter 11). Median onset age 6 years. Seizures of variable severity and some cognitive and speech disturbances. Rolandic discharges on EEG

The progressive neurological disturbance differentiates them from juvenile myoclonic epilepsy, which is a very common form of IGE. The causes of PME vary according to age of onset, pattern of inheritance, associated clinical features and prognosis. There is another group of conditions in which myoclonus and epilepsy may occur but are not key clinical features or are not present at first presentation. These include juvenile onset Huntington's disease, GM_2 gangliosidosis, Niemann-Pick disease type C, Gaucher's disease and Alzheimer's disease.

Table 3.3. Progressive Myoclonus Epilepsy Syndromes

Disease	Clinical Features	EEG	Prognosis	Genetics and Pathology
Unverricht-Lundborg disease	Onset age 8–13 with myoclonus, TCS, ataxia and mild dementia	Spike and wave when waking at 3–5 Hz with photosensitivity	Usually runs a benign course	Autosomal recessive mutation of cystatin B gene (protease inhibitor)
Dentatorubro-pallidoluysian atrophy (DRPLA)	Dominant disorder most common in Japan. Onset in late childhood to late adult with TCS and myoclonus. May also have a phenotype resembling Huntington's disease	Non-specific	Progressive disorder	Expanded triplet repeat of atrophin gene, function uncertain
Lafora body disease	Onset age 10–18 with TCS, occipital partial seizures myoclonus and progressive dementia	Spike and polyspike discharges with posterior abnormalities	Death in 2–10 years	Widespread Lafora body deposits. Autosomal recessive laforin mutation (tyrosine phosphatase)
Myoclonus epilepsy and ragged red fibers (MERRF)	Very variable phenotype, with myopathy, ataxia, seizures, myoclonus, deafness, optic atrophy and dementia	Spike-wave discharges with gradual slowing of the background	Prognosis very variable	Maternal inheritance of mitochondrial abnormality, commonly affecting tRNA Ragged red fibers usually present on muscle biopsy
Alper's disease	Initially normal development then psychomotor retardation with tonic clonic and focal seizures, myoclonus and focal motor status epilepticus	Anterior 1–3 Hz spike and wave which gradually declines	Progressive decline to death	Defects of mitochondrial complex IV causing defective oxidative phosphorylation

	Clinical features	EEG	Course/prognosis	Genetics/biochemistry
Sialidosis	Different onsets according to severity, including infantile, childhood and adolescent. Adolescent: angiokeratomas, severe myoclonus, tonic–clonic seizures, gradual visual failure and optic fundus cherry red spot. Younger onset less myoclonus but severe mental retardation, coarse facies, dysostosis, cardiac involvement and visceromegaly	Vertex positive spikes with myoclonus and in deep sleep	Infantile onset survival to second decade. Later onsets also progressive	Autosomal recessive. Neuraminidase deficiency, defective β-galactosidase and lysosomal protective protein activity. Milder in type I. Causes defective cleavage of oligosaccharides with accumulation and vacuolation
Neuronal ceroid lipofuscinosis	Visual loss, cognitive decline and seizures. The exact pattern depends on the type and age of onset. Seizures are common in all types and myoclonus in older variants, especially Kufs disease	Photosensitivity at low frequencies in young onset. Electroretinogram abolished	Progressive decline to death	Infantile CLN1, CLN2: autosomal recessive mutations of lysosomal enzymes. CLN3, CLN5 autosomal recessive mutations of membrane spanning proteins
Phenylketonuria	Mental retardation develops months after birth. Blonde hair, fair skin, eczema and vomiting in infancy, psychiatric disorders. Seizures and myoclonus are usually easy to control	EEG abnormalities in 80%.	Good prognosis with neonatal testing, and low phenylalanine diet	Autosomal recessive phenylalanine hydroxylase deficiency causes abnormal accumulation of phenylalanine and other normal substances
Biotinidase deficiency	Onset 3 months to 10 years. Dermatitis, stomatitis, episodes of hypertonia, coma, acidosis and ketosis. Seizures or myoclonus in 50%. Optic atrophy and hearing disturbances may occur	May be normal from outset or normalizes with biotin treatment	Seizures remit in 75% with biotin treatment. Fixed deficits persist	Autosomal recessive disorder of biotinidase which may be assayed in blood or liver. Reduced biotin and increased biocytin (precursor) result

THE GENETIC CONTRIBUTION TO SPORADIC EPILEPSY

A much commoner question is the genetic risks for relatives of probands with sporadic forms of epilepsy. A systematic approach is needed – the risk varies according to the epilepsy syndrome and the relationship to the proband (Table 3.4).

- A detailed family history of epilepsy or neurological disease is required. This should include living relatives and deaths as these may have been epilepsy-related, especially in young individuals. Several patterns may emerge: a clear genetic pedigree of epilepsy; a high genetic risk; a low genetic risk.
- What is the relationship of the proband to the individual? Sibling and offspring risks are different for different patterns of epilepsy (below).
- What is the epilepsy syndrome, including the EEG pattern? Idiopathic epilepsy is usually associated with higher familial risks than acquired epilepsy, for example after trauma.
- What is the age of the proband at presentation? Epilepsies with a strong genetic component tend to present before age 20.

Family Studies

- In a recent study the families of 1498 idiopathic epilepsy probands were compared with the families of 362 probands with epilepsy due to a postnatally-acquired cause.
- If the proband had generalized epilepsy, the prevalence amongst relatives was 4.2 percent. If the proband had focal epilepsy the prevalence amongst relatives was 2.2 percent.
- The risk of epilepsy is increased in twins of epilepsy sufferers, especially if the twins are monozygotic and the epilepsy is idiopathic. Concordance for epilepsy is 44 percent in monozygotic twins and 10 percent in dizygotic twins.

Table 3.4. Risk of Inheritance of Different Epilepsy Syndromes

Proband Diagnosis	Relationship	Risk of Epilepsy
Generalized epilepsy	All first degree	4.2%
Focal epilepsy	All first degree	2.2%
Idiopathic epilepsy	Monozygotic twin	44%
Idiopathic epilepsy	Dizygotic twin	10%
All unprovoked seizures	Sibling	2.7% by age 20
Acquired epilepsy	Sibling	1% by age 20
Idiopathic focal epilepsy	Sibling	12%
Epilepsy with generalized spike and wave	Sibling	6%
Mother with any epilepsy	Offspring	6%
Father with any epilepsy	Offspring	2%
Parent with onset before age 20	Offspring	9%
Parent with onset after age 20	Offspring	3%
Parent and one offspring with epilepsy	Second offspring	8%
Population risk		1% by age 20

Within the concordant pairs, at least 94 percent of monozygotic twins and 71 percent of dizygotic twins have the same epilepsy syndrome. The syndrome concordance is greater for generalized than for focal epilepsies.
- These data suggest a strong genetic contribution to epilepsy, probably with separate genes contributing to the overall epilepsy tendency and to the pattern of clinical expression.

Sibling Risks

- If a proband suffers an unprovoked seizure before the age of 15, then the risk to a sibling of seizures before the age of 20 is 2.7 percent, compared with a population risk of 1 percent. If the epilepsy of the proband is clearly due to a postnatally-acquired cause, then the risk for siblings is no greater than the population risk. Similarly the risks are not increased for siblings of probands with focal epilepsies, except idiopathic focal epilepsies such as benign epilepsy with centrotemporal spikes (12%).
- Mental retardation or cerebral palsy in the proband also increase the risk to about 3 percent – some of these cases may be due to an inherited cause of the handicap.
- Generalized spike and wave in the EEG is associated with a 6 percent risk of siblings developing epilepsy. If the sibling also has spike and wave but has not yet developed seizures, this risk rises to 15 percent.

Offspring Risks

- The overall risk to a child of having epilepsy if their mother has epilepsy is higher (8.7%) than if their father has epilepsy (2.4%). The risk is higher if the age of onset of the parent's epilepsy was under 20 years (9%), than if it was over the age of 20 (2.8%).
- The chance that a child of a parent with epilepsy will never experience a seizure is over 80 percent.
- The risk of epilepsy is higher if the proband has absence epilepsy (9%).
- Risk factors may combine, for example, where a sibling and a parent are affected by epilepsy then the overall risk for another sibling is about 8 percent.

THE GENETICS OF SPECIFIC, COMMON EPILEPSY SYNDROMES

Benign Epilepsy of Childhood with Centrotemporal Spikes (BECTS), Synonym Benign Rolandic Epilepsy

- BECTS is the commonest focal epilepsy in childhood (Chapter 11) and may account for as much as 15 percent of all childhood epilepsy. The typical EEG abnormality is found in 1 to 2.5 percent of healthy children, even though seizures may only be present in 0.24 percent.
- There appears to be autosomal dominant inheritance of the EEG trait, with the same risk in males and females. This would predict a sibling prevalence of 50 percent but penetrance is reduced and only 14 percent of siblings have the

epilepsy. Moreover, not all the sibling risk is for BECTS and some of the children may suffer other epilepsy syndromes, including generalized epilepsies. Linkage of BECTS has been proposed to chromosome 15q14.

- Other factors, most likely other genes, may determine epilepsy risk and alter the pattern of clinical expression.

Benign Occipital Epilepsy (BCOE)

- BCOE has two clinical phenotypes: younger and older onset (Chapter 11). Girls form 60 percent of cases of both variants. This suggests a somewhat different genetic profile from BECTS above. However, 40 percent of children with occipital EEG abnormalities go on at some time to have EEG abnormalities in the rolandic region, typical of BECTS.
- Some children with the young onset form of BCOE later develop typical clinical BECTS and in one family BCOE and BECTS were reported to occur in different siblings. The incidence of BCOE is probably only 30 to 40 percent of BECTS suggesting that additional genetic factors may be required for the expression of BCOE that are less prevalent.
- This has led to the concept of a benign partial epilepsy susceptibility syndrome, whose electrographic and clinical expression may be due to the combined effects of genes acting upon the dominantly inherited electrographic abnormality of BECTS.

Generalized Epilepsies

- Concordance rates of EEG traits are higher than concordance for seizure expression. Gibbs found two thirds of monozygotic twins were concordant for spike-wave discharges of IGE but only 47 percent of pairs both had seizures. This has implications for the genetics of epilepsy but also means one must not over-interpret EEG abnormalities in those with a family history of epilepsy.

Juvenile Myoclonic Epilepsy

- Juvenile myoclonic epilepsy (JME) accounts for 10 to 30 percent of all cases of IGE and division into four electroclinical syndromes has been suggested.
- JME occurs in roughly equal proportions in males and females. The condition has a strong genetic component with concordance in nearly all monozygotic twins. Up to 25 to 50 percent of patients give a family history of epilepsy; about 7 percent of first degree relatives suffer seizures and 15 percent have EEG abnormalities. Higher numbers seem to be found if the proband is female.
- No gene has yet been identified underlying these epilepsies but linkage has been demonstrated that differs between these sub-syndromes. Chromosome 6p in the region of the human lymphocytic antigen (HLA) gene has been implicated in classical JME. A candidate gene is the $GABA_B$ receptor in this region. Chromosome 1p has been implicated in childhood absence epilepsy evolving to JME.

Childhood Absence Epilepsy

- Classical childhood absence epilepsy (CAE) is three times more common in girls than in boys. A positive family history is found in 15 to 40 percent and the usual pattern in relatives is of absences or tonic–clonic seizures. There is a 10 percent risk of seizures amongst siblings of probands with absences and 25 percent of these will also suffer absences.
- Monozygotic twins are 100 percent concordant for the EEG trait but only 30 percent concordant for clinical absence seizures. The interpretation of the genetic data has varied but autosomal dominant inheritance with variable penetrance has been used as a model in genetic studies and linkage has been suggested to chromosome 8q24.
- A jerky gene has been identified at this site, as well as at chromosome 6p (JME above). In animals, abnormalities of jerky genes cause seizures as well as developmental and somatic abnormalities.

THE GENETIC CONTRIBUTION TO "ACQUIRED" EPILEPSY

- A number of studies suggest a significant effect of the individual's genetic makeup on the risk of developing epilepsy after environmental insults.
- The monozygotic twin of a patient with epilepsy associated with brain damage is at 17 percent risk of epilepsy, compared with 9 percent for dizygotic twins. Although some brain damage may be shared between twins, for example intrauterine catastrophes, these data imply that the risk of epilepsy after brain damage is loaded by genetic factors.
- The risk of epilepsy amongst the close relatives of patients with post-traumatic epilepsy is 1.8 percent, compared with a 0.5 percent population prevalence for epilepsy.
- Patients with brain tumors and infantile hemiplegia are more likely to suffer epilepsy if there is a family history of epilepsy. Epilepsy is also more common than expected in the families of those undergoing epilepsy surgery for refractory focal epilepsy supposedly due to acquired causes.

BIBLIOGRAPHY

Annegers JF, Hauser WA, Anderson VE, Kurland LT. The risks of seizure disorders among relatives of patients with childhood onset epilepsy. Neurology 1982;32174–179.

Baier WK, Doose H. Petit mal-absences of childhood onset: familial prevalences of migraine and seizures. Neuropediatrics 1985;16:80–83.

Berkovic SF, Howell RA, Hay DA, Hopper JL. Epilepsies in twins: genetics of the major epilepsy syndromes. Ann Neurol 1998;43:435–445.

Delgado-Escueta AV, Medina MT, Serratosa JM, Castroviejo IP, Gee MN, Weissbecker K, Westling BW, Fong CY, Alonso ME, Cordova S, Shah P, Khan S, Sainz J, Rubio-Donnadieu F, Sparkes RS. Mapping and positional cloning of common idiopathic generalized epilepsies: juvenile myoclonus epilepsy and childhood absence epilepsy. Adv Neurol 1999;79:351–374.

Eeg-Olofsson O. The genetics of benign childhood epilepsy with centrotemporal spikes. In: Berkovic S.F GPHEPF, (ed). Genetics of Focal Epilepsies. London: John Libbey and Co., 1999:35–41.

Lennox WG. The heredity of epilepsy as told by relatives and twins. JAMA 1951;146:529–536.

Neubauer BA, Fiedler B, Himmelein B, Kampfer F, Lassker U, Schwabe G, Spanier I, Tams D, Bretscher C, Moldenhauer K, Kurlemann G, Weise S, Tedroff K, Eeg OO, Wadelius C, Stephani U. Centrotemporal spikes in families with rolandic epilepsy: linkage to chromosome 15q14. Neurology 1998;51:1608–1612.

Neubauer BA, Sud H. The genetics of rolandic epilepsy and related conditions: multifactorial inheritance with a major gene defect. In: Berkovic S.F GPHEPF, (ed). Genetics of Focal Epilepsies. London: John Libbey and Co., 1999:57–66.

Ottman R, Lee JH, Hauser WA, Risch N. Are generalized and localization-related epilepsies genetically distinct? Arch Neurol 1998;55:339–344.

Panayiotopoulos CP. Benign childhood partial seizures and related epilepsy syndromes. London: John Libbey and Co.,1999.

Singh R, Scheffer IE, Crossland K, Berkovic SF. Generalized epilepsy with febrile seizures plus: a common childhood-onset genetic epilepsy syndrome. Ann Neurol 1999;45:75–81.

Tsuboi T, Endo S. Incidence of seizures and EEG abnormalities among offspring of epileptic patients. Hum Genet 1977;36:173–189.

Xiong L, Labuda M, Li DS, Hudson TJ, Desbiens R, Patry G, Verret S, Langevin P, Mercho S, Seni MH, Scheffer I, Dubeau F, Berkovic SF, Andermann F, Andermann E, Pandolfo M. Mapping of a gene determining familial partial epilepsy with variable foci to chromosome 22q11–q12. Am J Hum Genet 1999;65:698–710.

4

Epidemiology of Epilepsy

Epilepsy is paroxysmal: patients show no abnormality between seizures and there is no satisfactory diagnostic or prognostic test. This may make it very difficult to make decisions or prognosticate for individual patients. A clear understanding of what is likely to happen is crucial and the epidemiology of epilepsy is central to rational patient management.

The best epidemiological studies are based in the general population but relatively few studies have satisfied this simple criterion. Among the more robust epidemiological studies are the National General Practice Study of Epilepsy (NGPSE), the Rochester, Minnesota studies and studies from the South of France and Iceland. Although hospital-based studies have provided valuable information about specific issues in epilepsy, they suffer from inherent case ascertainment bias.

HOW COMMON IS EPILEPSY?

- Febrile seizures affect about 5 percent of the population under the age of five and a few of these individuals will go on to develop unprovoked seizures (below).
- Afebrile seizures affect 4 to 8 percent of the population at some point during their lives. The risk of developing seizures is highest in old age (Figure 4.1) and in Western, long-lived societies, this represents a substantial health burden. The second highest risk is in the first two decades but no age is exempt.
- The prevalence of epilepsy is 0.4 to 0.8 percent and is relatively consistent across different populations. The higher figures tend to come from populations in developing countries. This may reflect differences in population structure and different etiological factors. Antenatal care is usually poorer and infections such as neurocysticercosis are widespread in some countries.
- Age-related prevalence in Western populations is highest in the elderly, due both to the high incidence in this group and the effect of cumulative incidence that makes prevalence increase with age. In developing populations, the different population structure tends to make the second and third decades have the highest age-specific prevalence.

PATTERNS OF NEWLY DIAGNOSED EPILEPSY

- Tonic–clonic seizures are the clinical presentation in about 35 percent and focal seizures in 50 to 60 percent, sometimes evolving to tonic–clonic seizures. Other forms of idiopathic generalized epilepsy such as absence and myoclonus are less common overall but are relatively common between the ages of 5 and 20.

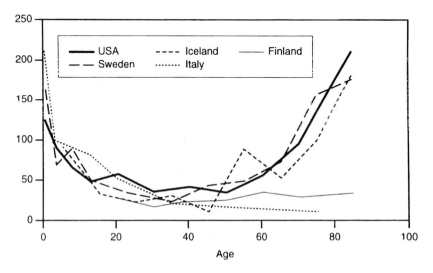

Figure 4.1. Epilepsy incidence and prevalence rates by age showing peaks in the young and the elderly incidence per 100, 000. (Reproduced with permission from Hauser W Allen, 1997.)

Table 4.1. Incidence of Different Syndromes in Southwest France

Syndrome	Annual Incidence Per 100,000 Population
Idiopathic partial epilepsy	1.68
Symptomatic partial epilepsy	17.11
Idiopathic generalized epilepsy	6.65
Symptomatic generalized epilepsy	1.15
Undetermined epilepsy	2.92
Acute symptomatic seizures	25.35
Isolated unprovoked seizure	11.70
Television epilepsy	0.26

(Reproduced with permission from Loiseau *et al.* 1990.)

- Focal epilepsy has the highest prevalence, reflecting a high incidence and a lower remission rate than for generalized epilepsy.
- Syndromic diagnosis has been attempted in community-based studies with varying success. Estimates of the incidence of different syndromic groups have been suggested for Southwest France (Table 4.1).

CAUSES OF EPILEPSY

- Exposure to different risk factors is age-related and means that the likely cause of the epilepsy depends on the age of the patient. Congenital brain insults and genetic idiopathic epilepsies usually cause seizures within the first two decades of life.
- In adults with newly diagnosed seizures in a hospital-based series, a cause may be found in up to 75 percent of cases, including stroke, intracranial infection, alcohol dependency and other metabolic causes.
- In the elderly, the overall likelihood of finding a cause is 60 percent in population-based studies. The causes are mainly cerebrovascular or neurodegenerative diseases or tumors (Figure 4.2).

Congenital Brain Injury

The pattern of brain damage produced by in utero insults is of cortical developmental abnormalities and the precise type depends on the timing of the pathology in relation to the stage of cortical development and the location of the damage (Chapter 2). Causes include:

- Genetic causes (Chapter 3)
- *In utero* infections with syphilis, toxoplasmosis, listeria, rubella, cytomegalovirus and Herpes zoster and occasionally other organisms
- Prenatal exposure to toxins such as heavy metals, drugs and alcohol
- Ischemic events due for example to placental disturbances, or eclampsia overlap with perinatal brain injury

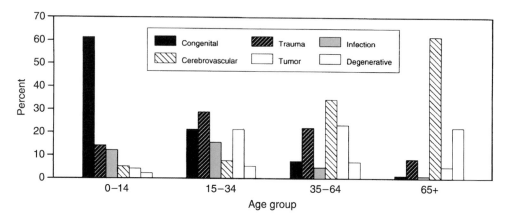

Figure 4.2. Proportion of incidence cases with known etiology by age (%). (Reproduced with permission from Hauser W Allen, 1997.)

Perinatal Brain Injury

- Only 10 to 20 percent of cerebral palsy in full term babies is due to perinatal trauma. Even in children who do suffer perinatal trauma, there is an excess of cases with minor congenital abnormalities, which may have predisposed to the problem. For example abnormal babies are more likely to be born by breech presentation, which carries a higher risk for the baby than normal cephalic presentation.
- The risk of cerebral palsy increases with decreasing gestational age and is 20-fold higher in babies whose birthweight is less than 1500 grams. About 5 to 15 percent of low birthweight babies are affected by cerebral palsy.
- Young children may develop a cerebral palsy-type picture after severe infection, ischemia or head trauma.
- Different causes of perinatal brain injury cause different patterns. Many are associated with epilepsy, especially those in which there is cortical or hippocampal damage.
- Focal epilepsy may arise from the region of damage.
- Symptomatic generalized epilepsies of childhood may be due to perinatal factors. These are among the most severe, refractory epilepsies (Chapter 11).

Febrile Seizures

- Febrile seizures are very common in childhood, affecting up to 5 percent of children. In one large study, 2 percent of children who had had a febrile seizure, developed epilepsy by the age of 7, compared to 0.5 percent of neurologically normal children who had not suffered febrile seizures.
- Convulsions with complex features: lasting longer than 15 minutes; multiple convulsions or convulsions with focal neurological features, carry a much greater risk. Children who were neurologically or developmentally abnormal before they developed febrile seizures, are at 18 times greater risk of developing epilepsy than normal children with simple febrile seizures.

- In the Rochester studies, the cumulative risk of developing epilepsy by the age of 25 was increased by febrile seizures. The risk was 2.4 percent for children with simple febrile seizures, 6 to 8 percent for children with a single complex feature and 49 percent for children with three complex features.
- Temporal lobe epilepsy due to mesial temporal sclerosis (MTS) is the form most closely associated with febrile seizures but there is a clear history of febrile seizures in only about one-third of patients with MTS. The relationship is probably complex (Chapter 2).
- A genetic association occurs occasionally between febrile seizures and other forms of epilepsy (Chapter 3).

Head Injury

- The mildest head injuries cause amnesia of less than 30 minutes around the time of the injury and minimal loss of consciousness. They do not increase the risk of epilepsy (Figure 4.3).
- The severest head injuries cause amnesia for more than 24 hours, focal neurological deficits or intracranial hematoma. These injuries result in epilepsy in over 15 percent of individuals. Although the maximal risk is early on, the increased risk does not disappear for 20 years. Penetrating missile injuries such as bullet wounds carry the very greatest risk.
- Intermediate injuries are those with amnesia for up to 24 hours, or skull fracture without evidence of major cerebral trauma. The cumulative risk of epilepsy for these cases is 2 to 3 percent over 20 years, about three times the background risk. All else being equal, a family history of epilepsy makes it more likely that a particular head injury will result in later seizures.
- Concussive seizures affect some patients instantaneously following head injury (Chapter 13). These are probably not epileptic and carry no increased risk of later epilepsy.

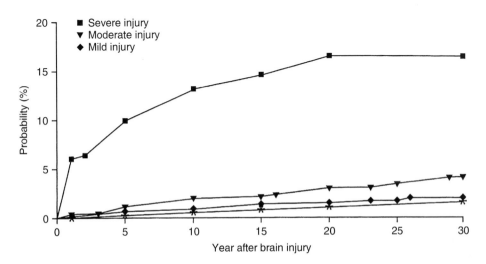

Figure 4.3. Cumulative incidence of seizures after different severities of head injury: see text for definitions. (Reproduced with permission from Annegers *et al.* 1998.)

- Early post-traumatic seizures occur within the first week following a severe head injury. These seizures do not increase a patient's risk of later epilepsy compared to other patients who have sustained similar injuries but have not had early post-traumatic seizures.
- Head injury causes focal epilepsy. The commonest sites are the anterior frontal or anterior temporal lobes, where the brain hits sharp bone as it moves within the skull.

Intracranial Infection

- Viral encephalitis and cerebral abscess carry the greatest risk (25 percent over 20 years) of later epilepsy as they directly affect the brain substance. The risk is greatest for those who experienced acute seizures at the time of their encephalitis or meningitis.
- Bacterial meningitis quadruples the risk of later epilepsy and aseptic meningitis doubles the risk.
- Most cases present within 5 years of the infection but an increased risk is present for at least 20 years. (Figure 4.4).
- Infections cause any form of focal epilepsy.

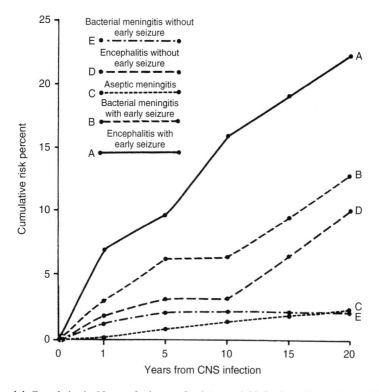

Figure 4.4. Cumulative incidence of seizures after intracranial infections. (Reproduced with permission from Annegers *et al.* 1988.)

- Specific infective causes of chronic epilepsy include tuberculosis (Figure 4.5) and parasitic infections such as neurocysticercosis or hydatid disease. Neurocysticercosis is acquired from pork infected with tapeworm larvae and is said to account for up to 50 percent of adult onset epilepsy in parts of the developing world where this parasite is not controlled.

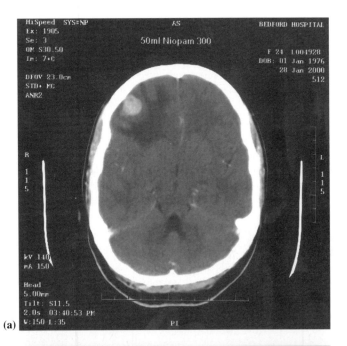

(a)

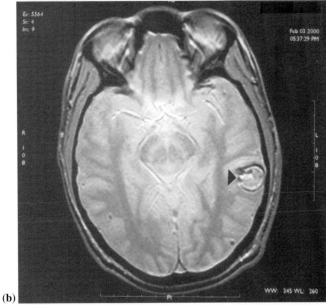

(b)

Figure 4.5. (a) CT scan of tuberculoma as a cause of epilepsy; common in the developing world. (b) MRI scan showing cortical lesion of cystercicosis, containing scolex of the organism.

Stroke

- Seizures are the first presentation of 5 percent of acute strokes, commonly as focal motor seizures, including focal motor status epilepticus. It may not be until after the seizures settle that it is apparent that the cause is a stroke (Chapter 11 and Case 4, Chapter 14).
- Chronic epilepsy affects 11 percent of stroke survivors, but the risk varies with different kinds of stroke (Table 4.2).
- If a patient is independent 1 month after the stroke, implying more minor cerebral damage, the risk is reduced (3% at 5 years).
- Most strokes cause focal epilepsy, but cerebrovascular disease may also unmask a tendency to idiopathic generalized epilepsy.

Alcohol and Illicit Drugs

- Alcohol is the commonest cause of seizures in young and middle-aged adults in some countries and is implicated in 10 to 40 percent of patients attending casualty departments with seizures. In many Western cultures, between 10 and 20 percent of adults are heavy drinkers and about 10 percent of these will suffer seizures.
- There is a dose-related effect. The risk of seizures increases progressively as alcohol consumption rises above 50 grams per day, to twenty times control levels at an intake of 300 grams per day. The seizures are usually tonic–clonic but 10 percent of alcohol-related seizures are focal and this may reflect different mechanisms whereby the epilepsy has arisen (Chapter 13).
- Both alcohol and illicit drugs were explored in a case-control study of underprivileged, young Afro-Caribbean males with a high incidence of drug-related problems in Harlem. Recent use of illicit drugs was more closely associated with seizures than remote use.
- Heroin increases the risk of seizures three to fourfold. Opiates may themselves trigger seizures and secondary consequences of intravenous injection such as bacteremia may predispose to seizures.
- Amphetamines carry a low risk of seizures at low doses, but the risk increases with dose.
- Ecstasy is associated with severe neuropsychiatric toxic effects and seizures. The frequency of these is difficult to estimate, but they are the major sources of its toxicity.

Table 4.2. Risk of Epilepsy Following Different Cerebrovascular Events

Type of Stroke	Risk of Epilepsy (%)
Total anterior circulation infarction	50
Partial anterior circulation infarction	5–7
Posterior circulation infarction	5–7
Lacunar infarction	5–7
Intracerebral hemorrhage	15–25
Subarachnoid hemorrhage	7–35

- Cocaine is a major cause of neurotoxicity and seizures, largely through vascular changes with infarction and intracerebral hemorrhage.
- Cannabinoids are reported to lower the risk of subsequent seizures compared to controls. There are also experimental data to support an anticonvulsant effect.

Neurodegenerative Disease

- Alzheimer's disease is the commonest neurodegenerative disease, accounting for over half of all dementias of old age. Seizures occur in about 5 percent of patients. They are usually convulsive and relatively easy to control.
- Lewy body dementia is less commonly associated with seizures but commonly causes parasomnias that are mistaken for epilepsy.
- Other rarer dementias such as classical Creutzfeldt-Jakob disease are more frequently associated with seizures.
- Seizures are uncommon in Huntington's disease except in the rare juvenile onset cases.

Systemic Disease

Hypertension

- Hypertension is the strongest risk factor for stroke, which is a common cause of epilepsy. Hypertension is however, a weak independent risk factor for epilepsy, increasing the risk 1.5 to 2 times.

Diabetes

- Diabetes is a strong risk factor for stroke and consequently for epilepsy.
- Hypoglycemia is a cause of acute symptomatic seizures and is probably also a cause of remote symptomatic epilepsy, possibly by causing mesial temporal damage.
- Non-ketotic, hyperosmolar hyperglycemia can be a cause of acute symptomatic seizures including status epilepticus, especially focal motor status (Chapter 13 and Case 8, Chapter 14).

Other Systemic Diseases

- Celiac disease is now thought to be associated with a wide variety of neurological complications, sometimes without obvious gastrointestinal involvement. The commonest is seizures. A CT scan often shows a typical pattern of calcification, following the sulci in the occipital region.
- Other autoimmune diseases may also be associated with cerebral involvement and seizures. The commonest is systemic lupus erythematosis (SLE) that may cause an acute fulminant encephalopathy or a more chronic seizure disorder.
- A wide variety of metabolic disturbances is also associated with seizures and may lead to status epilepticus.

Box 4.1. Metabolic Causes of Seizures

Hyponatremia/hypernatremia
Hypokalemia/hyperkalemia
Hypocalcemia/hypercalcemia
Hypoglycemia/hyperglyemia
Hypoxic states
Hepatic encephalopathy
Uremic encephalopathy
Severe hypothyroidism (myxedema coma)

Psychiatric Disease

- The association between epilepsy and psychiatric disease is complex (Chapter 17) and patients with epilepsy may develop a wide spectrum of psychiatric disease.
- Epilepsy also develops more commonly in patients with psychiatric disease, especially psychosis.

THE MORTALITY AND MORBIDITY OF EPILEPSY

- The overall mortality of epilepsy depends on the population being assessed. Important factors are the duration, type and severity of epilepsy. An important measure is the standardized mortality ratio (SMR). This is the number of deaths affecting patients with the condition of interest (epilepsy) in a given period compared to the number of deaths expected in a matched control group.

The Effects of the Epilepsy Syndrome on Mortality

- The SMR of recently diagnosed epilepsy is about 3 to 5, compared with only 1 to 1.5 for epilepsy of 20 years' standing. The likely explanation is that the early deaths are due to the cause of the epilepsy, for example tumors.
- The mortality of epilepsy is strongly age-related (Table 4.3).
- Childhood onset epilepsy with no identifiable cause, carries little increase in mortality. Where there is an identifiable cause of the epilepsy, the SMR may be as high as 115. In one third of these the death is directly attributable to the epilepsy. In most of the others it is due to an underlying condition or to

Table 4.3. Age-Related Mortality of Epilepsy

Age of Onset of Epilepsy	Ten Year Survival (%)
<1	69
1–19	99
20–59	82
>60	76

aspiration pneumonia in the context of severe handicap. Neurodegenerative disease and some rarer childhood epilepsies carry a significant mortality. For example only two-thirds of children with neonatal convulsions survive to the age of one year and the mortality of infantile spasms is 20 percent.

- Adult-onset epilepsy is often associated with a serious cause for example, stroke, alcohol or tumor, which in itself carries a significant mortality and morbidity.

The Effects of Seizures on Mortality and Morbidity

- Patients with only idiopathic generalized epilepsy (IGE) absence seizures are at minimally increased risk, but those with focal or convulsive seizures are at much higher risk.
- Severity of epilepsy is also important. The SMR for patients with severe epilepsy was 3.8 in one study, compared to only 1.8 for those in remission. This relates partly to the risk of status epilepticus, to accidents and to sudden unexplained death in epilepsy (SUDEP).
- There is a consistent elevation of morbidity and mortality from accidents amongst epilepsy sufferers, including road traffic accidents, drowning, falls, and burns, which is greatest for those with frequent seizures or tonic–clonic seizures.

Sudden Unexplained Death in Epilepsy

Epidemiology of SUDEP

When obvious causes, such as drowning or status epilepticus have been eliminated, there remains a group of patients, most commonly young, who die without a clear explanation, termed SUDEP. Many are found dead in bed.

- The overall risk of SUDEP is uncertain. Many studies are from specialized clinics and estimates cite SUDEP as affecting 0.5 percent of epilepsy sufferers per year or being the eventual cause of death in 10 percent of all epilepsy sufferers. A population study estimated the risk as about 0.035 percent of epilepsy sufferers per year. The risk has also been estimated at one in every 2000 to 3000 convulsive seizures.
- Childhood or adolescence onset epilepsy increases the risk of SUDEP for patients seven to eight times compared to patients with epilepsy onset over the age of 45.
- Age is usually 20 to 40 at death from SUDEP.
- Gender is probably not a factor.
- Seizure type is inconsistently reported to be a factor. IGE absences probably carry little risk and myoclonus the greatest risk. Other seizure types are intermediate in risk.
- Epilepsy severity is a strong risk factor. Although rare cases of SUDEP have been reported in patients with well-controlled epilepsy, a community-based study showed no increased risk in patients with 0 to 2 seizures per year. As seizure frequency increased to over 50 per year, the risk increased to 10 to 15 times control levels. Others have suggested much higher risks in patients who have been evaluated for but rejected from surgical programs or patients who are in drug trials for refractory epilepsy. These are amongst the most severe epilepsy

cases with the most frequent seizures and may be at 25 to 50 percent cumulative risk of SUDEP.

Possible Mechanisms of SUDEP

- The obvious assumption that SUDEP occurs during seizures has been surprisingly difficult to prove but strong evidence in favor of this hypothesis is accumulating.

  1. When SUDEP is witnessed it is almost always in the context of a seizure.
  2. SUDEP is more likely to occur away from a closely supervised environment where intervention during seizures may be delayed.
  3. The risk of SUDEP is closely related to epilepsy severity and successful epilepsy surgery eliminates the risk of SUDEP.

- Two mechanisms have been postulated for SUDEP. Both involve central disruption of autonomic control and probably both occur in different cases.

  1. Seizures induce apnea by interfering with descending autonomic control of respiration, resulting in sudden, severe abnormalities of oxygen and carbon dioxide concentrations. Arterial blood pressure suddenly rises, triggering acute pulmonary edema and fatal cardiac failure. A model in sheep has reproduced these events. In people dying from SUDEP, pulmonary edema has been found in many but not all on post mortem examination. Variations in respiration and apneic episodes are found quite frequently in patients with severe epilepsy admitted for video-EEG-telemetry.
  2. Seizures induce fatal arrhythmia through central autonomic influences on cardiac control. Severe bradycardias and occasionally tachycardias have been observed in spontaneous seizures (Case 6, Chapter 5). The autonomic control of cardiac rhythm arises from regions of the hypothalamus that are closely linked to the mesial temporal lobes that are commonly implicated in refractory focal epilepsy. Arrhythmia could explain some of the cases where death is at the onset of a seizure or where there is no pulmonary edema at post mortem.

Mortality from Other Causes

Most studies suggest an increase of morbidity and mortality in patients with epilepsy from causes not directly related to the epilepsy such as extracranial malignancy. It is difficult to control for other risk factors such as smoking and alcohol consumption in these data.

WILL A SINGLE SEIZURE RECUR?

The overall risk of having a second seizure after a first afebrile seizure is between 48 percent and 78 percent in the first 3 years. Some of the difference between studies probably relates to case ascertainment.

Seizure Type, Epilepsy Syndrome, Etiology and Recurrence (Strong Effect)

- Focal seizures nearly always recur, especially if due to a congenital insult or associated with an abnormal neurological examination (Figure 4.6).
- Tonic–clonic seizures without focal elements recur in three out of four patients by 3 years.
- Acute symptomatic seizures arising in the context of acute illness (acute provoked seizures) are least likely to recur (40%) at 1 year. Some acute causes are recurring, for example, alcohol-related.

Interval After the First Seizure and Recurrence (Strong Effect)

- Most seizure recurrence happens within 6 months of the first seizure (Figure 4.7) 75 percent recur within 1 year. Recurrence after 5 years is rare.

The Presence of EEG Abnormalities and Recurrence (Moderate Effect)

- The EEG may enable diagnosis of a specific epilepsy syndrome allowing a more precise prognosis to be made.
- The prognostic value of EEG is probably greatest in childhood, since the EEG is central to the diagnosis of many childhood epilepsy syndromes.
- All else being equal, an EEG with epileptiform abnormalities may double the risk of seizure recurrence, but in the study that evaluated this most clearly, there was a rather low overall recurrence rate, and the impact of the EEG may have been overestimated.

Age and Gender of the Patient and Recurrence (Moderate Effect)

- The risk of recurrent seizures is highest in children (52 to 83%), reflecting the epilepsy syndromes of childhood, although many ultimately remit.

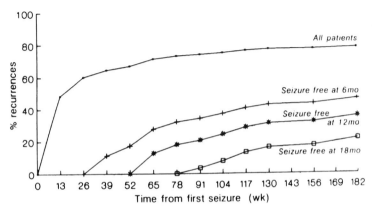

Figure 4.6. Risk of seizure recurrence after a first seizure in a general population. (Reproduced with permission from Hart *et al.* 1990.)

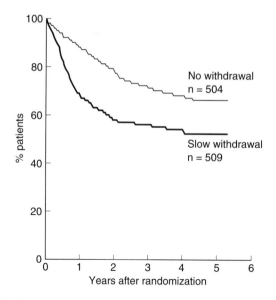

Figure 4.7. Risk of seizure recurrence after antiepileptic drug withdrawal. (Reproduced with permission from Medical Research Council antiepileptic drug withdrawal study group, 1991.)

- Epilepsy in the elderly also carries a high risk of recurrence, probably because many cases are due to focal (usually cerebrovascular) or progressive brain disease.
- Epilepsy in the middle years carries the lowest risk of recurrence. This is the commonest age group suffering acute symptomatic seizures through trauma or alcohol.
- Gender has no major effect on seizure recurrence.

WILL SEIZURES GO AWAY?

Overall Prognosis

- The overall prognosis of epilepsy is good. The prevalence is only 0.5 percent compared to a lifetime cumulative incidence approaching 5 percent. In developing countries, where the uptake of treatment may be very low, the prevalence is still similar to other countries with more developed health care. These figures can only be due to a high spontaneous remission rate or a very high mortality, which is not supported by other data.
- Over half of patients will have achieved a 3-year remission of epilepsy by 10 years after diagnosis and the NGPSE suggested this figure may be as high as 86 percent. In this study, by 9 years, two-thirds of patients had achieved a 5-year remission from their seizures.

Seizure Type, Epilepsy Syndrome and Remission (Strong Effect)

- Syndromic diagnosis is a major determinant of prognosis. In a large hospital-based study in adults with 1 to 7 years of follow-up, seizure control for at least

1 year was achieved for 82 percent of IGE, 45 percent with cryptogenic partial epilepsy and only 35 percent with symptomatic partial epilepsy. Syndromic diagnosis may be less precise in epidemiological studies, blurring the divisions between syndromes and under-emphasizing differences between them.

- The best prognosis epilepsies are the benign focal epilepsies of childhood, followed by some IGE syndromes.
- The worst prognosis epilepsies are symptomatic focal or generalized epilepsies.
- Within groups there are major differences. For example, childhood absence epilepsy often remits by age 20, whereas juvenile myoclonic epilepsy, another IGE syndrome, usually continues into adult life.
- The cerebral origin of focal epilepsy also has little impact on remission except temporal lobe epilepsy due to MTS, which remits in only 20 percent compared to 35 percent of extratemporal cases or extra-hippocampal temporal lobe epilepsy (TLE).

Epilepsy Etiology and Remission of Epilepsy (Strong Effect)

- The best prognosis is for patients who have suffered acute symptomatic seizures. As many as 80 percent will have been in remission for 5 years by 9 years after diagnosis.
- The worst prognosis is seen in epilepsy with a congenital cause. Even of these one-third of patients are likely to have had a 5-year and two-thirds a 3-year remission by 9 years after diagnosis.
- Intermediate in prognosis are other remote symptomatic and idiopathic epilepsies, with about 55 to 60 percent in 5-year remission by nine years. However, diagnostic labels in these groups are the least precise in epidemiological studies. Remote symptomatic epilepsies are usually focal and probably have a poorer prognosis than idiopathic epilepsies that are more commonly generalized.
- The worst pathologies for seizure remission are MTS, with 1-year remission in only 11 percent of cases; cortical dysgenesis, with remission in 24 percent of cases and dual pathology (MTS and another lesion) remission in only 3 percent of cases.
- The best prognosis focal epilepsy is due to vascular disease, with remissions of 50 to 75 percent depending on the type of lesion and the population studied. If the epilepsy is due to a tumor then studies vary according to the likelihood of remission. In the hospital-based study, a one-year remission was seen in a similar number to vascular disease (46%). Three-year remission in the community-based study was 60 percent but 5-year remission was only 40 percent. Post-traumatic epilepsy only achieved a 1-year remission in 30 percent of patients.

Effect of Age and Gender on the Remission of the Epilepsy (Moderate Effect)

- Gender has no effect on the remission of epilepsy.
- Age is a determinant of remission of epilepsy, mainly because different epilepsy syndromes manifest at different ages.

- About half of children under the age of 16 will achieve a five-year cumulative remission by 9 years after diagnosis. This masks two categories: a small group with onset of epilepsy under 1 year of age with a very poor prognosis and a larger group of older children with a much better prognosis. Very long-term follow-up over 30 years into adulthood suggests that over 81 percent may achieve remission but that 47 percent of these subsequently relapsed and just under half had been in remission for the last 20 years of the study. The epilepsy syndrome was a key factor. Idiopathic epilepsy achieved over 80 percent remission, cryptogenic 60 percent and symptomatic 30 percent.
- In the 16 to 39-year age group in the NGPSE study, over 70 percent achieved a 5-year remission by 9 years after diagnosis. Some more refractory causes of epilepsy may manifest in this age group: cortical dysplasia, post-traumatic and tumor-related epilepsy.
- In middle age over 80 percent achieved 5-year remission by 9 years after diagnosis.
- In the elderly, mortality increases from all conditions and this makes the prognosis of epilepsy more difficult to assess but there is probably no major difference from other adult patients.

Early Treatment and Remission of Epilepsy (Effect Uncertain)

It is not clear whether anti-epileptic drug (AED) treatment merely suppresses seizures or also reduces the underlying seizure tendency. Two main lines of evidence provide opposing views.

- Animal models of epilepsy, such as kindling support the concept that abnormal discharges within the hippocampus promote the development of epilepsy and blocking this process with drugs may reduce the epileptic tendency. There is some human evidence that refractory TLE causes progressive hippocampal atrophy, perhaps predisposing to further epilepsy.
- In developing countries patients often have suffered seizures for many years before starting treatment. The remission rates among these patients seems to be just as good as for patients with recently developed epilepsy, suggesting that treatment has little impact on the underlying processes.

WILL THE EPILEPSY COME BACK AFTER TREATMENT IS STOPPED?

Overall Prognosis

- In a large Medical Research Council study of drug withdrawal, over 1000 patients were randomized to continuing therapy or to withdrawing treatment after varying periods of seizure freedom, from 2 to more than 5 years. Drug withdrawal was undertaken very slowly over 6 months or more. At 2 years, 78 percent of patients still taking treatment were seizure-free, compared to 59 percent of those who had withdrawn treatment (Figure 4.7). About 40 percent of recurrences were just single seizure episodes, with patients subsequently becoming free of attacks. About half the recurrences in the drug withdrawal arm occurred during the drug withdrawal period.

- Recurrence after drug withdrawal probably depends on rather similar factors to those governing whether they will recur in the first place, but there are some differences.

Seizure Type, Epilepsy Syndrome and Recurrence Risk (Strong Effect)

- Tonic–clonic seizures, whether idiopathic or focal onset are associated with a significantly greater risk of recurrence after drug withdrawal.
- Once in remission, focal seizures that have never secondarily generalized tend to recur less frequently than other seizure types. This group includes the common benign partial epilepsies of childhood, which have a particularly good prognosis.
- Epilepsy associated with myoclonic seizures is also particularly likely to recur. Myoclonic seizures are most commonly seen in juvenile myoclonic epilepsy, a persistent IGE syndrome and also in several malignant epilepsies and neurodegenerative conditions.

Duration of Seizure Freedom Prior to AED Withdrawal and Recurrence Risk (Strong Effect)

- The relative risk of a patient suffering recurrent seizures if medication is withdrawn more than 10 years after becoming seizure-free is only a quarter the risk if withdrawal is started after 2 to 3 years of seizure-freedom.

Etiology of the Epilepsy and Recurrence Risk (Moderate Effect)

- Epilepsy associated with mental retardation or abnormal neurological signs increased the risk of recurrence in some studies of children but may have a more modest effect in adults.
- Other symptomatic epilepsies also seem to be associated with an increased recurrence, again more in children than in adults.

Age and Gender and Recurrence Risk (Moderate Effect)

- Age at first seizure has a very limited effect on the chances of maintaining a remission.
- Age at attempted drug withdrawal seems to have somewhat more of an impact. Children fare better than adults, but within the adult population, the elderly have the lowest risk of recurrence once they are seizure-free.
- Females may have a slightly higher risk of recurrence after AED withdrawal.

Duration and Severity of the Epilepsy and Recurrence Risk (Moderate Effect)

- A long duration of epilepsy or of treatment prior to becoming seizure-free does not necessarily make it any less likely that a patient will remain seizure-free after treatment is withdrawn.

- More severe epilepsy prior to becoming seizure-free does make it less likely a patient will remain seizure-free. Measures of the severity of the epilepsy include occurrence of status epilepticus, persistence of seizures after the initiation of treatment and requirement for more than one anti-epileptic drug, although none of these alone reach statistical significance.

EEG Characteristics and Recurrence Risk (Moderate Effect)

- A normal EEG throughout the patient's seizure history increases the chances of remaining seizure-free after AED withdrawal.
- Generalized paroxysmal EEG abnormalities on any EEG taken during the patient's seizure history probably increase the risk of seizure recurrence. These abnormalities correlate with the presence of tonic–clonic seizures, which themselves are a risk factor for recurrence.
- The significance of focal EEG paroxysms is less clear-cut. In the MRC study of all ages they were not a significant risk factor, but in other studies they have been associated with poorer prognosis in children.
- Many clinicians would be cautious about drug reduction in patients with very active EEGs but would not consider a normal EEG to mean a clear green light to withdraw AED, as the EEG is often normal at diagnosis when the epilepsy is known to be active.

BIBLIOGRAPHY

Annegers JF, Hauser WA, Lee JR-J, Rocca WA. Factors prognostic of unprovoked seizures after febrile convulsions. N Engl J Med 1987;316:493–498.

Annegers JF, Hauser WA, Beghi E, Nicolosi A, Kurland LT. The risk of unprovoked seizures after encephalitis and meningitis. Neurology 1988;38:1407–1410.

Annegers JF, Hauser WA, Coan SP, Rocca WA. A population-based study of seizures after traumatic brain injury. N Engl J Med 1998;338:20–24.

Annegers JF, Shirts SB, Hauser WA, Kurland LT. Risk of recurrence after an initial unprovoked seizure. Epilepsia 1986;27:43–50.

Arts WF, Visser LH, Loonen MC, Tjiam AT, Stroink H, Stuurman PM, Poortvliet DC. Follow-up of 146 children with epilepsy after withdrawal of antiepileptic therapy. Epilepsia 1988;29:244–250.

Blom S, Heijbel J, Bergfors PG. Incidence of epilepsy in children: a follow-up study three years after the first seizure. Epilepsia 1978;19:343–350.

Burn J, Dennis M, Bamford J, Sandercock P, Wade D, Warlow C. Epileptic seizures after a first stroke: the Oxfordshire Community Stroke Project. BMJ 1997;315:1582–1587.

Camfield PR, Camfield CS, Dooley JM, Tibbles JA, Fung T, Garner B. Epilepsy after a first unprovoked seizure in childhood. Neurology 1985;35:1657–1660.

Cockerell OC, Johnson AL, Sander JW, Shorvon SD. Prognosis of epilepsy: a review and further analysis of the first nine years of the British National General Practice Study of Epilepsy, a prospective population-based study. Epilepsia 1997;38:31-46.

Cockerell OC, Johnson AL, Sander JWAS, Hart YM, Shorvon SD. Remission of epilepsy: results from the National General Practice Study of Epilepsy. Lancet 1995;346:140–144.

Earnest MP, Thomas GE, Eden RA, Hossack KF. The sudden unexplained death syndrome in epilepsy: demographic, clinical, and postmortem features. Epilepsia 1992;3:310–316.

Falconer M. Surgical treatment of drug-resistant epilepsy due to mesial temporal sclerosis. Arch Neurol 1968;19:353–361.

Ficker DM, So EL, Shen W, Annegers JF, O'Brien P, Cascino G, Belau PG. Population-based study of the incidence of sudden unexplained death in epilepsy. Neurology 1998;51:1270–1274.

Gilchrist JM. Arrhythmogenic seizures: diagnosis by simultaneous EEG/ECG recording. Neurology 1985;35:1503–1506.

Harvey AS, Nolan T, Carlin JB. Community-based study of mortality in children with epilepsy. Epilepsia 1993;34:597–603.

Hauser WA, Kurland LT. The epidemiology of epilepsy in Rochester, Minnesota, 1935 through 1967. Epilepsia 1975;16:1-66.

Hopkins A, Garman A, Clarke C. The first seizure in adult life. Lancet 1988;i:721–726.

Johnston SC, Horn JK, Valente J, Simon RP. The role of hypoventilation in a sheep model of epileptic sudden death. Ann. Neurol 1995;37:531–537.

Klenerman P, Sander JWAS, Shorvon SD (1993). Mortality in patients with epilepsy: a study of patients in long term residential care. J Neurol Neurosurg Psychiatry 1993;56:149–152.

Loiseau J, Loiseau P, Guyot M, Duche B, Dartigues JF, Aublet B. Survey of new seizure disorders in the French Southwest. I. Incidence of epileptic syndromes. Epilepsia 1990;31:391–396.

Manford M, Hart YM, Sander JWAS, Shorvon SD. The National General Practice Study of Epilepsy: The syndromic classification of the International League Against Epilepsy applied to epilepsy in a general population. Arch Neurol 1992;49:801–808.

Matricardi M, Brinciotti M, Benedetti P. Outcome after discontinuation of antiepileptic therapy in children with epilepsy. Epilepsia 1989;30:582–589.

Nashef L, Fish DR, Garner S, Sander JW, Shorvon SD. Sudden death in epilepsy: a study of incidence in a young cohort with epilepsy and learning difficulty. Epilepsia 1995;36:1187–1194.

Nashef L, Walker F, Allen P, Sander JW, Shorvon SD, Fish DR. Apnoea and bradycardia during epileptic seizures: relation to sudden death in epilepsy. J Neurol Neurosurg Psychiatry 1996;60:297–300.

Nelson KB, Ellenberg J. Predictors of epilepsy in children who have suffered febrile seizures. N Engl J Med 1976;295:1029–1033.

Ng KS, Brust JCM, Hauser WA, Susser M. Illicit drug use and the risk of new-onset seizures. Am J Epidemiol 1990;132:47–57.

Ng KS, Hauser WA, Brust JCM, Susser M. Alcohol consumption and withdrawal in new-onset seizures. N Engl J Med 1990;319:666–673.

Ng KS, Hauser WA, Brust JCM, Susser M. Hypertension and the risk of new-onset unprovoked seizures. Neurology 1993;43:425-8.

Nilsson L, Farahmand BY, Persson PG, Thiblin I, Tomson T. Risk factors for sudden unexpected death in epilepsy: a case-control study. Lancet 1999;353:888–893.

O'Donoghue M, Sander JWAS. Does early anti-epileptic drug treatment alter the prognosis for remission of epilepsies. J Roy Soc Med 1996;89:245–248.

Sander JWAS, Hart YM, Johnson AL, Shorvon SD. National General Practice Study of Epilepsy: newly diagnosed epileptic seizures in a general population. Lancet 1990; 336:1267–1274.

Semah F, Picot M-C, Adam C, Broglin D, Arzimanoglou A, Bazin B, Cavalcanti D, Baulac M. Is the underlying cause of epilepsy a major prognostic factor for recurrence? Neurology 1999;51:1256–1262.

Sillanpaa M, Jalava M, Kaleva O, Shinnar S. Long-term prognosis of seizures with onset in childhood [see comments]. N Engl J Med 1998;338:1715–1722.

Spitz MC. Injuries and death as a consequence of seizures in people with epilepsy. Epilepsia 1998;39:904–907.

Tardy B, Lafond P, Convers P, Page Y, Zeni F, Viallon A, Laurent B, Barral FG, Bertrand JC. Adult first generalized seizure: etiology, biological tests, EEG, CT scan, in an ED. Am J Emerg Med 1995;13:1–5.

Todt H. The late prognosis of epilepsy in childhood: results of a prospective follow-up study. Epilepsia 1984;25:137–144.

BIBLIOGRAPHY

Annegers JF, Hauser WA, Beghi E, Nicolosi A, Kurland LT. The risk of unprovoked seizures after encephalitis and meningitis. Neurology 1988;38:1407–1410.

Hauser WA. Incidence and Prevalence. Indidence and prevalence. In Engel J Jr and Pedley TA (eds). Epilepsy: A Comprehensive Textbook. Philadelphia: Lippincott Raven, 1997;Chapter 5.

Hart YM, Sander JWAS, Johnson AL, Shorvon SD. National General Practice Study of Epilepsy: recurrence after a first seizure. Lancet 1990;336:1271–1274.

Medical Research Council Antiepileptic Drug Withdrawal Study Group. Randomised study of antiepileptic drug withdrawal in patients in remission. Lancet 1991;337:1175–1180.

SECTION 2
Diagnosis

5

Differential Diagnosis of Epileptic Seizures

- The differential diagnosis of epileptic seizures depends on the age of the patient and the clinical manifestations of the attack. Convulsive episodes are the commonest presentation but there are many other types.
- Misdiagnoses are common (20%), most frequently syncope, with convulsive features and psychogenic non-epileptic seizures (PNES) that can mimic any seizure type. All the component symptoms of a seizure need to be considered before making a clinical diagnosis.
- The gold-standard investigation is to capture an attack with appropriate investigations – EEG, video, ECG and if necessary blood tests, for example to detect hypoglycemia. Home videos of attacks may be invaluable.
- Clinical diagnosis may be the only method available as many patients have infrequent attacks, and investigations obtained between episodes are frequently non-contributory.

GENERAL PRINCIPLES IN EPILEPSY DIAGNOSIS

- The limitations of diagnostic precision are probably greater in these paroxysmal disorders than in any other conditions.
- A witnessed account should be obtained in all cases; the telephone is an invaluable tool. The account of the patient and a witness are complementary: only the patient can give the symptoms of their aura, which may be diagnostic

of epilepsy or of another disturbance such as migraine but a witness's account is vital in gleaning details of which the patient is not aware and for which the patient's own account may be frankly misleading.

Case History 1 (58-year-old businessman)

Patient's history: "I was sitting discussing work with a colleague, when I suddenly felt disorientated. I was trying to remember the building where we do this work but I couldn't remember the layout. I told my colleague and I remember he walked me through the department to the nurse's office where an ambulance was called and I was sent to hospital. I don't think I had any problem talking to people on the way, it was just knowing where I was. I don't remember the ambulance, I was just told that. After 35 minutes I was back to normal."

Witness's history: "We were sitting talking when he became muddled. He didn't seem to remember anything. He couldn't remember what we were talking about. I tried to tell him but he didn't seem to take anything in. He just kept asking the same questions. There was never any physical problem. He was taken to hospital and recovered after about 2 hours."

The patient's history suggests a brief and very focal right temporal disturbance, perhaps related to a seizure or a transient ischemic attack. The witness's history is more typical of transient global amnesia. MRI scan and EEG were normal and the patient was reassured and allowed to continue driving. There were no recurrences.

- No clear diagnosis may be better than an incorrect diagnosis of epilepsy with all its psychosocial consequences. The diagnosis may become clear in time.

Case History 2

A 32-year-old woman gave a two-year history of occasional stereotyped episodes. She would develop a strange butterfly feeling in her stomach that rose up to her neck and she felt hot and flushed for a few seconds. There were no objective changes during these episodes. On one occasion her husband had noted that she appeared agitated in sleep and woke up a little confused, before going back to sleep a minute or two later. She had been under some domestic pressure. An MRI scan, EEG and sleep-deprived EEG were normal. She was told that there was a possibility these were epileptic seizures but there was no definitive proof. In the absence of objective changes or altered awareness during the episode, no treatment was instituted. Nine months later, she had a witnessed tonic–clonic seizure. Medication was started on the basis that the previous episodes had indeed been epileptic and that this was therefore not an isolated seizure.

The patient had been informed of the possibility of epilepsy and had been prepared to some degree for when the diagnosis was confirmed. Equally a diagnosis had not been imposed without good clinical evidence: the early episodes could have turned out to be psychogenic as she had thought.

- The diagnosis should be kept under review, especially if the clinical course or response to treatment are atypical.
- Diagnostic trials of anti-epileptic therapy are unreliable because of high placebo responder rates or alternatively a 30 percent rate of epilepsy refractory to treatment.

- Patients should be informed early that the diagnosis may be made on clinical criteria alone and that investigations are often non-contributory.

THE STAGES OF A SEIZURE

In taking the history, all four stages of an epileptic seizure should be sought, but only sometimes are all four present (Figure 5.1).

1. Prodrome. A period of non-specific malaise lasting minutes to a day or two prior to the seizure. There may be reduced concentration, altered mood, altered sleep pattern and even sometimes a change in appearance such as looking pale or drawn. Very often it is those around the patient (sometimes even pets) rather than they themselves that recognize these changes.
2. Aura. Those seizure symptoms at the onset of the attack that only the patient can recognize, such as odd stereotyped sensations or thoughts. Many patients experience the aura alone without progression to an overt seizure.
3. Ictus. The overt seizure as seen by witnesses.
4. Postictal state. The period after the ictus prior to returning to the normal interictal state.

USE OF INVESTIGATIONS IN DIAGNOSING EPILEPSY

- Dynamic investigations, for example ECG or EEG, change with the attack and are used to diagnose the nature of the attack. They may also give diagnostic clues between attacks.
- Static investigations, for example brain scan or echocardiogram, are the same between and during attacks and do not prove the nature of the attack. They may give supportive diagnostic evidence and also explain the underlying cause.

Electroencephalography (Chapter 7)

- All epileptic seizures have an electrophysiological correlate – but it is not always detectable. Interictal (EEG) has a high false negative and a lower but significant false positive rate.

Case History 3
A 27-year-old man with mild learning disability was seen with a history of blank spells. An EEG elsewhere had shown a type IV photosensitive response and he had been treated with valproate without success. Treatment was changed to clonazepam and the episodes had reduced. The episodes had never occurred in his mother's company, only when out alone. He described one in detail. He had been out at the shops when he felt a little unwell. He had gone to sit in a doorway when he saw two friends whom he called to. They helped him into a shop, where he recovered with a cup of tea. They confirmed he was conscious. The patient was anxious throughout the consultation and hyperventilation reproduced the onset of one of his attacks with no alteration of awareness. He continued to hyperventilate for several minutes after being asked to stop.

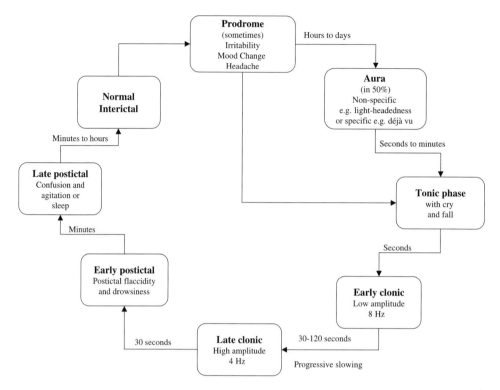

Figure 5.1. The sequence of events in a typical tonic–clonic seizure.

This case illustrates the potential false positive rate of EEG. Photosensitivity puts the patient at risk of seizures in the future but the clinical episodes described were not epileptic. Improvement in his clinical state was probably due to the anxiolytic effect of benzodiazepines and not their anti-epileptic effect.

- Ictal electroclinical correlation is the gold-standard diagnostic test. It is often said that epilepsy is a clinical diagnosis but that is only because seizures are usually too infrequent to obtain ictal electrophysiological corroboration. The great majority of seizures cause an ictal scalp EEG abnormality. When the diagnosis is in doubt, the key is to record the ictus, ideally with video-EEG, but alternatively with ambulatory EEG monitoring and home video recording.
- A minority of seizures do not cause ictal EEG changes (auras and frontal lobe seizures) and these are often predictable from the clinical seizure type. A video recording is especially important for these types.

Neuroimaging (Chapter 8)

- Normal neuroimaging is common in patients with epilepsy and does not exclude a diagnosis of epilepsy.
- Abnormal neuroimaging makes epilepsy more likely but does not prove the diagnosis. Some abnormalities such as glioma strongly suggest epilepsy but others such as arachnoid cysts are a common coincidental finding.

Table 5.1. Key Questions in Assessing Seizures

Patient	Witness
Triggers: physical or emotional	Triggers: physical or emotional
Prodrome	Prodrome
Stereotyped attacks	Stereotyped attacks
Attacks from sleep	Attacks from sleep
Aura	"Blow-by-blow account"
Tongue biting (which part of tongue)	Changes in color or sweating
Incontinence of urine	Awareness or ability to respond
Injury	Duration of recovery or confusion
Myoclonus	Focal postictal deficit e.g. weakness or aphasia
Specific symptoms e.g. déjà vu or olfactory hallucinations	

Serum Prolactin

Serum prolactin rises to at least double within 20 minutes of most convulsive epileptic seizures, probably because the seizure interferes with dopaminergic pathways that inhibit prolactin release. It has a significant error rate.

- False negatives occur in 10 percent of tonic–clonic seizures; in many focal seizures mimicking convulsions; in status epilepticus and in many cases where the timing of the sample is incorrect.
- False positives occur in a proportion of PNES, as a result of normal diurnal variation and in those taking dopamine antagonists.
- A baseline prolactin measurement is needed to interpret any postictal result.

Case History 4

A 34-year-old woman had suffered epilepsy with learning disability since age 2. After a prolonged seizure, she was taken to casualty where a physician found her postictal prolactin was 1500 mIU/ml. A baseline prolactin was performed some weeks later and was also 1500 mIU/ml. An MRI brain scan showed a large pituitary tumor compressing the optic nerves that was subsequently removed.

DIFFERENTIAL DIAGNOSIS OF DIFFERENT SEIZURE TYPES

Convulsive Episodes

The timing of the main causes of convulsive episodes is helpful in diagnosis but sometimes an EEG is required to confirm that the onset is truly from sleep (Figure 5.2).

Syncope – Clinical Features

- Presyncopal symptoms are blurring of vision, sweatiness, pallor and buzzing in the ears that most individuals have felt at some time and are similar irrespective

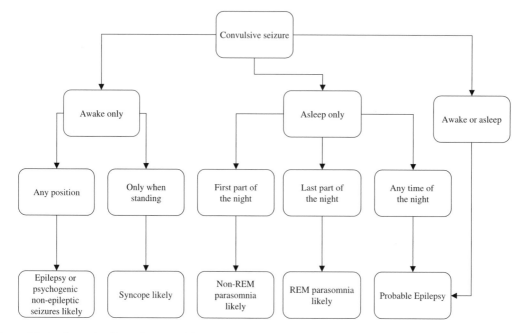

Figure 5.2. A scheme for diagnosing convulsive episodes.

of the cause. The visual symptoms may resemble simple hallucinations with colored patches or lights. Presyncope may be so rapid as not to be identified or recalled and the patient may just present with collapse.

- The situation of the episode often gives the diagnosis, especially if there has been more than one attack under similar circumstances (below).
- Tonic stiffening of the trunk is commoner than floppiness in video recordings of syncope.
- Convulsive movements occur in 70 to 90 percent of patients. These vary from minor twitching to violent myoclonic jerks. The myoclonus is usually asymmetric and asynchronous but may be symmetric. It rarely lasts more than a few seconds.
- Recovery of neurological function after syncope is usually complete by 30 seconds after the end of the attack but head injury may delay recovery.
- The diagnosis is especially important in order to avoid inappropriate treatment and driving restrictions (Chapter 18).

Reflex Anoxic Seizures

- A faint may occasionally evolve into a full-blown convulsive episode. This is most likely to occur if the patient is unable to collapse to the ground during the faint – for example passing out standing in a hot, packed crowd.
- The convulsion itself may be indistinguishable from an epileptic convulsion, although recovery is usually more rapid.

Causes of Syncope

1. Postural hypotension. Typically the patient rises and suffers the symptoms after 30 to 60 seconds. Symptoms are especially likely to occur on rising from a warm bed when the patient is warm and vasodilated (Case 5). Drugs are a common contributory cause, including antihypertensive medication and others such as neuroleptic drugs or dopamine agonists. A less common cause is an autonomic neuropathy.
2. Vasovagal syncope occurs in the context of acute emotion or in response to pain.
3. Neurocardiogenic syncope. Abnormal CNS responses to changes in posture may lead to syncope or more commonly drop attacks without premonitory symptoms (below). This condition is under-diagnosed in all age groups.
4. Micturition syncope, cough syncope and defecation syncope are suggested by the stereotyped circumstances.

Case History 5
A 67-year-old man had a history of hypertension and mild prostatism. One night he awoke and went to the lavatory, where he passed urine, having to strain a little. His wife found him collapsed and unconscious on the toilet. He had been incontinent of urine. He recovered consciousness after a few seconds and was dazed but not confused. It was clear that he had bumped his head in the fall.

This is a typical scenario for micturition syncope. Antihypertensive agents and straining contributed to a drop in blood pressure. The head injury delayed his recovery and as he had a full bladder, he was incontinent. He was advised to wait for 30 seconds before getting up and to pass urine sitting. Antihypertensive and prostatic treatments were reviewed.

5. Serious causes are suggested by absence of these obvious triggers. Of special concern is if faints happen when a patient is lying down. This suggests a primary failure of cardiac output such as arrhythmia or hypovolemia. Exertional syncope may point to cardiac disease such as aortic stenosis.
6. Rarely and confusingly, epileptic seizures can trigger alterations in heart rhythm that present with clinical syncope.

Case History 6
A 44-year-old housewife presented with three unwitnessed episodes of loss of consciousness over a 3-month period. On each occasion she had been seated when she briefly felt her head starting to spin, followed by loss of consciousness. She was not incontinent and did not bite her tongue but on one occasion she bit the inside of her cheek and cut her lip, requiring suturing. On recovery she felt shaky with a headache but was not confused. Between the first and second episodes, she had felt odd and detached and had prolonged episodes of numbness of her right hand and foot, lasting days at a time.

She suffered an episode during routine EEG recording (Figure 5.3a,b). This showed a focal epileptic seizure triggering cardiac sinus arrest, leading to a reflex anoxic seizure.

An MRI brain scan (Figure 5.3c) revealed a lesion in the left temporal lobe with signal characteristics typical of a cavernous angioma.

A dual chamber rate-responsive pacemaker was implanted. She had no further collapses over the following two years but brief episodes of altered awareness later came to light. A typical temporal lobe complex partial seizure was recorded of 30 seconds duration. Treatment was started with carbamazepine.

This patient illustrates a complex interplay between neurological and cardiovascular changes. More severe episodes were prevented by cardiac pacing, unmasking focal seizures.

Examination and Investigation in Syncope

- Pulse for irregularities
- Blood pressure supine and after 5 minutes of standing. (Postural hypotension may be delayed after standing)
- Cardiac murmurs
- Routine ECG for example for evidence of prolonged Q–T interval, predisposing to arrhythmia
- Investigations are often non-contributory but ambulatory ECG, echocardiogram, tilt table test, exercise ECG or EEG may be indicated in recurrent cases.

Concussive Seizures

- Head injury may cause immediate convulsive attacks, especially in contact sports. The circumstances make the diagnosis obvious.

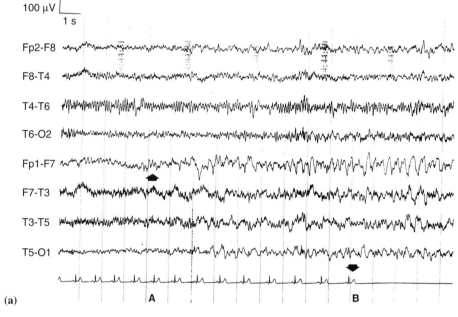

(a)

Figure 5.3 (a) and (b), EEG in Case 6. EEG changes preceded any symptoms. (A) alpha rhythms attenuated over the left hemisphere followed by left-sided slow activity over a period of 20 seconds. (B) the ECG showed heart rate slowing followed by sinus arrest, with only two beats over 14 seconds. (C) the patient became unresponsive with dilated pupils and the EEG slowed bilaterally, then became isoelectric for 7 seconds (D) normal cardiac rhythm returned (E) with high amplitude delta activity on the EEG, accompanied by irregular clonic arm jerks. Consciousness returned after 10 seconds and there was no obvious postictal slowing on the EEG. Prior to the event there were frequent runs of left frontotemporal delta activity. (c) T$_2$-weighted MRI scan from Case 6 showing a large cavernous haemangioma in the left temporal lobe.

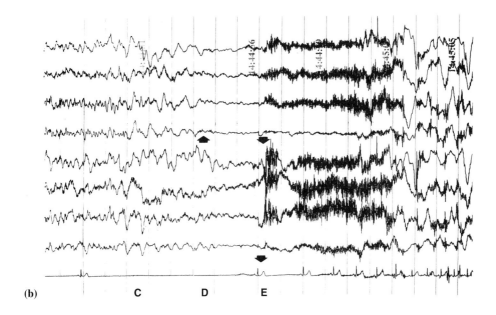

(b)   C   D   E

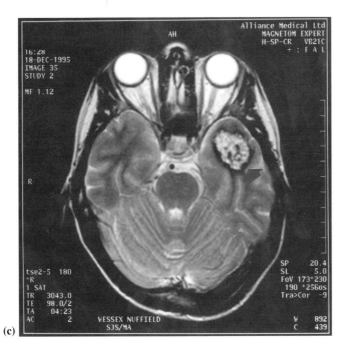

(c)

- A typical attack causes loss of consciousness immediately after impact. Within 2 seconds there is stiffening and posturing of the limbs, sometimes with head deviation and rapidly leading onto convulsions. Even though they may last 2 to 3 minutes, recovery is often rapid, sometimes within seconds of the end of the convulsions. Post-traumatic amnesia may however be as long as 45 minutes. All investigations are normal and there appears to be no increased risk of later, unprovoked seizures.

Tonic–Clonic Seizures (Synonyms: Convulsive Seizures, Grand Mal)

Clinical Features of Tonic–Clonic Seizures

- Tonic–clonic epileptic seizures are usually easy to recognize.
- There may be a prodrome lasting hours with irritability, elation, headache or hunger. Sometimes there may be fragments of seizures building up to the convulsion such as a crescendo of myoclonic jerks, absences or recurrent auras.
- An aura occurs at the onset of half of all seizures and usually lasts less than 30 seconds. The symptom may be non-specific such as a light-headedness or a vague feeling of unease or it may suggest a more specific focal brain activation such as an olfactory sensation.
- The convulsive phase has a characteristic evolution (Figure 5.1). It starts with a tonic phase characterized by stiffening and flexion of trunk and limbs, followed by tonic extension. With this there may be a cry, probably due to the forced expulsion of air followed by apnea. If standing, the patient will fall and there may be injury and incontinence. The patient's head and eyes may turn to one side or look upwards. The seizure then enters the clonic phase starting with low amplitude limb jerks at about 8 hertz and evolving into higher amplitude jerks at 4 hertz. The jerks then slow and stop. The pupils contract and dilate with each jerk but this is rarely noted. During and after the seizure there may be cyanosis. Most convulsions last 1 to 2 minutes.
- After the seizure the patient becomes flaccid. Their breathing is labored and noisy and their tongue may obstruct respirations. As consciousness is recovered, they may be confused and agitated, with non-directed violence, especially if attempts are made to restrain them. Sometimes there are focal deficits such as focal paresis or dysphasia, usually lasting 20 to 60 minutes. The patient often sleeps off the attack and may suffer prolonged postictal changes such as headache, drowsiness or loss of concentration, lasting a day or more.
- Variations on the theme of tonic–clonic seizures include attacks in which the tonic component is minimal or absent and tonic–clonic–tonic seizures, both of which are much less common.

The So-Called Classical Symptoms of Epilepsy

There are several symptoms that have the reputation of being diagnostic of epilepsy. The clinical picture of the blackout must be viewed as a whole; no single symptom is diagnostic but some are helpful.

1. Tongue-biting is the single strongest predictor of epilepsy, where it is usually the side of the tongue that is affected and the damage may be severe. The mouth should be inspected. Occasionally the tip of the tongue is bitten in PNES.
2. Incontinence of urine is commoner in convulsive epileptic seizures than in other sorts of blackout but is not specific and may occur in up to 50 percent of syncope or any cause of collapse if the patient's bladder is full at the time (Case 5).
3. Incontinence of feces is a rare symptom that usually suggests epilepsy.
4. Cyanosis implies an organic cause of the attack but a witnessed description of facial color may be misleading. If a patient strains performing a Valsalva manoeuvre

prior to syncope or in PNES, the purple discoloration of their face may mimic cyanosis.

5. Injuries may occur in any type of blackout if the circumstances are appropriate, for example causing a major fall. Colles fractures or similar injuries of the outstretched hand imply retained consciousness and make epilepsy less likely.

6. Significant burns and scalds are usually only seen if there is deep loss of consciousness, most commonly in epileptic seizures. Carpet burns to face or trunk happen when the patient rubs against the carpet and are almost always due to PNES.

Examination and Investigations

- The examination is usually normal between seizures. Any focal neurological sign suggests focal pathology.
- Positive Babinski responses are often noted immediately after an epileptic attack but return to normal within minutes.
- Neuroimaging and EEG are key investigations. Blood tests may be helpful if there is evidence of an acute symptomatic cause.
- Hypoxia is common during epileptic seizures but rare during PNES.
- Postictal serum prolactin may be helpful.

Psychogenic Non-Epileptic Convulsions

- No single feature reliably distinguishes epilepsy from psychogenic convulsions.
- There are a number of pointers that may help, including the timing of seizures, reproducibility of seizures and their clinical features (Table 5.2).
- Associated psychopathology is common and is usually different from the psychiatric complications of epilepsy. Anxiety, histrionic behavior and a history of childhood sexual abuse are common (Chapter 17).

Nocturnal Convulsive Episodes

Common causes are benign parasomnias, nocturnal epilepsy and psychogenic episodes (Table 5.3). A witnessed account may be less reliable than with diurnal attacks.

Pointers in the History

- Episodes truly arising from asleep are organic but not necessarily epileptic.
- A history of waking episodes or awareness of the episodes effectively excludes a primary sleep disorder.
- The timing of episodes during the night is important in diagnosis (Figure 5.2).
- A prolonged hangover effect is consistent with epilepsy although may be caused by some sleep disorders, including sleep apnea and narcolepsy.
- Waking in the morning having been incontinent or with blood on the pillow suggest epilepsy.
- A family history of similar episodes is common in somnambulism, sleep terrors and some forms of epilepsy.

Table 5.2. Clinical Differentiation of Tonic–Clonic Seizures

Clinical Feature	Epilepsy	Psychogenic Seizures	Syncope
Attacks from sleep	Common	No (but may awake from sleep prior to attack)	No
Stereotyped attacks	Yes	Usually more variable	Yes
Prolonged episodes	Rare	Common	No
Incontinence of urine	Common	Uncommon	Fairly common
Tongue-biting	Common, side of tongue	Uncommon, tip of tongue	Rare
Major injury or burns	Common	Uncommon	Uncommon
Carpet burns	Rare	Common	No
Motor activity	Tonic–clonic but may be atypical in focal epilepsy	Often tremulous or thrashing	Brief asynchronous convulsive movements
Bizarre manifestations	Pelvic thrusting, complex automatisms but none is specific	Opisthotonic posturing, pelvic thrusting, but none is specific	No
Postictal state	Minutes to hours, drowsy, stertorous respiration and sometimes confused with automatisms	Often tearful and appears vague, minutes to hours	Brief, seconds unless head injury or reflex anoxic seizure
Previous illness	Sometimes organic brain disease e.g. encephalitis or prolonged febrile convulsions	Often other somatic disorders with no cause e.g. abdominal pain	Cardiac sometimes
Seizure triggers	Photosensitivity and occasionally others (Chapter 1)	Acute emotional stresses	Postural change, pain, cough, acute emotion, micturition
Associated psychopathology (Chapter 17)	Depression common. Sometimes psychosis	Histrionic behavior, history of childhood abuse including sexual abuse	No

Parasomnias

Sleep Structure

- There are five stages of sleep that occur in cycles through the night.
- Rapid eye movement (REM) sleep is a deep stage in which most dreaming occurs and is most prominent in the later part of the night, towards waking. In normal REM sleep there are rapid movements of the eyes but only minor twitches elsewhere. The descending motor pathways are "switched off" to prevent more gross movements. Lesions or diseases affecting the locus ceruleus in the brainstem may prevent this switching causing hyperactivity during REM sleep.
- Non-REM sleep goes through phases of light sleep (stages 1 to 2) into deep sleep (stages 3 to 4). In these deeper stages, non-REM parasomnias occur especially in the first half of the night. There is a broader spectrum of these conditions than of REM sleep disorders and some conditions are much commoner in children, for example sleep terrors.
- A sleep laboratory is required for accurate diagnosis of paroxysmal nocturnal events. Here the parasomnia can be observed on video and EEG can link it to specific sleep stages and help to exclude epilepsy. Additional tests of oxygenation and respiratory function can exclude sleep apnea.

Table 5.3. Differential Diagnosis of Nocturnal Convulsions

Diagnosis	Age of Onset	Time of Night	Waking Episodes?	Associated Disease	Clinical Features
Epilepsy	Any	Any	Yes	Various	Tonic–clonic seizures, frontal lobe attacks, BECTS
REM parasomnia	Usually >50	Towards waking	No	Commonly Parkinsonism	Thrashing and violent movements lasting minutes
Sleep walking	Children or young adults	Early part of night	No	None	Glassy eyed and purposeless activity
Periodic movements of sleep	Adults (frequency increases with age)	Any	When resting or drowsy in severe cases	Restless legs syndrome	Characteristic triple flexion movement occurring periodically throughout sleep
Psychogenic non-epileptic seizures	Adolescents and young adults commonest	Various, sometimes on retiring	Always awake at onset but may appear asleep	Psychiatric, epilepsy coexists in 20%	Panic attacks and various patterns of PNES
Hypnic jerks	All ages	Sleep/wake transitions	Timing is pathognomonic	None	Sudden massive jerk with feeling of fear

REM Parasomnia in Adults

- REM parasomnias usually occur in the middle-aged and elderly. They are associated with neurodegenerative disease, most commonly Parkinsonism. Some cases are familial.
- REM sleep disorders predominate in the second half of the night and may represent acting out of dreams. The duration of the motor disorder is typically minutes and it may occur occasionally or more than once each night.
- The activity is normally vigorous or even violent and may appear semi-coordinated. Patients may injure themselves or attack a sleeping partner, including attempting to strangle them and there are reports of fatal assaults. There may be some speech during the episode.
- Patients are typically very difficult to rouse from this behavior and have no recollection of it. They may recall the accompanying dream, the content of which is often violent and entirely consistent with the observed behavior.
- Treatment with clonazepam is often helpful.

Case History 7
A 72-year-old man with moderate Parkinsonism developed episodes of agitation in sleep. During these there were thrashing movements and he would shout out. On several occasions he had hit out at his wife and once had grabbed her by the throat. After a few minutes he settled back to sleep and had no recall the next day but did remember experiencing vivid dreams. His wife bought twin beds which resolved her problem.

Non-REM Parasomnias

- Sleep terrors and sleep walking (commonest in children)
- Periodic limb movements (commonest in the elderly)
- Benign neonatal sleep myoclonus
- Nocturnal head banging (commonest in children)
- Hypnic jerks (all ages)

Sleep Terrors and Sleep Walking

- Sleep terrors affect 4 to 5 percent of adults and sleep walking 1 to 2 percent of adults. Adult cases are generally those that persist from childhood. There is a high familial incidence and concordance in twins, suggesting a strong genetic component to the condition.
- They generally only present in adults if they cause harm such as falls, inconvenience others, such as a partner, cause daytime sleepiness or secondary problems such as excess alcohol consumption, in an attempt to improve sleep.
- In a sleep terror, the individual sits up, looks frightened and may call out. They are unaware of their surroundings and settle back to sleep rapidly. These episodes occur no more than once per night – more frequent episodes suggest a different diagnosis. Sleep walking and sleep terrors arise mostly from stage four sleep so occur most commonly in the first hour of sleep.
- When sleep walking, the individual typically appears glassy eyed and motor activity is purposeless. They may pluck at objects or get up and walk around. There may be extreme autonomic discharges and if the patient is restrained, they

may become agitated and resist violently. Occasionally dreaming and a hallucinatory content may be associated with somnambulism, making it more difficult to differentiate from REM sleep disorder and in some patients, especially secondary rather than idiopathic cases, there may be an overlap with REM sleep disorder.

- Treatment with benzodiazepines or tricyclic antidepressants may help but the mainstay of treatment is to adjust the environment to protect the patient from harm.

Case History 8

A 17-year-old boy suffered episodes nearly every night from sleep, usually in the first part of the night. He would rise from his bed, walk down the stairs and attempt to leave by the front door. On several occasions he had tried to climb out of his upstairs window. The episodes lasted several minutes and were not associated with any obviously epileptic movements. His parents were terrified and conducted a night-time vigil to stop him from harming himself. He had no recall of these attacks, which stopped with a small dose of clonazepam.

The timing was typical of somnambulism and the semi-purposeful "escape" activity is much commoner than in epilepsy. The response to clonazepam was unusually good.

Periodic Movements of Sleep

- These are very common, stereotyped movements, usually of one leg that occur at regular intervals at night. They are most prominent in non-REM sleep but may occur at any time, even during waking in severe cases. They increase in prevalence with age, affecting 5 percent of normal individuals from age 30 to 50 and 44 percent over age 65. The movements also become more severe with age.
- Periodic movements occur in association with any cause of peripheral nerve damage such as neuropathy or sciatica and radiculopathy. They may also be due to drugs such as tricyclic antidepressants or due to withdrawal of sedatives such as benzodiazepines but in many cases the cause is unknown. Up to 60 percent of cases give a history of an affected first degree relative.
- Triple flexion is the typical movement, affecting hip, knee and ankle that lasts one to two seconds and recurs at very regular intervals, usually 20 to 30 seconds. The longer duration distinguishes it from other conditions such as hypnic jerks and sleep myoclonus.
- Periodic movements are associated with restless legs syndrome, a condition in which the patient feels that they have to keep their legs moving and they may have to get out of bed to satisfy the urge to move. These symptoms may lead to non-restorative sleep and daytime somnolence.
- Treatment is difficult but the condition may respond to clonazepam, dopamine agonists or codeine.

Nocturnal Head Banging

- This is a behavior of children and adults with learning disability.
- It may recur nightly for years in some individuals lasts for several hours, which readily distinguishes it from epilepsy.

Benign Neonatal Sleep Myoclonus

See Chapter 11

Hypnic Jerks

These movements are a benign, universal experience, which occasionally come to medical attention. They are the sudden massive myoclonus that individuals experience on falling asleep (hypnagogic jerks) and less often on waking up (hypnapompic jerks). They are typically described as being associated with a feeling of falling off a cliff.

Nocturnal Epilepsy

The phrase nocturnal epilepsy is often used for seizures arising from sleep at any time of day. Any form of epilepsy may occur during sleep but certain syndromes are more likely to be restricted to sleep. Seizures most commonly arise from the deeper stages of non-REM sleep but can arise at any time and are not usually restricted to one part of the night.

- Frontal lobe epilepsy has two patterns that may occur largely or exclusively from sleep (Chapter 6) and may be inherited (Chapter 3).

  1. Attacks of limb posturing, sometimes proceeding to tonic–clonic seizures. The attacks are often very brief with rapid recovery and may occur many times each night.
  2. Attacks with complex automatisms and bizarre motor activity. These are also often brief, with rapid recovery.

- Benign epilepsy of childhood with centrotemporal spikes presents in young children with focal motor attacks and tonic–clonic seizures, mostly from sleep (Chapter 11). The characteristic EEG changes may also only occur in sleep.
- Some patients experience focal seizures when awake, which only ever evolve into tonic–clonic seizures when asleep.
- Nocturnal temporal lobe epilepsy is also described.

Psychological Phenomena Arising from Sleep

- Panic attacks are associated with autonomic phenomena and a feeling of fear that overlap with partial seizures. There may be a history of specific thoughts or fears at these times that point to a psychological cause. EEG recording may help to show that the patient wakes up before the attack occurs. The symptoms overlap with those of post-traumatic stress disorder in which the patient may experience flashbacks of the event triggering the disturbance.

Case History 9
A 34-year-old man presented with episodes of shaking, soon after going to sleep. His partner described him as unresponsive for several minutes and shaking all over. The patient described an odd smell before the attacks occurred. On closer

questioning, he associated the smell with his memory of sexual abuse he had suffered as a child at the hands of his father. He described his memories of that experience coming back to him at these times. A diagnosis of non-epileptic seizure disorder was made and supported by an ictal EEG recording showing arousal but no other abnormality. He declined psychiatric treatment.

Odd smells and tastes may be manifestations of PNES, especially if they are associated with hyperventilation. This case illustrates the importance of also making a positive psychiatric diagnosis. A history of sexual abuse is common but may be concealed.

Drop Attacks

Sudden, unexplained falls are a common problem especially in the elderly. There are many potential factors, which may combine to cause drop attacks, including loco-motor, visual and cardiovascular disturbances (Table 5.4, Figure 5.4). Drop attacks are rarely due to epilepsy unless there is also a history of other kinds of epileptic attacks. Recovery from the fall is often very rapid and even with a witnessed account it may be difficult to establish whether there has been alteration of awareness.

Clinical Features

- Other kinds of attacks may be a clue to the diagnosis.
- Physical disabilities may cause a locomotor disturbance.
- Similar attacks occurring when sitting or especially when lying down make a postural cause such as syncope or locomotor much less likely.
- The circumstances of the falls may give a clue to environmental triggers for example, loose carpets or physiological triggers such as hypotension.
- Medication may predispose to hypotension or ataxia.

Table 5.4. Causes of Drop Attacks

Type of Drop Attack	Specific Causes
Locomotor disturbance	Parkinsonism, hemiparesis, visual disturbance, ataxia, gait apraxia, weakness Arthritis, bone disease Inappropriate environment e.g. loose floor covers
Cardiovascular	Arrhythmia, neurocardiogenic syncope, aortic stenosis
Cerebrovascular	Vertebrobasilar TIA (rare and only with other symptoms e.g. ataxia, or diplopia)
Intermittent hydrocephalus	Blocked ventricular shunt, Chiari malformation, intraventricular tumours e.g. Colloid cyst. Recurrent collapses associated with sudden, severe headache
Vestibular	Sudden and disabling vertigo may present with drop attacks but there is usually no loss of awareness
Cataplexy	Usually associated with narcolepsy
Medication	Hypotensive, sedative, hypoglycemic and ataxic e.g. AED
Epilepsy	Almost always in the context of other seizure types
Psychogenic	Swoons are a moderately common form of PNES
Startle disease	Rare abnormality of glycine receptor with infantile hypertonia and falls triggered by startle. Responds to clonazepam

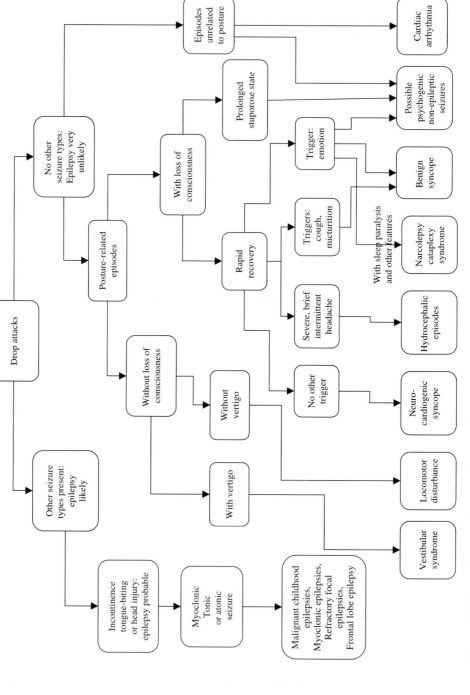

Figure 5.4. Scheme for approaching the diagnosis of drop attacks.

Examination

Examination can be informative with special attention to:

- Gait disorders
- Focal neurological deficits, especially vestibular function
- Cardiovascular examination, including carotid sinus massage, erect and supine blood pressure
- Rheumatological abnormalities affecting back, hips, knees and feet

Case History 10

A 65-year-old woman presented with a history of several years of drop attacks refractory to a wide variety of anti-epileptic drugs (AED). Repeating the history suggested that her left leg always gave way at the onset of the fall. Examination revealed brisk reflexes in her left leg with an extensor plantar response and loss of temperature sensation in the right leg extending up to the right side of her umbilicus. A diagnosis of a mild Brown-Sequard syndrome was made but MRI of her spine and brain failed to reveal a cause. Her falls stopped after she was provided with a walking stick and AEDs were withdrawn.

Cardiovascular Causes of Drop Attacks

- Neurocardiogenic syncope (NCS) may occur at any age but is probably the commonest cause of drop attacks in the elderly. It is defined as a drop in systolic blood pressure of more than 50 mm Hg (vasodepressor) or asystole of more than three seconds (cardioinhibitory) produced by carotid sinus stimulation.
- Presyncopal symptoms occur in less than 10 percent of patients with neurocardiogenic syncope.
- On standing, there is venous pooling in the legs, which triggers an abnormal overactive sympathetic response. Secondary changes from atrial stretch receptors cause reflex bradycardia and hypotension, which may be delayed by many minutes. A tilt table test often reproduces the cardiovascular abnormality. Treatment is with beta blockers, disopyramide or serotonin reuptake inhibitors, which block the central mechanism of NCS.

Case History 11

A 53-year-old headmistress developed episodes at the age of seven. These only occurred when standing and some were associated with migrainous headaches. At the age of 20 she had further attacks. These started with a frontal headache and a feeling of depersonalization. She then fell to the ground and "struggled to regain her senses" for several minutes. She received phenytoin and the attacks stopped after 6 months. She then withdrew medication. Recent episodes occurred every three to four days. They comprised a feeling of light-headedness, that went on to transient loss of vision, usually without loss of awareness but with a feeling of unsteadiness. On five occasions in the last year she had fallen. A baseline ECG was normal. A tilt test was performed. After nine minutes she had a period of asystole lasting 34 seconds. Her eyes rolled up and she became floppy. She was successfully treated with a beta blocker.

Narcolepsy–Cataplexy Syndrome

Narcolepsy–cataplexy syndrome affects 0.02 to 0.18 percent of the population. A canine genetic form of the disorder is related to abnormalities of the hypocretin gene. The condition usually starts in adolescence or in early adult life but may remain undiagnosed for some time. There is a breakdown of the coordination of REM sleep and REM atonia and the separation of sleep and waking states. The resulting symptoms are:

1. Cataplectic falls (REM sleep and atonia intruding into wakefulness)
2. Excessive daytime sleepiness with irresistible urges to sleep
3. Poor nocturnal sleep
4. Hypnagogic visual hallucinations (an abnormal dream-like state on going to sleep)
5. Sleep paralysis (atonia without sleep): a terrifying sensation in which the patient may feel unable to move for seconds to a minute, usually upon waking.

- Cataplectic falls are characteristic of the condition. They may occur spontaneously or they may be triggered by sudden emotion, whether laughter, crying or fear. The patient feels a sudden sensation of "wobbliness" and their legs give way. This is often preceded by a typical tremulous muscular contraction around the mouth and face that may be perceived by the patient or noticed by others. Recovery from the fall is usually rapid but injuries may occur. Occasionally cataplexy may appear before the other features of the condition.
- HLA antigen HLA2/DQW1 is present in 95 to 98 percent of patients and 12 to 35 percent of the general population. Its absence makes narcolepsy–cataplexy syndrome very unlikely.
- The REM sleep latency test looks for the characteristic feature of abnormally early onset of REM sleep in the sleep cycle.
- Treatment: cataplexy usually responds to tricyclic drugs such as clomipramine.

Case History 12
A 22-year-old pharmacist had a secure diagnosis of juvenile myoclonic epilepsy. Her condition was well controlled with sodium valproate but she became increasingly sleepy. Alteration of her medication to lamotrigine had no effect on her symptoms and some seizures recurred. She then developed new, brief drop attacks, with rapid recovery, that were preceded by tremulous movements around her mouth. These became very frequent and when she was undergoing an attack there were almost continuous tremulous movements around her mouth. Blood tests showed HLA2/DQW1 genotype consistent with narcolepsy–cataplexy syndrome. Small doses of clomipramine abolished her drop attacks but led to a recurrence of myoclonic jerks and had to be withdrawn. Her sleepiness was well controlled with modafanil.

This complex case illustrates the symptoms of narcolepsy–cataplexy syndrome and that the patient herself was able to distinguish cataplectic episodes from coincidental myoclonic jerks.

Epileptic Drop Attacks

Drop attacks without aura usually affect patients with established, severe epilepsy. There is almost always a history of other seizure types that readily gives the diagnosis. The previous attacks may be convulsive seizures, absence attacks or partial seizures. Drop attacks are especially common in:

- Malignant epilepsies of childhood, West syndrome or Lennox-Gastaut syndrome
- Refractory focal epilepsy, especially frontal lobe epilepsy
- Myoclonic epilepsies

  - Atonia, myoclonus or hypertonia may cause drop attacks. They are brief and a video recording may be needed to distinguish between them. Atonic seizures are rare, myoclonic and tonic seizures are commoner.
  - In tonic seizures there may be some degree of posturing before the fall occurs or the tonic contraction may persist for some while after the patient has fallen. Tongue-biting and urinary incontinence are common.
  - Myoclonic drops are rarely isolated and the diagnosis can be made from the presence of other myoclonic jerks that do no lead to falls.
  - Injuries are common and severe, including intracranial hemorrhage.
  - Rapid recovery with minimal confusion is usual, providing there has been no head injury. Fear may cause patients to lay on the ground for some minutes to regain their composure, prolonging the episode.
  - Similar episodes when seated or lying can often be revealed by careful questioning.

Case History 13
A 33-year-old woman with moderate learning difficulty had developed epilepsy in early childhood. She suffered frequent absence episodes, tonic–clonic seizures and drop attacks. In the drop attacks, her body stiffened and she fell without warning. She was often incontinent and sometimes suffered severe injury. If she didn't hurt herself, she was confused only for a few seconds and was rapidly able to get up and continue as normal. The injuries were such that she took to wearing a protective helmet. An interictal EEG showed frequent bifrontal spike and slow wave complexes and an MRI showed bilateral thickening of the frontal cortex consistent with cortical developmental abnormality (Figure 5.5)

Epileptic drop attacks only occur in the context of pre-existing, severe epilepsy. Recovery is usually rapid. The severity of epilepsy in these patients means that the interictal EEG is usually abnormal. The EEG at the time of the drop attack usually shows a brief paroxysmal disturbance that is commonly widespread or frontally predominant.

Psychogenic Drop Attacks

- Sudden collapse is a moderately common form of psychogenic episode. The typical patient crumples to the ground without sustaining severe injury, but occasionally they may fall downstairs.
- Patients often lie motionless on the ground for many minutes, as if asleep. The recovery from organic drop attacks is usually much quicker.
- Incontinence of urine is rare (common in epileptic drop attacks).
- Injuries such as Colles fracture of the outstretched hand suggest retained awareness and differentiate these attacks from epilepsy.

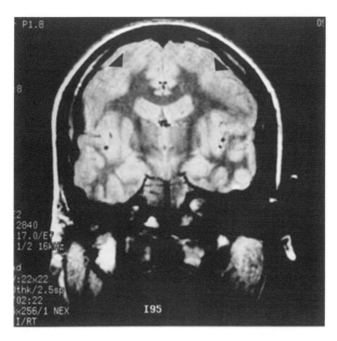

Figure 5.5. Proton density MRI from Case 13 scan showing bilateral frontal cortical thickening due to a developmental abnormality.

Case History 14

A 22-year-old woman had first developed episodes at the age of 16. In a typical attack she felt tired for minutes to hours. Then without warning she fell to the ground and lay motionless and unresponsive, as if asleep for up to 10 minutes. There was no incontinence or injury. Afterwards she felt drained and went back to sleep. Routine EEGs were normal and an ambulatory EEG recorded two episodes. During these she appeared asleep but the EEG showed normal waking rhythms.

Giddy and Dizzy Episodes

- Giddy episodes are common. The term giddiness is used to describe a variety of different feelings with different clinical significance (Table 5.5). It is important to define the symptom the patient is suffering.
- Non-specific auras such as disorientation or lightheadedness are common in epilepsy.

Table 5.5. Meanings of "Giddiness"

Sensation	Term	Significance
A feeling of relative motion of the patient and their environment	Vertigo	Peripheral or central vestibular disorder
A feeling of light-headedness and remoteness	Light-headedness	Presyncope, epilepsy aura, hyperventilation, psychogenic
Unsteadiness	Ataxia	Disorder of locomotion

- Paroxysmal vertigo is characterized by a sensation of relative movement. There are numerous causes (Table 5.6) but epilepsy is rare.

Vestibular Epilepsy

- Vertigo with a sense of relative motion may occur in 3 percent of auras. A feeling of vertigo may be due to movement of eyes or head in the seizure or to involvement of cortical vestibular centers in the seizure.
- Epileptic vertigo may remain undiagnosed for many years. Attacks are usually frequent, from weekly to several times daily.
- Other epileptic symptoms are usually present, helping in diagnosis: auditory or olfactory hallucinations, déjà vu or other psychic phenomena. Seizures usually evolve to motor manifestations of focal epilepsy, especially oroalimetary automatisms or tonic–clonic seizure (TCS).

Blank Spells

Blank spells are a relatively common problem in neurological practice. Usually an observer reports a period of altered mental function, often with reduced responsiveness. Sometimes the patient may be completely unaware that a blank spell has occurred but occasionally the patient may report a period when they lost track of time. Figure 5.6 and Table 5.7 show a simplified diagnostic scheme for the common causes:

- Epilepsy
- Syncope

Table 5.6. Differential Diagnosis of Paroxysmal Vertigo

Diagnosis	Frequency	Causes	Clinical Features
Peripheral vestibular syndromes	Very common	Benign paroxysmal postioning vertigo, Menière's disease, neurovasucular compression of the vestibular nerve	Vertigo often triggered by head movement or associated with hearing loss or tinnitus. BPPV has characteristic positive Hallpike's test
Central vestibular disturbance	Common	Brainstem lesions including demyelination and tumors.	Abnormal neurological examination including nystagmus without vertigo, head tilt, alteration of patient's perception of visual vertical or other neurological signs.
Migraine	Common	Usually idiopathic	Typical timing of migrainous aura and may be associated with other features of migraine
Hyperventilation syndrome	Common	Anxiety	Fluctuating feelings of floatiness rather than discrete attacks of giddiness. May have other features, e.g. tingling or alteration of awareness. Often reproduced by forced hyperventilation in the clinic.
Vestibular epilepsy	Rare	Temporal lobe lesions	Vertigo usually associated with alteration of consciousness and other epileptic features.
Paroxysmal ataxias	Very rare	Ion channel disorders	Bouts of nystagmus and vertigo lasting minutes or hours. No loss of consciousness.

- Psychogenic disturbance
- Hypoglycemia (rare)

Clinical Features

Is there Altered Consciousness?

- Focal deficits may be mistaken for unconsciousness. Breaking down the process of assessing consciousness into its component elements may uncover a more focal neurological deficit.

1. The patient fails to recall the attack, but could respond at the time. This suggests an amnesic episode, most commonly in transient global amnesia but occasionally in pure amnesic seizures or psychogenic amnesia.
2. The patient does not respond during the episode, but is able to describe their symptoms and some events around them. They may have had unpleasant or preoccupying symptoms but they must have been at least partly conscious at the time, usually in epileptic or psychiatric episodes.
3. The patient is unable to talk during the attack but recalls it fully. The main symptom may be aphasia, usually in epilepsy, transient ischemic attack or migraine.
4. Ictal automatic behavior may suggest the patient is responding to their environment in a semi-coordinated fashion and yet is unaware of what they are doing, usually in epilepsy or PNES.

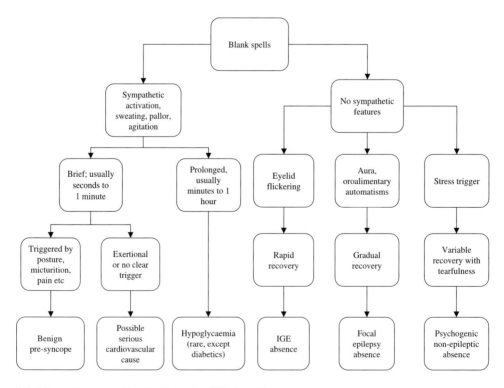

Figure 5.6. Scheme for approaching the diagnosis of blank spells.

Table 5.7. Differential Diagnosis of Absences

Diagnosis	Duration of Attack	Amnesia	Other Clinical Features	Ictal EEG
IGE absences	Usually 5–20 seconds	Usually complete	Usually childhood onset. Staring, sometimes eyelid fluttering or automatisms. Rapid recovery	Generalized epileptiform abnormalities
Focal epilepsy absences	Usually 30–90 seconds	Usually complete	Aura, oroalimentary automatisms, manual automatisms. Recovery in seconds to minutes	Focal epileptiform abnormalities
Status epilepticus with absences	Minutes to hours, occasionally days	Usually complete	Confusional state with partial responsiveness. Automatisms, eyelid fluttering or myoclonic jerks	Epileptiform abnormalities
Psychogenic absences	Minutes to hours, occasionally days	Usually complete	Often triggered by emotional stress and associated with coordinated but incongruous behavior	Normal
Hypoglycemia	Minutes to hours	Usually partial	Agitation, sweating and pallor	Generalized slowing
Syncope	Seconds to a minute	Minimal	Pallor, sweating, blurred vision and relation to posture. Rapid recovery	Generalized flattening. Rapidly normalizes

Case History 15

A 58-year-old man had developed posttraumatic epilepsy at the age of 40. He had had a severe head injury with frontal lobe damage at the age of 30. All his seizures arose from sleep. On one occasion his wife saw him awake from sleep in his garden chair and chase her around the garden, trying to grab her and push her into their swimming pool. She escaped into their kitchen but was followed by him where he started to fumble with objects around him in a purposeless fashion. He recovered awareness of his surroundings and noted that he had been incontinent of urine. He sought urgent medical attention, fearful that he would harm his wife.

Patients are usually amnesic for automatisms. Agitation of this kind is seen especially in frontal lobe epileptic seizures. It is exceptionally rare, however, for the patient to act in a fashion suggesting a coordinated mental strategy.

Blank Spells Due to Syncope

- Syncope that is too mild to cause a collapse may lead to a brief blank episode, with typical presyncopal symptoms of sweating, blurred vision and tinnitus but no amnesia.
- There may be the classical precipitants of syncope (above).

Blank Spells Due To Epilepsy

- Absence seizures cause brief blank spells. Absences in idiopathic generalized epilepsy (IGE) or in malignant childhood epilepsies may occur many times each day. Longer episodes may be due to postictal states or absence status epilepticus.
- The brief absences of IGE are generally associated with marked alteration of awareness but not necessarily complete loss of consciousness; staring or eyelid fluttering are common.

- Focal epileptic absences often start with a focal aura, for example olfactory and are often associated with stereotyped automatisms. Chewing, swallowing or other mouth movements are common.
- Patients with absence status epilepticus may suffer fugues lasting 30 minutes to several days. In this state the patient may be nearly normal: responding to simple commands, eating and dressing themselves. They are unable to perform more complex tasks and are usually amnesic for the event. There are often subtle features of epileptic seizures such as fluttering of the eyelids, mild myoclonus or automatisms (Chapter 14). Occasionally patients may suffer very brief and subtle seizures with a postictal confusional state that dominates the clinical picture.
- Ictal EEG is always abnormal during epileptic absences.

Blank Spells Due to Hypoglycemia

- Hypoglycemia is rare except in diabetics taking hypoglycemic medication. The diagnosis is usually obvious from the context and from blood sugar measurements.
- Attacks tend to be prolonged, lasting many minutes and sometimes an hour or more. Typical symptoms of sympathetic activation (sweating, agitation and pallor) usually occur but may be reduced if the patient suffers frequent hypoglycemic episodes.
- Severe hypoglycemia may cause acute symptomatic seizures and recurrent hypoglycemia damages the hippocampus predisposing to epilepsy.

Psychogenic Blank Spells

- Psychogenic blank spells are often dissociative episodes triggered by acute emotional distress for example, domestic conflict. The unresponsiveness may be difficult to differentiate from minor epileptic episodes but the context is usually suggestive. Patients may occasionally suffer prolonged fugue states.
- A normal EEG in an apparently unconscious patient rules out epilepsy and strongly points to a psychogenic cause.

Case History 16

A 55-year-old woman described episodes in which she would lose touch with the outside world. They typically occurred after a hard day's work when she was relaxing in a chair. Her husband described her as being in a dream-like state for up to two minutes with no abnormal motor activity and quickly coming back to normal. She was putting in many hours of overtime and finding work particularly stressful. EEG, including during an attack was normal.

These attacks occurred under stereotyped circumstances when she was not being distracted by her busy job. They seem to represent a combination of exhaustion and a stress reaction and they improved when her workload reduced.

Paroxysmal Focal Neurological Symptoms

Paroxysmal focal neurological symptoms arise as a result of four main causes:

- Epilepsy
- Migraine

- Transient ischemic attacks (TIA)
- Psychological causes

Table 5.8. Other Cause of Paroxysmal Focal Neurological Symptoms

Symptom Type	Causes	Clinical Features
Memory disturbance	Transient global amnesia	Episodes of hours of anterograde memory loss (unable to store new information) with no alteration of awareness or physical. Patients often appear agitated and repeat questions over and over
Motor disturbance	Paroxysmal choreoathetosis (due to channelopathies)	Different disorders with paroxysmal episodes lasting seconds or minutes to hours
	Periodic movements of sleep	See sleep disorders above
	Tonic spasms of multiple sclerosis	Sudden tonic spasms lasting seconds may occasionally be the presenting feature of MS. They respond to carbamazepine, paradoxically much better than most dystonic seizures
Visual hallucinations	Ocular disorders Lewy body dementia Visual pathway disorders Peduncular hallucinosis (brainstem disorder)	Visual hallucinations are similar in all these conditions. They may be simple patches or complex figures and scenes where there is visual loss, they may be restricted to the abnormal visual field. There may be marked diurnal variation of hallucinations, worst on falling asleep or in poorly illuminated environments
	Hallucinogenic drugs e.g. LSD, cocaine and amphetamines	Commonest cause is ocular pathology especially senile macular degeneration
		Peduncular hallucinosis is usually associated with other brainstem signs
		Drug-related hallucinations often occur in more than one modality and may be associated with thought disorder
Sensory symptoms	Nerve compression e.g. carpal tunnel syndrome	Sensory symptoms usually last minutes and lack the typical Jacksonian progression of epilepsy and may be triggered by focal compression
	Multiple sclerosis	Timing similar to tonic spasms of MS above and no alteration of awareness

Table 5.9. Discriminatory Features of Focal Neurological Symptoms of Epilepsy, Migraine or TIA

Clinical Feature	Epilepsy	Migraine	Transient Ischemic Attack
Age	Any	Any, but skewed to younger	Usually older
Duration	<5 min	20–60 min	Usually minutes to 1 h, occasionally hours
Onset	Sudden	Gradual	Sudden
Nature of symptoms	Positive	Positive or negative	Negative
Triggers	Sleep deprivation, hyperventilation, stress	Hunger, stress, specific foods, fatigue	None specific
Examination	Usually normal	Usually normal	Usually normal
Consciousness	Usually impaired	Usually normal	Usually normal
Fall	Common	Rare	Rare
Memory of episode	Often impaired	Usually normal	Usually normal

Some other neurological conditions may present with focal neurological symptoms and the differential diagnosis depends on the pattern of the neurological symptom (Tables 5.8–5.10).

The whole event needs to be evaluated but some specific features may be useful.

1. Timing, especially the speed of onset and the duration of the symptoms (Figure 5.7)
2. The quality of the symptoms; are they positive (an extra symptom such as jerking of a limb or tingling or negative (a loss of a function such as paresis or loss of sensation)
3. The specific symptoms, for example déjà vu is not a symptom of migraine or vascular disease, whereas diplopia is an exceptionally rare symptom of epilepsy
4. Associated clinical features such as alteration of awareness (epilepsy) or headache (migraine)
5. Are episodes multiple and stereotyped (migraine or epilepsy)?
6. Do symptoms conform to a single vascular territory (TIA) or spread beyond it (epilepsy, migraine, psychogenic)?

Focal Symptoms of Epilepsy

- A wide variety of focal neurological symptoms that may arise from focal epileptic activation of the brain (Chapter 6).
- The onset is usually abrupt and symptoms are predominantly positive: tonic or clonic limb movements; hallucinations in any sensory modality; odd fragmentary thoughts, memories or experiences, such as déjà vu.
- Duration of focal seizures is usually one to three minutes but very brief seizures lasting only seconds are common in frontal lobe epilepsy. Focal status epilepticus may occasionally cause prolonged focal symptoms (Chapter 14).
- Evolution of the symptoms of a focal seizure usually follows one of four general patterns that reflect different pathways from the same initial process.

1. Resolution without additional symptoms.
2. Local spread due to local activation of the cerebral cortex. For example

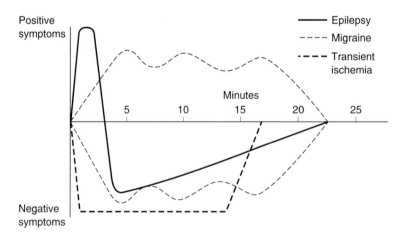

Figure 5.7. Differences in the timing of symptoms in migraine, transient ischemic attack and epilepsy.

Table 5.10. Patterns of Specific Symptoms in Epilepsy, Migraine and TIA

Symptom	Epilepsy	Migraine	Transient Ischemic Attack
Visual	Simple or complex visual hallucinations. May be restricted to one field. Sometimes ictal blindness	Usually bright spots of light or tesselated patterns, blurring of vision. May be one eye, one field or non-anatomical	Loss of vision, like a curtain coming down. Monocular or hemifield
Somatosensory	Tingling and occasionally pain, may spread with Jacksonian march. Usually cannot use limb	Tingling and heaviness affecting one side. Can often still use limb for some tasks	Loss of sensation and occasional tingling. Usually cannot use limb
Motor	Jerking or posturing of limb, sometimes with Jacksonian march. Usually cannot use limb. Todd's paresis common	Heaviness and mild weakness. Major hemiparesis uncommon, can often still use limb	Paresis
Speech	Speech arrest followed by dysphasia in some focal seizures. Usually accompanied by other ictal manifestations	Speech disturbances rare but occasional dysphasia	Dysphasia or dysarthria according to location of TIA
Hearing	Occasional auditory hallucinations, simple or complex	Rarely affected	Rarely affected
Smell/taste	Hallucinations, usually unpleasant	Occasional hypersensitivity to smell	Rarely affected
Emotion	Involuntary fear is common. A range of other emotions seen less frequently	Rarely affected	Rarely affected
Cognition	Altered awareness and sometimes focal deficits postictally	Rarely affected	Dyspraxia, dyscalculia or other manifestations according to location
Autonomic	Tachycardia or bradycardia, pallor or flushing are common	Nausea, pallor and gastric stasis common. Sometimes diarrhea	Rarely affected
Automatisms	Oroalimentary, simple or complex motor automatisms	Not a feature	Not a feature

jerking may start in one corner of the mouth and progress down one side of the body, usually over about 30 seconds, reflecting spread of the discharge down the motor homunculus (Jacksonian motor seizures).

3. Distant spread of symptoms reflecting activation of distant cerebral cortex, via long intercortical pathways. For example, olfactory hallucinations, from anterior temporal seizure discharges evolving into dystonic posturing of the contralateral limb from motor pathway involvement.

4. Rapid evolution to a typical tonic–clonic seizure (secondary generalization).

All four patterns may affect the same patient at different times and may be described as different seizure types until a careful history often shows that they are related. For example temporal lobe seizures more commonly evolve into tonic–clonic seizures when the patient is asleep than when they are awake and any focal onset may not be detected by the patient or an observer

Seizures may also evolve over years and with different treatments. Auras may only appear when the seizures are slowed down by treatment and sometimes they may disappear later in the course of the epilepsy as seizure spread becomes more rapid.

- Alteration of awareness and amnesia are common in epilepsy, even if the other symptoms suggest quite localized discharges within the cerebral hemispheres.
- Patterns of symptom evolution do not reflect vascular territories of the cerebral cortex.
- Following a seizure the patient may notice a temporary reduction in function of the parts of the brain that were activated at the onset of the attack (Todd's phenomenon). Focal motor seizures may result in focal paresis or dominant temporal lobe seizures may cause temporary dysphasia. These symptoms usually resolve within 30 minutes, unless there are serial seizures, in which case they may cause a more persistent disturbance (Case 4, Chapter 14). Headache and drowsiness are common.

Focal Migrainous Symptoms

- Migraine affects around 10 percent of the population, of whom about 20 percent suffer migraine with aura. The onset is commonest in the first three decades, but it may occur at any age. Occasionally the neurological symptoms may be severe or may dominate the clinical picture.
- A prodrome may occur, lasting hours to days in which there is alteration of mood with depression or euphoria and sometimes autonomic symptoms such as hunger or repetitive yawning.
- Neurological symptoms of migraine aura typically evolve to their maximum over 5 to 15 minutes (Figure 5.7). They usually last 20 to 60 minutes before resolving and are usually followed by a throbbing, migrainous headache that may be unilateral and is often associated with nausea or photophobia.
- Aura without headache is a common presentation in older patients; many have suffered more typical migraines in young adult life.
- Visual phenomena are the commonest neurological symptoms. The aura comprises spots, zig-zag lines or patterns. These are usually in one eye rather than in one part of the visual field, although either may occur. The patient often

describes being able to see round or through the abnormality "like looking through a heat haze."

- Mixed positive and negative neurological symptoms are common. For example shining patches of light with patches of visual loss or tingling down one side of the body, associated with difficulty using the arm and some unsteadiness in walking.
- Neurological symptoms of migraine do not obey vascular territories.
- Altered awareness and amnesia are rare.

Transient Ischemic Attack

- The incidence of TIA is around 30 per 100, 000 population. They are commonest in the elderly mirroring the prevalence of atheromatous vascular disease.
- A typical episode has an abrupt onset associated with loss of function attributable to a single vascular territory, for example, left middle cerebral artery TIA causing dysphasia and right hemiparesis. By definition, a TIA has recovered within 24 hours and most recover within one hour. Some TIAs cause a mild headache.
- Loss of consciousness is rare, except in brainstem TIA, when it is almost always associated with other symptoms of brainstem disturbance such as ataxia or diplopia.
- Frequent recurrences of very similar TIAs over a long period are rare without developing a stroke, except for amaurosis fugax. Many similar events should make one think of an alternative diagnosis such as migraine or epilepsy (Case 17).

Case History 17
A previously fit, right-handed 58-year-old man suffered an intracerebral hemorrhage, leaving him with a right superior quadrantanopia. Over the next seven years he suffered attacks 2 to 3 times per year. These comprised a feeling of being slightly unwell and developing a fluent aphasia of which he was not aware. He would sleep off these episodes. They were diagnosed as TIA. At the age of 65 he suffered a typical aphasic episode that evolved into TCS.

The episodes of aphasia arose from the left temporal lobe, consistent with the site of his previous hemorrhage. They were highly focal and stereotyped but it was not until they evolved into a typical TCS that the diagnosis of TIA was revised to epilepsy. Seizures complicate about 15 percent of cerebral hemorrhages.

Atypical Features in The Differential Diagnosis of Epilepsy, Migraine and TIA

Positive Symptoms of Cerebrovascular Disease

- Shaking of the contralateral arm is sometimes seen as a symptom of very high grade carotid stenosis. Perfusion insufficency is thought to be the mechanism.
- The movements are coarse and irregular and last several minutes. They may be triggered by maneuvers that affect cerebral perfusion such as alteration of posture. They lack the other typical feature of focal motor seizures: tonic head and eye deviation; a march of motor activity; other seizure manifestations and alteration of awareness.

- Strong vascular risk factors, such as diabetes, hypertension and smoking are usually present.

Negative Symptoms of Seizures

- When seizures cause negative symptoms, the evolution of the seizure, associated symptoms, presence of other seizure types and results of investigations may give a clue to the diagnosis.
- Loss of vision may be the main aura symptom in one quarter of occipital epilepsy. The loss of vision may be abrupt and bilateral leading to other seizure manifestations. Associated loss of consciousness and headache may lead to an erroneous diagnosis of a basilar ischemic episode or basilar migraine.
- Focal paresis is an uncommon isolated manifestation of seizures. It is usually associated with lesions of the sensorimotor cortex and can be reproduced by electrical stimulation just anterior to the lateral motor cortex.
- Negative myoclonus; sudden, transient loss of tone of an individual limb may be associated with electrophysiological evidence of myoclonus.
- Atonic drop attacks are usually seen in association with other seizure types.
- Dysphasia is a common symptom of seizures and may rarely occur in isolation.
- Amnesia is usual in any seizure in which there has been alteration of awareness (see below) but very occasionally may occur as an isolated seizure manifestation (Chapter 16).

Psychogenic Focal Neurological Symptoms

The symptoms attributable to psychological causes overlap with those due to epilepsy and include: abnormal smells and tastes, abnormal memories (Case 9), jerking of one arm or leg, focal sensory symptoms.

- Forced hyperventilation for 1 minute is worth attempting as a diagnostic test in any patient with unexplained paroxysmal neurological symptoms. It can, however, occasionally trigger epileptic seizures, especially in children with IGE absences.
- Hyperventilation commonly causes sensory symptoms, light-headedness and altered awareness which may progress to carpopedal spasm or convulsive movements (Case 1, Chapter 17).

Dual Diagnosis

Some patients suffer two kinds of episodes. The clinician and the patient have to identify which attacks are which and how to distinguish them. A separate treatment strategy has to be developed for each type. If seizure control deteriorates, the clinician must identify which kind of attack is responsible and target treatment appropriately.

Epilepsy and Psychogenic Non-Epileptic Seizures

- About 20 percent of patients with PNES also have epilepsy. The proportion of patients with epilepsy who also have non-epileptic attacks is probably very small. PNES should be considered in any patient with previously stable epilepsy, where there is a sudden change in their condition.

- Interictal EEG abnormalities are unhelpful as they are expected in these patients who are known to have epilepsy.
- Ictal EEG is required and must be correlated with each clinical seizure type. Home video recording of each of the seizures may be invaluable.
- The combination of epilepsy and psychogenic seizures may arise in various ways.

1. PNES in a patient with a past history of epilepsy.

Case History 18
A 21-year-old nurse developed attacks of daytime convulsions that became increasingly frequent over a period of weeks. There was a past history of convulsions occurring exclusively in sleep, about once a year from the age of 12 to 18. EEGs were normal and when she was admitted to hospital with a crescendo of attacks, clinical observation and ambulatory EEG confirmed non-epileptic seizures. She received counseling and remained seizure-free two years later.

The previous history of rare attacks just at night certainly suggests epilepsy that was coincidental in this case.

2. Epilepsy and PNES may coexist.

Non-epileptic attacks often arise in situations of stress as an avoidance mechanism and the timing of the new seizures linking them to external events often gives the diagnosis. The stress may be a change of home environment or an extra demand placed upon the individual.

Case History 19
A 47-year-old man with learning disability lived with his elderly parents. He had a long history of well-documented focal epileptic seizures occurring two or three times per year, for which he took carbamazepine. He was admitted acutely to hospital with a cluster of convulsions. A CT brain scan was performed that showed compensated hydrocephalus. Forced hyperventilation for one minute caused a convulsive episode with thrashing and flailing movements of his limbs lasting three minutes that settled with reassurance. This was identical to spontaneous episodes that had been witnessed by nursing staff.

The presence of significant learning disability often implies structural brain disease. In this context it is especially important that the diagnosis of PNES is secure. He was continued on maintenance carbamazepine and referred to learning disability services for behavioral therapy for his new attacks.

3. PNES may occasionally arise out of epileptic attacks.

If the patient has preserved awareness during the attack, they may find the experience so distressing as to trigger a reaction manifesting as a non-epileptic attack (Case 2, Chapter 14). Hyperventilation and panic may play a role in these circumstances.

Migraine-Epilepsy Overlap Syndrome

- There is an epidemiological association between migraine and epilepsy. The frequency of epilepsy in individuals with migraine has been estimated as

5.9 percent, more than ten times the general prevalence of 0.5 percent. The frequency of migraine in patients with epilepsy may be 25 percent, compared with a general prevalence of 10 to 15 percent. The mechanism of the association is not clear and probably includes genetic and environmental factors such as trauma. Some conditions are well recognized to cause both problems, such as arteriovenous malformations or mitochondrial diseases but these cases form the minority.

- Boundary cases with features of epilepsy and migraine present diagnostic problems, especially differentiating basilar migraine and occipital epilepsy. Both conditions may cause headache, visual disturbance, vomiting and blackouts. Some patients suffer frequent migraines that occasionally evolve into seizures and there may be EEG abnormalities in migraine.
- The visual auras of migraine are typically white or silver and shiny and linear and appear concentrically around the center of fixation in one eye then expand. Those of epilepsy with visual aura are characteristically multi-colored, more circular and appear in one hemifield. These distinctions are sometimes difficult to establish and the EEG during migraine may also show spikes and waves suggesting epilepsy, although there is not usually the evolution of the discharge seen in epileptic seizures.

BIBLIOGRAPHY

Andermann E, Andermann F. Migraine–epilepsy relationships: epidemiological and genetic aspects. In Andermann F, Lugaresi E (eds). Migraine and Epilepsy. Boston: Butterworths, 1987;281–292.

Andermann F. Clinical features of migraine-epilepsy syndromes. In Andermann F, Lugaresi E (eds). Migraine and Epilepsy. Boston: Butterworths, 1987;3–30.

Beaumanoir A, Jekiel M. Electrographic observations on the attacks of classical migraine. In Andermann F, Lugaresi E (eds). Migraine and Epilepsy. Boston: Butterworths, 1987;163–180.

Benbadis SR, Wolgamuth BR, Goren H, Brener S, Fouad TF. Value of tongue biting in the diagnosis of seizures. Arch Intern Med 1995;155:2346–2349.

Dey AB, Kenny RA. Drop attacks in the elderly revisited [editorial; see comments]. QJM.1997;90:1–3.

Fisher CM. Concerning recurrent transient cerebral ischaemic attacks. Can J Neurosci 1962;86:1091–1099.

Fisher CM. Transient paralytic attacks of obscure nature: the question of non-convulsive seizure paralysis. Can J Neurol Sci 1978;5:267–273.

Gowers WR. Epilepsy and Other Chronic Convulsive Diseases: Their Causes Symptoms and Treatment. London: J. and A. Churchill;1881.

Hoefnagels WAJ, Padberg GW, Overweg J, Roos RAC, Van Dijk JG, Kamphuisen HAC. Syncope or seizure? The diagnostic value of the EEG and hyperventilation test in transient loss of consciousness. J Neurol Neurosurg Psychiatry 1991;54:953–936

Selected Writings of John Hughlings Jackson Vol. 1. Nijmegen: Arts & Boewe, 1996;312–313.

Kales A, Soldatos C, Bixler EO. Hereditary factors in sleepwalking and night terrors. Br J Psychiatry 1988;137:111–118.

King MA, Newton MR, Jackson GD, Fitt GJ, Mitchell LA, Silvapulle J, Berkovic S. Epileptology of the first-seizure presentation: aclinical electroencephalographic and magnetic resonance imaging study of 300 consecutive patients Lancet 1998;352:1007–1011.

Kogeorgos J, Scott DF, Swash M. Epileptic dizziness. BMJ 1981;282:687–689.

Lempert T. Recognizing syncope: pitfalls and surprises. J RoySoc Med 1996;89:372–375.

Lennox WG, Cobb S. Epilepsy. Aura in epilepsy: a statistical review of 1359 cases. Arch Neurol Psychiatr 1933;30:374–87.

Lipton RB, Ottman R, Ehrenberg BL, Hauser WA. Comorbidity of migraine: the connection between migrane and epilepsy. Neurology 1994;44(Suppl. 7.):S28–S32.

Luchins DJ, Sherwood PM, Gillin JC, Mendelson WB, Wyatt RJ. Filicide during psychotropic-induced somnambulism: a case report. Am J Psychiatry 1978;135:404–405.

Mahowald MW, Schenck CH. REM sleep behavior disorder. In: Kryger AI, Roth B, Dement W, (eds). Principles and Practice of Sleep Medicine. Philadelphia: WB Saunders, 1994:574–588.

Marks DA, Ehrenberg BL. Migraine-related seizures in adults with epilepsy, with EEG correlation. Neurology 1993;43:2476–2486.

McCrory PR, Bladin PF, Berkovic SF. Retrospective study of concussive convulsions in elite Australian rules and rugby league footballers: phenomenology, aetiology and outcome. BMJ 1997;314:171–174.

McIntosh S, Lawson J, Kenny RA. Clinical characteristics of vasodepressor, cardioinhibitory and mixed carotid sinus sensitivity in the elderly. Am J Med 1993;95:203–208.

Montplaisir J, Godbout R, Pelletier G, Warnes H. Restless legs syndrome and periodic limb movements during sleep. In: Kryger AI, Roth B, Dement W (eds). Principles and Practice of Sleep Medicine. Philadelphia: W.B. Saunders, 1995:589–597.

Palmini A, Gloor P, Jones-Gotman M. Pure amnestic seizures in temporal lobe epilepsy. Definition, clinical symptomatology and functional anatomical observations. Brain 1992;115:749–770.

Penry JK, Porter RJ, Dreifuss FE. Simultaneous recording of absence seizures with video tape and electroencephalography. Brain 1975;98:427–440.

Salanova V, Andermann F, Olivier A, Rasmussen T, Quesney LF. Occipital lobe epilepsy: electro-clinical manifestations, electrocorticography, cortical stimulation and outcome in 42 patients treated between 1930 and 1991. Brain 1992;115:1655–1680.

Schenck CH, Boyd JL, Mahowald MW. A parasomnia overlap disorder involving sleepwalking, sleep terrors and REM sleep behavior disorder in 33 polysomnographically confirmed cases. Sleep 1997;20:402–405.

Tatemichi TK, Young WL, Prohovnik I, Gitelman DR, Correll JW, Mohr JP. Perfusion insufficiency in limb shaking transient ischaemic attacks. Stroke 1990;21:341–347.

Ward C, Kenny RA. Reproducibility of orthostatic hypotension in symptomatic elderly. Am J Med 1996;100:418–422.

Yanagihara T, Piepgras DG, Klass DW. Repetitive involuntary movements associated episodic cerebral with ischaemia. Ann Neurol 1999;18:244–250.

6

Principles of Syndromic Diagnosis and Focal Epilepsy Syndromes

An epileptic seizure is a symptom; the next stage in diagnosis is to classify the epilepsy syndrome (Figure 6.1). The key criteria are clinical seizure type, EEG and etiology.

- Acute symptomatic seizures are provoked by acute insults, either direct, for example, stroke, or indirect, for example, alcohol withdrawal (Chapter 13). These are defined as seizures not necessarily requiring a diagnosis of epilepsy.
- Epilepsy is usually defined as recurring, unprovoked seizures.
- In generalized onset epilepsy, the electrical discharge appears to start over the whole brain at the same time. This produces a limited repertoire of seizure types: tonic–clonic seizures, absences, myoclonic seizures, tonic seizures and atonic seizures. Onset is usually in childhood or adolescence (Chapter 11).
- In focal onset epilepsy, the electrical discharge appears to start in one cortical region and then may remain localized or may spread over the whole brain. This produces a more varied repertoire of focal (partial) seizures, whose manifestations are often a corruption of the normal functions of the cortical region of onset of the seizure. The terms complex partial seizure (awareness is impaired during the seizure) and simple partial seizure (awareness is preserved) are widely used but have been dropped from the latest classification. When the discharge spreads, the seizure may evolve into a tonic–clonic (secondarily generalized) seizure, a tonic or an atonic seizure.
- Epileptic encephalopathies are malignant syndromes of childhood in which epileptic abnormalities contribute to progressive neurological or cognitive decline. They are not easy to classify as either focal or generalized and are considered separately (Chapter 11).

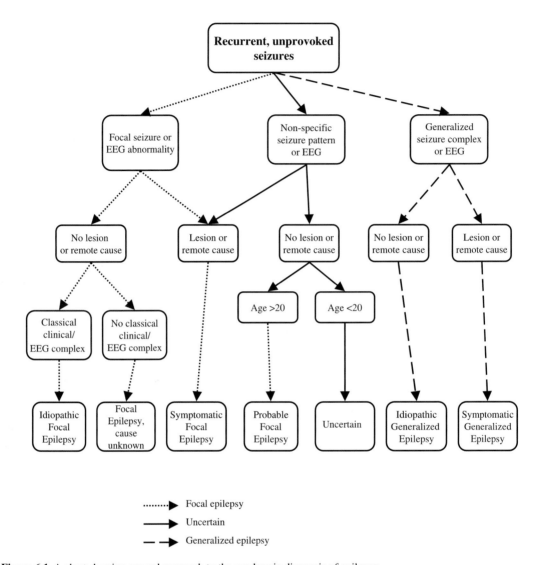

Figure 6.1. A chart showing general approach to the syndromic diagnosis of epilepsy.

- The etiology of the epilepsy provides the next layer of classification. In symptomatic epilepsies, the etiology is known, for example a tumor. Until recently the term cryptogenic epilepsies was used where there is presumed to be a focal lesion but it has not been identified. The new term is probably symptomatic epilepsies.
- In idiopathic epilepsy a polygenic cause is presumed with no identifiable structural lesion. Idiopathic epilepsies tend to have onset in childhood or adolescence and have characteristic electroclinical features (Chapter 11). The benign focal epilepsies of childhood and most generalized epilepsies are idiopathic but some severe childhood generalized epilepsies are usually symptomatic for example Lennox-Gastaut syndrome associated with tuberose sclerosis.

DIFFERENTIATING FOCAL AND GENERALIZED EPILEPSIES

- Age of onset: most generalized epilepsy starts below the age of 20. Focal epilepsies may start at any age (Figure 6.2).
- Focal epilepsy is likely if seizure symptoms suggest focal activation of the cerebral cortex, such as sensory auras, focal motor activity or psychic phenomena or if there is a focal neurological deficit after the seizure, most commonly focal paresis or dysphasia. However, many focal epilepsies do not cause focal seizure manifestations.
- Generalized epilepsies usually cause seizures without major focal elements. Often a number of seizure types cluster together in a typical syndrome, for example juvenile myoclonic epilepsy (Chapter 11).
- Interictal EEG is commonly normal especially in focal epilepsies. Usually focal epileptiform discharges can be differentiated from generalized ones but it may be difficult, especially in frontal lobe epilepsy. Photosensitivity nearly always implies a generalized epilepsy but occurs in some normal individuals and in occipital epilepsy.
- Neuroimaging may point to an epileptogenic lesion, implying a focal epilepsy.
- Overlap occurs between clinical manifestations of focal and generalized epilepsies. For example absence seizures due to focal or generalized discharges may cause similar automatisms and a similar EEG abnormality. It may only be the presence of an epileptogenic frontal lesion on MRI that enables one to make a diagnosis of focal epilepsy (Case 8). Equally some generalized epilepsies such as juvenile myoclonic epilepsy may include some elements of focal motor activity such as head turning and focal features in the EEG. Even after full evaluation the classification may remain uncertain in some patients.

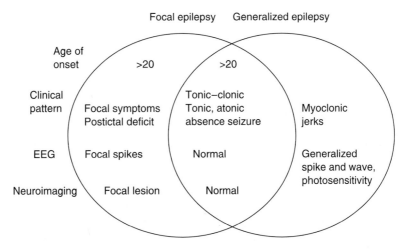

Figure 6.2. A Venn diagram showing the relationship of clinical features and investigations to the diagnosis of generalized and focal epilepsies.

FOCAL SEIZURE PATTERNS: PRINCIPLES OF SEIZURE LOCALIZATION

What is Seizure Localization and What does it Mean?

- The concept of a restricted electrical "focus" where seizures arise is supported by the observation that focal surgical resection may render patients seizure-free. However, some seizures are generated by a network of neurons, which is distributed widely in the brain and focal epilepsy is often not amenable to surgery because it is not focal enough. Clinical localization is the method of identifying the region of onset of focal seizures from clinical patterns and investigations. It is of most value in evaluating patients for epilepsy surgery (Chapter 15).
- Clinical seizure patterns may be highly characteristic of epilepsy arising in one brain region or they may be quite non-specific (Table 6.1).

The Analysis of Focal Seizure Symptoms

- Some considerations are helpful in determining the region of origin of focal epileptic seizures.
- The earliest seizure symptoms are the most useful, as they are more likely to reflect the region of seizure onset, before discharges have spread.
- Seizure symptoms are a corruption of the normal functions of the part of the brain from which they arise and their location can be predicted from a knowledge of cerebral localization of function.
- Some aura symptoms are pathognomonic of focal epilepsy, for example olfactory hallucinations, but others may also occur in generalized epilepsy, for example light-headedness.
- Primary motor and sensory seizures are the easiest to localize. They relate to a single part of the brain that is devoted to a single function and in some cases there is a cortical map of localization, for example the motor homunculus.
- The spread of abnormal electrical activity may follow predictable patterns probably dictated by local and distant intercortical connections but inevitably the later components of the seizure are of less value in clinical localization. Statistical analysis has been helpful in delineating typical patterns of seizure evolution in temporal lobe epilepsy (TLE) but has also shown that seizures from many origins have similar symptoms later in the attack (convergence) and seizures from one region may end in a variety of different ways (divergence). An absence with oroalimentary automatisms may be due to epilepsy from either temporal lobe. If it evolves to dystonic posturing of the right arm, then a left temporal onset is likely (Table 6.2).
- Tonic–clonic seizures are the "ultimate convergence" of seizures from different regions and may be caused by seizures arising in any part of the brain; they have no localizing value.
- Multiple seizure types can sometimes be viewed as variations on a theme. In other cases, different seizure types may be arising from different cortical regions. In some patients, an aura that is valuable in clinical seizure localization may only be present for part of their seizure history. It may disappear if seizures

Table 6.1. The Localizing Value of Different Seizure Symptoms

Symptom		Localization	Comments
Primary sensations	Olfaction[1]	Temporal (uncinate)	Smells are unpleasant and difficult to define
	Taste[2]	Temporal, orbitofrontal or opercular	Tastes are unpleasant and difficult to define
	Simple visual[1]	Occipital	Usually colored blobs. May be loss of vision. Sometimes restricted to one visual field
	Somatosensory[1–2]	Parietal, sometimes motor cortex or supplementary motor area (SMA)	More highly localizing when there is a Jacksonian march
	Epigastric sensation[3]	Temporal, frontal or parietal	Rising sensations are more typically temporal
Complex perceptual phenomena (rare and often polymodal, Case 2)	Complex auditory hallucinations[1]	Temporal	These may be speech or music
	Complex visual hallucinations[2]	Temporal, parieto-occipital junction, occasionally frontal	Images of people, animals scenes
	Distortions of body shape or image[2]	Parietal association, or temporal	Includes out of body experiences.
Emotions	Fear[3] (Case 1)	Temporal especially amygdala, cingulate, frontal or parietal	Fear may be an involuntary seizure symptom or a reaction to the onset of a seizure
	Anger[2], sadness[2], elation[2], sexual arousal[1]	Mostly temporal or temporo-parietal	These emotions are much rarer than fear. Epileptic orgasm is restricted to women
Experiential[1] phenomena	Déjà vu, déjà entendu, déjà vécu, jamais vu, jamais entendu, jamais vécu (Case 2)	Temporal lobe	Highly specific sensations are different from a vague feeling of familiarity that is of much less value. Déjà vu, if strictly visual, is probably right temporal
	Forced thoughts[2]	Frontal or temporal	A recurring irresistible thought
Motor phenomena	Clonic jerks[1–2]	Sensorimotor cortex	Most valuable are focal clonic jerks in clear consciousness, with Jacksonian progression
	Tonic posturing and head or eye deviation[2–3] (Case 6)	Contralateral motor cortex, supplementary motor area, lateral premotor area	Brief tonic seizures in clear consciousness are usually SMA or lateral premotor
	Complex repetitive motor activity[3] (Case 8)	Frontal if at seizure onset	Tapping or plucking movements common. Sometimes bicycling or other bizarre patterns. Mostly they are late in a seizure and of little localizing value
	Complex behavioral automatisms[2]	Orbitofrontal, anterior cingulate, but may reflect spread of TLE	Actions are often very bizarre and there may be semi-purposeful interaction with the environment (Case 9)
	Oroalimentary automatisms[1]	Operculum activation, usually from TLE	Typically chewing or swallowing movements
Vocalizations	Non-specific noise[3]	Non-specific	Often part of a tonic or tonic–clonic seizure
	Musical noises[2]	Frontal	Often bizarre humming
	Speech[1]	Temporal	Distinct from post-ictal speech and voluntary speech, ictal speech is often followed by postictal dysphasia

[1] = highly localizing, [2] = moderately localizing, [3] = poorly localizing.

Table 6.2. Lateralizing Symptoms in Temporal Lobe Epilepsy

Symptom	Relation to Ictal Discharge	Reliability
Unilateral dystonic posturing	Contralateral	High
Unilateral manual automatisms	Ipsilateral	High
Nose rubbing	Left sided discharge	High
Unilateral blinking	Left sided discharge	High
Postictal anomia	Dominant hemisphere	Very high
Déjà vu	Non-dominant hemisphere	Moderate

evolve more rapidly as the epilepsy progresses, or it may be modified by treatment.

- A postictal phenomenon may reliably point to the region of onset of the seizure, for example focal weakness "Todd's paresis" from contralateral motor cortex seizures, or dysphasia from dominant temporal lobe seizures.

Problems in Localizing Seizure Onset in Focal Epilepsy

- Alteration of awareness or amnesia for the seizures may mask some manifestations. Symptoms that occur when a patient is conscious are more valuable in localization. For example, if consciousness is lost before one half of the body starts to jerk then the discharge has spread beyond the contralateral motor cortex.
- Seizure activity may spread rapidly from one part of the brain to another, so that there is no clinical manifestation from the region of onset and onset is falsely attributed to a secondary region. For example, temporal lobe and frontal lobe epilepsies can be very difficult to differentiate, which may be explained by the close functional and anatomic relationships between these regions.
- Some regions of seizure onset (for example, frontopolar) may be clinically silent and the seizure only becomes clinically manifest when it has spread to other regions.
- Rapid secondary generalization with no focal features is also common in frontal lobe epilepsy.

The Focal Epilepsies

Focal seizures are symptoms of focal epilepsies (Figure 6.3). The focal epilepsies are syndromes characterized by:

1. Epidemiology, especially age of onset
2. Etiology
3. Seizure patterns
4. EEG patterns

Most focal epilepsy is symptomatic with a clear cause in the patient's history or on neuroimaging. Other cases are presumed to have a specific cause that cannot be proven and some are benign focal epilepsies of childhood, thought to be primarily genetic (Chapter 11).

Frontal lobe epilepsy

Epidemiology	Second commonest focal epilepsy 25-40%
Aetiology	Tumours, vascular malformations, dysplasia, post-traumatic. Various patterns are more frequent from particular regions of the frontal lobes (below) but delineation is not sharp. Seizures are often brief, with rapid recovery, occur with high frequency and are predominantly nocturnal. Status epilepticus is common both convulsive and non-convulsive.
Clinical seizure types	
EEG	Often unhelpful in localization and may be completely normal interictally. Ictal EEG may be masked by prominent motor activity.

Type of frontal epilepsy	Features
Supplementary motor area (mesial)	Tonic posturing of limbs, sometimes painful with forced head and eye deviation. Occasionally bilateral motor activity with preserved awareness. Interictal EEG is often normal and ictal EEG masked by artefact with no postictal changes.
Sensorimotor cortex	Focal motor seizures with head and eye deviation to the contralateral side. Seizures may have typical Jacksonian progression with postictal paresis of affected limbs; Todd's paresis (case 7).
Frontopolar cortex	Pseudo-generalized epilepsy: absences and tonic clonic seizures with no focal features. EEG may show secondary bilateral synchrony, mimicking IGE
Orbitofrontal cortex	Auras are common including fear, abdominal sensations, smell or taste. Autonomic phenomena common: mydriasis; tachycardia; facial flushing; urinary incontinence. Motor activity is often bizarre: thrashing movements; flailing; rolling; running and is often misdiagnosed as non-epileptic. Ictal EEG is usually required and may need orbitofrontal electrodes.

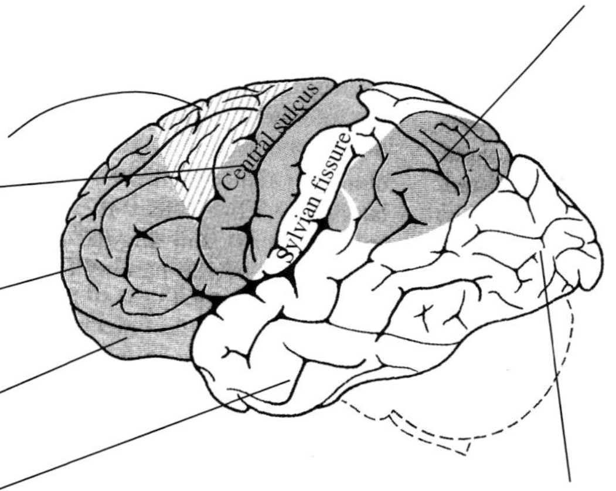

Temporal lobe epilepsy

Epidemiology	Commonest focal epilepsy. 50-60%.
Aetiology	Mesial temporal sclerosis commonest, associated with previous complex febrile convulsions (chapter 2) also foreign tissue lesions, developmental abnormalities and dysembryoplastic neuroepithelioma
Clinical seizure types	Commonly auras including experiential, fear or other emotions, complex perceptual (especially from neocortical onset) smell and taste. Absences with oroalimentary automatisms evolving to contralateral dystonic posturing, ipsilateral manual automatisms. Secondary generalization less common than frontal lobe epilepsy.
EEG	Commonly focal interictal and ictal discharges over one or both frontotemporal regions. Sometimes only detectable with special electrodes, such as superficial or deep sphenoidal electrodes.

Parietal lobe epilepsy

Epidemiology	About 5% of focal epilepsy
Aetiology	Tumours, vascular malformations, dysplasia
Clinical seizure types	Somatosensory, including pain from primary sensory cortex, sometimes with Jacksonian march. Often evolves to focal tonic or clonic seizures. Complex visual auras with formed hallucinations and perceptual such as distortion of body parts, out of body experience or anosagnosia from parietal association cortex. Evolution to absence seizures.
EEG	Parasagittal abnormalities common

Occipital lobe epilepsy

Epidemiology	About 5% of focal epilepsy
Aetiology	Structural lesions common, vascular, tumor, dysplasia. Also benign occipital epilepsy of childhood (chapter 11)
Clinical seizure types	Typically simple visual hallucinations, but ictal blindness at onset in 25%. Spread to temporal lobes with absence and automatisms or to frontal lobes with head and eye deviation and clonic movements
EEG	Often non-specific, sometimes with posterior quadrant interictal an ictal abnormalities

Figure 6.3. Focal epilepsy syndromes.

BIBLIOGRAPHY

Anonymous. Proposal for revised classification of epilepsies and epileptic syndromes. Commission on Classification and Terminology of the International League Against Epilepsy. Epilepsia 1989;30:389–399.

Engel J Jr. ILAE Commission report. A proposed diagnostic scheme for people with epileptic seizure and with epilepsy: report of the ILAE task force on classification and terminology. Epilepsia 2001;42:1–8.

Fish DR, Gloor P, Quesney LF, Olivier A. Clinical responses to electrical brain stimulation of the temporal and frontal lobes in patients with epilepsy. Brain 1993;116:397–414.

Kotagal P, Luders HO, Williams G, Nichols TR, McPherson J (1995). Psychomotor seizures of temporal lobe onset: analysis of symptom clusters and sequences. Epilepsy Res 1995;20:49–67.

Manford M, Fish DR, Shorvon SD. An analysis of clinical seizure patterns and their localizing value in frontal and temporal lobe epilepsies. Brain 1996;119:17–40.

Hughlings-Jackson J. A study of convulsions. In: Taylor J, Holmes G, Walshe FMR (eds). Selected Writings of John Hughlings Jackson Volume One. Nijmegen: Arts & Boeve 1996:8–36.

Wieser HG. Ictally active pathways in psychomotor seizures: a stereo-EEG study. In: Dam M, Gram I, Penry JK (eds). Advances in Epilepstology: XIIth International Symposium. New York: Raven Press 1981:305–312.

APPENDIX: FOCAL SEIZURE HISTORIES

Case History 1

A 28-year-old woman developed seizures 2 weeks after severe measles infection at the age of 5. At the onset of her seizures she felt an intense fear and guilt, associated with a rising epigastric sensation. She became tachycardic and flushed and her pupils dilated. She looked frightened and clutched on to her mother's arm if she was near. Her limbs stiffened slightly and she would swear, before recovering after about 15 seconds. Her interictal EEG showed bilateral frontal slow wave disturbances without spikes. Neuroimaging was not available. This case illustrates how the feeling of fear may be accompanied by appropriate facial appearance and autonomic changes and may cause motor activity consistent with the emotion.

Case History 2

A 30-year-old man was undergoing evaluation for epilepsy for mesial temporal sclerosis. His seizures comprised a blank spell preceded by the same thought that took the form of a flashback. He recalled the sensation when he had fallen into a river at the age of 5. He didn't feel as if he was falling he just recalled the sensations that he associated with the accident, combined with the same feeling of fear. In this case the flashback was not a recollection of a specific event but a recurrence of the feelings associated with that event – a common type of experiential flashback.

Case History 3: Occipital Epilepsy

A 27-year-old man experienced seizures since the age of 19. The seizures occurred several times per month. The onset was with flashing colored lights in his left visual field. This was followed by loss of consciousness and head and eye deviation to the right. Secondary generalization was moderately common. Interictal EEG showed occasional spikes in the right posterior quadrant and MRI showed a right occipital arteriovenous malformation. This was a typical occipital seizure. Head and eye movement are usually contralateral to seizure onset but may be ipsalateral, especially when a later seizure manifestation.

Case History 4: Parietal Lobe Epilepsy

A 25-year-old woman presented with seizures starting with pain and tingling down her left arm. The feeling had been recurrent over several weeks but was not brought to medical attention until she had a secondarily generalized attack. This seizure had evolved into jerking of the left arm then spread to the opposite side with loss of consciousness. An interictal EEG was normal but MRI showed a right parietal lesion thought to be a low grade glioma.

Case History 5: Temporal Lobe Epilepsy

A 50-year-old woman had developed seizures soon after mastoid surgery for chronic suppurative ear disease at the age of 30. Seizures tended to cluster three to four times per month. They started with an odd smell and taste and then she had the irresistible thought that she was a bald-headed, little old man. Her husband described her going pale during these attacks, with hypersalivation and some grunting noises. Then her head would turn to the right and her right arm twist up. Following the seizure she was dysphasic for several minutes. An EEG during the episode showed rhythmical left sided slow wave activity, maximal in the left temporal region, consistent with a unilateral seizure discharge but not highly localized.

This case illustrates the bizarre nature of some phenomena and how different types of aura may occur together. It illustrates the deviation and posturing that co-localizes with postictal dysphasia to the left hemisphere.

Case History 6: Supplementary Motor Area Epilepsy

A 45-year-old man developed very frequent seizures with up to 200 per day. His eyes and head deviated slowly to the left and his left arm usually rose into the air. During the attack he appeared less responsive. The seizures finished within 10 to 20 seconds and within another 5 seconds he was back to normal. Interictal EEG showed occasional left frontal spikes at F3 to F7. Ictal EEG showed brief, widespread slow waves, followed by muscle artefact and rapid recovery. MRI showed a developmental abnormality centered on the left premotor cortex but extending anteriorly and back to the primary motor cortex.

Case History 7: Motor Cortex Epilepsy, from Selected Writings of Hughlings-Jackson

Elizabeth F., 9 years old. June 25, 1866. The child was brought to the outpatient room by her mother on account of fits. Before I spoke to her, the mother made a statement to the following effect, which I give as nearly in her words as I could write it down. "This child has fits. The first was two months ago. It begins in the right eye; then her mouth opens; the face draws up to this side" (pointing with her finger to the child's right cheek). "Her hand draws up to her head and her leg works. She cannot talk when it begins and it has altered her speech a good deal." In reply to a question the mother said the child was not at all insensible in the attacks. I asked her how she knew that, as the child could not talk. She replied, because the child could tell her what had happened during the fits, instancing without questioning that the child knew who was there and what was done. She also said that during one fit she (the mother) being distressed shed tears, and when the fit was over the child spoke of her crying. In reply to an enquiry, she said the fits would last 10 minutes, and on my expressing incredulity she very quietly added she had "timed them by the clock". I now made enquiries as to the details of the fit. It would begin in the midst of talking or singing. Although the face was the first to twitch, the fit began by an aching in the hand, and the arm "dropped". After the face had begun to twitch the arm drew up. She never bit her tongue. Hughlings-Jackson noted that Elizabeth F. suffered mild dysarthria and suggested a structural lesion of the left hemisphere. This case illustrates the long duration of some focal motor seizures, the characteristic evolution, that bears Jackson's name, the tonic features and also describes rarer ictal paresis.

Case History 8: Frontopolar Cortex Epilepsy

A 35-year-old woman had developed epilepsy at the age of 22. Her seizures were tonic–clonic with just a brief abdominal aura or absences with brief manual automatisms but no focal features. An interictal EEG when she was 20 showed bilateral frontally-predominant spike and wave discharges, consistent with a generalized epilepsy. A CT scan was normal. An MRI 10 years later showed a lesion extending from the orbitofrontal to the frontopolar cortex (Figure 6.4). This case illustrates a deceptive pseudo-generalized epilepsy arising from the frontal cortex.

Case History 9: Orbitofrontal Cortex Epilepsy

A 31-year-old man had suffered seizures since a road traffic accident at the age of 12. Seizures were at day or night. With the seizures, he first experienced an abdominal sensation and he became tachycardic with facial flushing. A few seconds later he sat up and screamed. His limbs flailed violently for a few

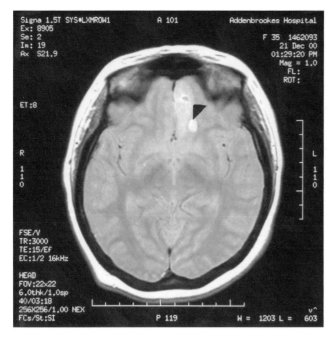

Figure 6.4. Proton density MRI scan of an orbitofrontal/frontopolar lesion in a patient with pseudo-generalized epilepsy (Case 8).

seconds and when sitting he threw himself off his chair. This violent motor activity ceased and he returned fully to normal within seconds. These seizures had been misdiagnosed as non-epileptic. Ictal EEG showed rhythmic bifrontal activity and an MRI showed atrophy in the right orbitofrontal region. Orbitofrontal seizures often manifest with bizarre motor activity and are commonly misdiagnosed as psychogenic non-epileptic seizures.

7

Electroencephalography

INTRODUCTION AND TECHNIQUES OF ELECTROENCEPHALOGRAPHY

Collectively, the electrical activity of many nerve fibers generates fields big enough to be detected at a distance and even on the surface of the head. Electroencephalography (EEG) is the usual technique whereby this spontaneous electrical activity of the brain is recorded. The commonest recordings use a standard array of scalp electrodes (Figure 7.1). The recording is undertaken and supervised by highly trained electroencephalographers. They interact with the patient, note any clinical events occurring during the recording, correct some recording artifacts arising during the recording and may tailor the recording to identify abnormalities as it is proceeding.

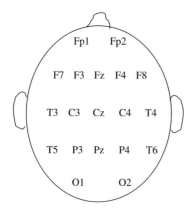

Figure 7.1. Scheme showing standard electrode placements.

USES OF EEG

- Diagnosis of epilepsy
- Classification of epilepsy syndromes (Chapter 6)
- Localization of epilepsy for the purpose of planning surgical treatment, including intracranial EEG recording (Chapter 15)
- The management of status epilepticus (Chapter 14)
- Non-epilepsy uses especially the diagnosis of Herpes simplex encephalitis and certain neurodegenerative conditions such as Creutzfeldt-Jakob disease.

PRINCIPLES OF EEG RECORDING

- The montage is the pattern of connections between the electrodes. There are two kinds of recording montage: referential (monopolar) and bipolar. Most montages have 16 or more recording channels.
- Upward deflection, at an electrode in the recording trace means a net negative field at that electrode.
- In referential recording the electric field at a particular electrode is compared against a point thought to be electrically neutral such as the earlobe or against an average of all the electrodes. This gives a deflection that is proportional to the field at that electrode. Background rhythms are usually easiest to interpret in referential recordings.
- In bipolar recordings, the field at each electrode is compared to its neighbor. If there is a similar field generated at each, no matter how big, the net output is zero. This montage thus detects differences between electrodes. If an electric field is generated over the scalp, the nearer the electrode to its peak, the more negative it will become. The electrodes are linked in a chain of pairs. A common pattern is to compare electrodes in chains front to back, in the parietal and temporal regions on each side and also in a chain across the middle of the head. Modern equipment allows one to recreate any chain from the raw, electronically recorded data. Bipolar recordings are better for localizing paroxysmal abnormalities by detecting phase reversal (Figure 7.2).

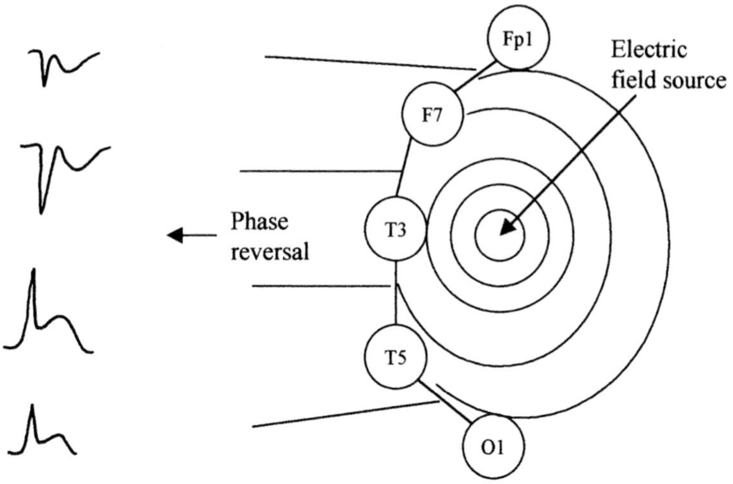

Figure 7.2. The discharge of neurons generates a negative electric field. As the electrode pairs approach the peak of an electric field, there will be a positive (downward deflection) because the first electrode of the pair is less negative than the next. When the electrode chain passes the peak, the field starts to decline, and each electrode will be more negative than the next in the chain: the direction of the deflection will be up. At the peak of the electric field the deflection changes direction "phase reversal."

- Additional electrodes may be used at specific sites under certain circumstances, for example superficial sphenoidal electrodes to detect temporal lobe epilepsy (TLE) or orbitofrontal electrodes to detect orbitofrontal epilepsy.
- Intracranial electrodes are sometimes needed in presurgical evaluation if extra-cranial electrodes do not give a very specific localization of the region of onset of the patient's epilepsy.

ROUTINE INTERICTAL RECORDING

A routine interictal recording lasts about half an hour with the patient comfortable and at rest. Several procedures are standard during the recording:

1. The patient opens and closes their eyes to assess the normal waking alpha rhythm.
2. The patient hyperventilates for approximately 3 minutes.
3. The patient is exposed to stroboscopic stimuli from 1 hertz to up to 50 hertz to assess photosensitivity (Chapter 1). This may trigger seizures in susceptible individuals and requires specific consent.

PATTERNS OF EEG ACTIVITY

EEG activity is defined by its frequency in hertz, duration in milliseconds or seconds and amplitude in microvolts. The electroencephalographer records the patient's clinical state throughout the EEG so that the tracing may be interpreted in clinical context. The normal EEG varies according to:

- Age: the normal EEG is very different in infants and young children and is much more difficult to interpret.
- Arousal: the EEG slows down through stages 1 to 4 of non-REM sleep and specific features appear that give clues to the sleep stage (Table 7.2).
- Medication may slow down or speed-up the background EEG.
- Pathological states.

Background EEG Activity in Adults

Background EEG activity comprises and is divided into four frequency ranges (Figure 7.3).

- Alpha activity is in the range 8 to 13 hertz. It is the normal rhythm of the waking patient. It is usually most prominent over the occipital regions and is commonly slightly asymmetric. Alpha rhythm occurs when the subject shuts their eyes and disappears on eye-opening. It disappears progressively with deeper sleep stages.
- Theta activity is from 4 to 7 hertz and is normal in light sleep.
- Delta activity is below 4 hertz and is normal in deep sleep.
- Beta activity is above 13 hertz. Some beta activity is often seen normally.

Paroxysmal EEG Activity

- Paroxysmal EEG activity comprises occasional features. Some paroxysmal discharges are seen in the normal EEG, especially in sleep (Tables 7.1 and 7.2).

Abnormal Features of the EEG

- Abnormalities in the EEG may be localized or generalized.
- Abnormalities in the EEG may be paroxysmal or affect background activity. Many paroxysmal abnormalities are pathological. Disturbances of the

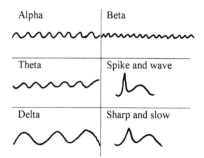

Figure 7.3. Typical waves of an EEG, boxes are 1 second across.

Table 7.1. Benign EEG Variants

Variant	Appearance	Significance
Mμ rhythm (10%)	Arc-shaped rhythm over rolandic region, around 10 Hz	Involved in cortical motor function
Lambda waves 80% in children 35% age 30–50	Sharpened, biphasic wave 2 300 ms over occipital cortex	Involved in visual exploration
Occipital 6 Hz spike and wave (0.5–1%)	Strongly positive wave may occur at any stage of arousal	Not associated with epilepsy (frontal variant sometimes associated with epilepsy)
Rudimentary spike-wave complex (mostly children)	Slow wave discharge with a positive spike in the trough between slow waves at 3–4 Hz	Probably relates to hypnagogic (pre-sleep) state and is benign
Small sharp spikes (up to 8% of age 30–60)	Sharp positive and negative components mainly over frontal and temporal areas	Associated with drowsiness and light sleep
Occipital spikes of the blind	Needle-like spikes seen in congenital blindness	Cause unclear but no relation to epilepsy
14 and 6 Hz positive spike discharge. Commonest in children.	Bursts of arch-shaped waves over one or both temporal regions in sleep	No relation to epilepsy but sometimes seen in metabolic coma
Rhythmical temporal theta bursts Commonest in young and middle-aged adults	Rhythmical activity 5–6.5 Hz lasting 10–60 s over mid-temporal region often in drowsiness	No clear pathological association
Temporal minor transients of old age and wicket spikes	Mixed delta, theta and alpha over temporal regions, sometimes with spikes and sharp waves	Associated with cerebrovascular disease and not a marker for epilepsy

Table 7.2. Paroxysmal sleep changes in the EEG

Variant	Appearance	Significance
Vertex waves	Sharp waves at vertex	Compound evoked potentials in deep drowsiness
Positive sharp transients of sleep (POSTS)	Positive spike-like waves in stage II–III sleep	Very common but function unknown
K complexes, largest in adolescents and young adults	Sharp wave then slow wave followed by fast activity over vertex or frontal midline	Generated by arousal from stage 2 sleep

background are very dependent on the state of arousal of the patient. Normal fluctuations in background activity are symmetric and any asymmetry of activity raises the possibility of a pathological cause.

Background Abnormalities

- Generalized slow waves are most commonly due to drowsiness. This may be normal or may reflect pathological processes affecting arousal including drugs, severe metabolic disturbance, lesions of the ascending reticular activating system or diffuse cortical disease such as encephalitis.
- Focal slow waves suggest a localized pathological abnormality but are not more specific. This can include tumors or vascular lesions in the underlying region.

- Fast activity is most commonly due to drugs such as barbiturates or benzodiazepines.

Paroxysmal EEG Abnormalities

- Spikes are negative (upward) deflections of the EEG lasting less than 70 milliseconds. They represent the simultaneous depolarization of large groups of neurons and are the interictal hallmark of epilepsy. Sharp waves have a similar appearance but last slightly longer (up to 200 milliseconds). They have a similar significance to spikes. Both sharp waves and spikes are usually followed by slow waves that represent synchronized neuronal repolarization after the discharge. Spikes and sharp waves are "interictal epileptiform abnormalities."
- Spikes may be focal or generalized, reflecting focal or generalized epilepsy.
- Spikes may be spontaneous or triggered (activation procedures below).

The EEG Diagnosis of Epilepsy

- The hallmark of epilepsy is abnormal electrical discharges. The value of the EEG in the diagnosis of epilepsy depends on when the EEG is done and the clinical pattern of the event under question. It is useful to divide EEG recordings into interictal (between seizures) and ictal (during seizures).
- Epilepsy cannot be diagnosed from an EEG alone. There must be a clinical description of episodes that are compatible with epilepsy. Because many EEGs are equivocal and because the test has a false positive rate, an EEG should only be requested if the demonstration of epileptiform abnormalities would lead to a diagnosis of epilepsy.
- Interictal epileptiform discharges imply a potential to generate seizures but do not on their own mean a patient has epilepsy.
- False positive interictal EEGs occur in up to 0.5 percent of healthy young adults. Patients with a strong family history of epilepsy are much more likely to have coincidental and irrelevant epileptiform EEG abnormalities.
- False negative interictal EEGs are common. Half of all patients with epilepsy will have no sign of it on a single interictal EEG. If the EEG is repeated the number of false negatives falls to 30 percent. In a sleep-deprived recording the patient's night's sleep is reduced by several hours. A sleep-deprived recording increases the yield of abnormalities, reducing the false negative rate to 20 percent.
- Ictal EEG recordings are needed to diagnose epilepsy with absolute certainty. Attacks must be frequent and attempts at ictal recording are generally unhelpful if the frequency of seizures is less than one per week. The diagnostic appearance is an evolving discharge during the clinical event (Figure 7.4). The EEG may change prior to the clinical seizure onset, during the seizure or afterwards enabling a diagnosis of epilepsy to be made. The pattern may include spikes or sharp waves or just a slow wave discharge. If the background EEG is very abnormal, it may be difficult to tell exactly when seizures occur, for example in some severe epilepsy syndromes of childhood.

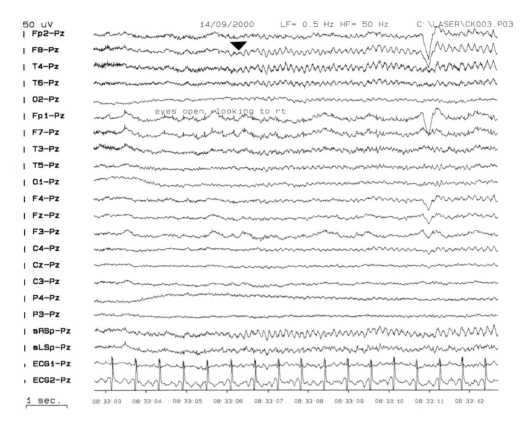

Figure 7.4. An evolving focal seizure discharge showing rhythmical 8 Hz discharge building up over the right temporal and sphenoidal electrodes.

- An ambulatory EEG may be used to detect ictal events. Electrodes are attached to the patient's head and connected to a portable tape recorder. The patient can be at home with this system. If the patient has an attack whilst wearing the system, they or a relative can press an event marker that marks the recording tape and they can note it in a diary. The tape records for 24 to 48 hours and can then be analyzed with particular attention to the marked regions. The number of electrodes used in many ambulatory systems is less than for a resting record and spatial sensitivity is less. Not all epileptic seizures can be detected with this system (Case 1).
- Video-EEG-telemetry can be undertaken if the diagnosis remains in doubt and in presurgical evaluation of epilepsy (Chapter 15). The patient is admitted to hospital and continuous EEG recording is combined with video recording in a specially tailored room. The patient's medication may be reduced if that makes attacks more likely to occur. The EEG is abnormal during most kinds of seizure. It is important to anticipate the occasional seizure types, such as frontal lobe epilepsy, for which even an ictal EEG may be normal (Case 1 and Table 7.3). For these, it is the video recording of the patient's clinical attack that enables a diagnosis to be made. A home video of the seizures may be helpful, even if the EEG is non-diagnostic.

Table 7.3. Ictal EEG Patterns

Focal seizures with no loss of consciousness	Focal abnormalities may be detectable but up to 50% of patients with focal motor seizures or just auras have no EEG abnormalities, before, during or after the seizures.
Focal seizures with prominent motor activity for example frontal lobe epilepsy	The ictal EEG is often obscured by movement artifact and postictal recovery is rapid. There may be no scalp EEG change during the seizure.
Convulsive seizures	Build-up of abnormal rhythms may be seen but they may be obscured by muscle artifact. In the postictal state widespread slow activity is prominent.
Focal seizures with early loss of consciousness for example TLE	Focal seizure discharge should be apparent but may require special electrodes, for example sphenoidal electrodes. During the period of altered consciousness, EEG abnormalities should be apparent.
Primary generalized epilepsy	Generalized spike and wave is always present during clinical seizures but may be masked by muscle artifact in convulsive episodes.

Italics – seizures that may manifest with no diagnostic ictal EEG abnormality.

Case History 1

A 26-year-old woman had suffered epilepsy since the age of 5. Seizures occurred mostly at night and comprised movement of her legs with stiffening. Sometimes seizures occurred serially and she developed generalized convulsions. Clinicians had viewed her as an immature woman, heavily dependent on her mother and the question of non-epileptic seizures was raised. She underwent ambulatory EEG monitoring and several of her attacks were recorded. The EEG onset was masked by movement artifact and no epileptiform changes occurred through the course of the attack. She provided a home video of several daytime attacks. This showed that the attacks started with a flapping movement of the left leg for a few seconds. The leg then stiffened and lifted above the right leg. Her left arm also stiffened. The attack subsided after 20 seconds but then soon recurred in identical fashion.

The clinical pattern of the attack suggests frontal lobe epilepsy (Chapter 6). This is a pattern that may relatively frequently be associated with normal ictal EEG. In this case the home video confirmed the diagnosis and laid to rest the suspicion of psychogenic non-epileptic seizures.

The EEG in Syndromic Diagnosis

- The EEG forms a key element in the syndromic diagnosis of epilepsy (Chapter 6). The main differentiation is between focal and generalized epilepsies and each category has a number of subdivisions.
- Focal epilepsy is suggested by epileptiform EEG abnormalities during or between seizures that are restricted and consistent in their extent. For example they may appear over only one electrode, or over a whole hemisphere.
- Generalized epilepsy is suggested by epileptiform abnormalities that appear simultaneously over a wide extent of both hemispheres. They may be asymmetric and are commonly maximal over the midfrontal regions, electrodes F3 and F4. Photosensitivity usually suggests generalized epilepsy, but is occasionally seen in focal occipital epilepsy.

- Childhood epilepsy syndromes often have specific EEG features that are the neurophysiological signature of the condition, for example benign epilepsy with centrotemporal spikes (Chapter 11).
- Differentiating focal and generalized EEG patterns may be difficult. Some generalized syndromes, especially juvenile myoclonic epilepsy may have significant focal EEG elements. As patients get older the generalized epilepsies tend to contain more focal EEG elements. Some forms of focal epilepsy are associated with widespread or generalized EEG patterns. Frontal lobe epilepsy may generate both ictal and interictal abnormalities that spread rapidly across the corpus callosum over both hemispheres and may resemble generalized EEG abnormalities – termed secondary bilateral synchrony (Case 8, Chapter 6). The issue then becomes to decide whether the epilepsy is a rapidly spreading focal type or a generalized type with marked focal elements and other clues from the clinical history or neuroimaging may be needed.

EEG VARIANTS

- Normal variants are common in EEG recordings and may be misinterpreted as being abnormal (Case 2).
- Asymmetric changes are more likely to be abnormal than symmetric changes.
- The age and state of arousal of the individual determine the patterns that can be considered normal. For example, sharp waves appearing over the vertex in an awake patient are likely to be abnormal but are common in normal individuals who become drowsy. The rest of the EEG and the technician's comments may give clues to the context.

Case History 2
A 35-year-old woman presented with nocturnal convulsive episodes and diurnal fugue states with loss of memory. There was a strong suspicion that these were psychogenic non-epileptic seizures. She had been abused as a child and had been beaten in a previous marriage. An EEG showed 6 hertz occipital spikes that were initially interpreted as epileptiform. This led to an initial diagnosis of epilepsy but on re-evaluation the EEG was felt to show a normal variant and her management was redirected towards psychiatric services.

Table 7.4. Common EEG Artifacts

Artifact	Appearance on EEG
Electrical mains	Distorted baseline with regular 50 Hz or 60 Hz (USA) waves
Eye movement	Waves on anterior electrodes appear to come together and separate again according to direction of eye movement
ECG	Regular spikes coincide with ECG
Head movement in patients with tremor or slight bobbing with each pulse	Usually seen as slow waves posteriorly as these electrodes move against the pillow
Muscle	Irregular high frequency muscle spikes without slow waves, that may obliterate the EEG
Sweating	Gradual fluctuation in skin conductivity may give an appearance like very slow waves

ACTIVATION PROCEDURES WITH THE EEG

- Special stimuli can be used to activate the EEG. Stroboscopic stimulation and hyperventilation are standard procedures used in many recordings but others may be tailored to the patient's history. For example, if there is a history of seizures triggered by reading then one can ask the patient to read during the recording.
- Hyperventilation is usually performed for three minutes and the technician usually notes how strenuously it was performed. If a patient finds the procedure uncomfortable and makes half-hearted attempts at hyperventilation, the results have to be interpreted more cautiously. The normal response is a generalized slowing of the EEG that is most marked in children.

Abnormal Responses to Hyperventilation

1. Slow wave asymmetry implies localized cerebral pathology.
2. Interictal epileptiform spike discharges may appear or become more prominent.
3. Idiopathic generalized epilepsy (IGE) syndromes often manifest spike-wave discharges especially the characteristic 3 hertz discharge of childhood absence epilepsy.
4. Seizures may also be triggered, most commonly in IGE but sometimes in focal epilepsies.

- Visual stimulation may be with stroboscopic lights at 1 to 50 hertz (usually with eyes closed) or by exposing the patient to flickering patterns of lines or dots. An abnormal response is probably genetically determined but is not on its own diagnostic of epilepsy (Chapter 1). The normal "photic driving response" is a rhythm at the same frequency or at a harmonic of the photic stimulus, usually maximal posteriorly but sometimes more frontally.

Abnormal Responses to Photic Stimulation

1. Asymmetry of the response may reflect a unilateral destructive occipital lesion.
2. A photomyoclonic response is more common in adults and is usually seen with stimulation frequencies of 12 to 18 hertz. Brief repetitive muscle spikes are seen anteriorly with flutter of the eyelids and eyeballs. They stop as soon as the stimulation stops. It is associated with brainstem lesions and with psychiatric disorders but not epilepsy.
3. A photoparoxysmal (PPR, photoconvulsive) response is characterized by spike-wave and polyspike-wave complexes that are bilateral and outlast the stimulus by a few seconds (see Figure 1.3). There may be associated clinical phenomena such as muscle jerks of the head and neck and sometimes of the whole body. The effect is usually seen at 15 to 20 hertz. The response has been subdivided:

Type 1: spikes with the occipital rhythm
Type 2: parieto-occipital spikes with a biphasic slow wave

Type 3: as type 2 with spread to the frontal regions
Type 4: generalized spikes or polyspikes and waves

4. Only type 4 is strongly associated with epilepsy. It is almost always associated with IGE. It occurs in 2 percent of all new cases of epilepsy and 10 percent of new cases presenting in their second decade, reflecting the frequency of IGE in this age group. Rarer causes of a PPR are inherited diseases such as neuronal ceroid lipofuscinosis, progressive myoclonus epilepsies (Chapter 3) and Creutzfeldt-Jakob disease.

5. Closely spaced lines or dots that oscillate may trigger a PPR. The response is maximal if both of the patient's eyes are open; the stimulus fills as much of the patient's visual field as possible and the visual contrast, spacing and movement of the pattern are optimized. Most patients are sensitive to both pattern and stroboscopic stimulation but rare patients may respond to only one.

- Other stimuli triggering seizures see Chapter 1.

SPECIALIZED EEG TECHNIQUES

- Intracranial EEG recording is used in the evaluation of some patients for epilepsy surgery. It is used to answer specific questions concerning the location of onset of seizures. An example is if extracranial ictal EEG fails to differentiate between left and right temporal lobe epilepsy. As non-invasive methods of evaluation increase, the need for intracranial EEG is declining.
- Stereotactic intracranial EEG involves the placement of wires into the brain substance. Each wire has a number of electrode contacts. These are useful for detecting deep, inaccessible sites but only sample a small volume of the brain.
- Subdural electrode grids can be placed over the surface of the brain and sample a much greater volume but cannot access the deep parts.
- Per-operative EEG recording "electro-corticography" is undertaken in some centers during epilepsy surgery. It is used to delineate the region of seizure onset in order to tailor cortical resection. Whilst it is not a primary prognostic indicator, the chance of seizure remission is better if the brain left behind is electrically normal during the operation.
- Magnetoencephalography (MEG) is the recording of the magnetic fields generated by the electrical activity of the brain. The advantage of magnetic recording over EEG is that the magnetic field is not so heavily influenced by all the tissues between the brain and the recording system. The disadvantage is that the magnetic field is very weak and very sophisticated (and expensive) equipment is needed to record it. For this reason, MEG is currently a research tool.
- Mathematical models of analysis of electrical recordings are used to try and enhance the specificity of EEG. None is yet standard.

HOW TO READ A ROUTINE INTERICTAL EEG REPORT

1. What is the clinical epilepsy pattern? Some epilepsies normally manifest with interictal EEG changes for example childhood absence epilepsy. This alters the interpretation of a negative result.

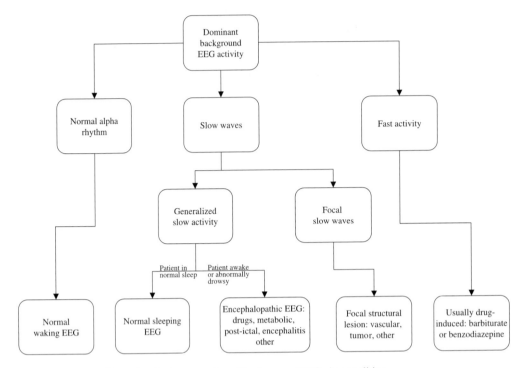

Figure 7.5. A flow chart illustrating the interpretation of background EEG abnormalities.

2. The background EEG activity is interpreted in the context of the patient's state of arousal. Drowsiness is the commonest cause of symmetrical slowing, otherwise consider pathological causes of reduced arousal for example drugs or systemic illness (Figure 7.5). A brain scan may be indicated if focal abnormalities are found.

3. Is there paroxysmal activity supporting a diagnosis of epilepsy? This is usually spikes or sharp waves but occasionally a slow wave seizure discharge may be recorded by chance.

4. Are epileptiform abnormalities generalized or focal?

5. Are there epileptiform abnormalities on photic stimulation? If this fits with the clinical history, it almost always implies IGE.

BIBLIOGRAPHY

Blume WT, Pillay N. Electrographic and clinical correlates of secondary bilateral synchrony. Epilepsia 1985;26:636–641.

Gregory RP, Oates T, Merry RTG Electroencephalogram epileptiform abnormalities in candidates for aircrew training. Electroencepahlogr Clin Neurophysiol 1993;86:75–77.

Hopkins A, Garman A, Clarke C. The first seizure in adult life. Value of clinical features, electroencephalography and computerised tomographic scanning in predicting seizure recurrence. Lancet 1988;2:721–726.

Jeavons PM, Harding GFA. Photosensitive epilepsies: a review of the literature and a study of 460 patients. London: Heinemann, 1975

Niedermeyer E. Abnormal EEG patterns: epileptic and paroxysmal. In Niedermyer E, Lopes da Silva F (eds). Electroencephalography Basic Principles, Clinical Applications and Related Fields. 4th Edition. Philadelphia: Lippincott, Williams and Wilkins, 1999:235–260.

Quesney LF. Intracranial EEG investigation in neocortical epilepsy. In: Williamson PD , Siegel AM, Roberts DW, Thadani VM, Gazzaniga MS (eds). Advances in Neurology 84: Neocortical Epilepsies. Philadelphia: Lippincott Williams & Wilkins, 2000.

Wolf P. Epileptic Seizures and Syndromes. London: John Libbey, 1994.

8
Neuroimaging

Before the 1970s the structural basis of a patient's epilepsy remained uncertain unless they underwent epilepsy surgery. CT scanning allowed a radiological diagnosis to be made in 10 to 20 percent of patients. MRI increased the yield to around 50 percent of patients with refractory partial epilepsy. Since then, more sophisticated techniques have made it possible to visualize structural abnormalities in 80 percent of focal epilepsy, revolutionizing the management of epilepsy patients (Tables 8.1 and 8.2).

Table 8.1. Comparison of Detection Rates of CT and MRI

Lesion	CT Detection	MRI Detection
Mesial temporal sclerosis	Rarely	Usually
Cortical dysplasia	Rarely except gross forms	Commonly
Tumors	Most	Nearly all
Arteriovenous malformations	Many	Nearly all
Cavernous hemangioma	Rarely	Nearly all
Post-traumatic change	Sometimes	Commonly
Calcification	Nearly all	Sometimes, nearly all with spin-echo MRI
Fracture	Nearly all	Rarely

USES OF STRUCTURAL NEUROIMAGING

- Neuroimaging may be used to assess brain structure – looking for a pathological cause for epilepsy – and to assess dynamic brain function – looking for evidence of altered brain function due to epilepsy.
- In the first presentation of epilepsy, neuroimaging is used to identify the underlying cause for the epilepsy that in itself might require treatment. For example tumors, vascular malformations or strokes.
- Syndromic diagnosis may be helped by neuroimaging. An epileptogenic lesion points to a symptomatic epilepsy, usually focal but occasionally generalized, even if clinical seizure types or EEG are not diagnostic (Chapter 6).
- Subtle lesions underlying epilepsy may be identified by modern neuroimaging. These may have management implications, other than simply the treatment of the patient's epilepsy for example, genetic counseling for subependymal heterotopia.
- For refractory epilepsy, neuroimaging is a vital instrument in selecting those most likely to benefit from epilepsy surgery. Numerous studies have shown that surgery is most likely to be successful if there is a visible lesion to resect (Chapter 15).

Who Should Have a Structural Brain Scan?

- Status epilepticus or acute, severe epilepsy merits urgent neuroimaging
- All patients over 20 years old who develop seizures
- Any patient with focal epilepsy unless the electroclinical syndrome is typical of a benign focal epilepsy syndrome of childhood (Chapter 11)
- Refractory epilepsy affecting patients at any age
- Children with epilepsy and developmental delay or evidence of a neurocutaneous syndrome.

What Sort of Structural Scan?

- Magnetic Resonance Imaging (MRI) is better than computerized X-ray tomography (CT) in nearly all situations.
- CT is usually adequate if the purpose is to exclude larger tumors but a normal CT does not rule out a focal lesion and a highly focal clinical seizure pattern or EEG, increases the chance that MRI will detect a focal abnormality (Case 1).
- MRI does not involve ionizing radiation so carries less risk. MRI probably does not affect the fetus in pregnant women undergoing imaging but is nevertheless avoided if possible.

Case History 1

A 27-year-old man presented with a tonic–clonic seizure. In retrospect, he recalled episodes of intense déjà vu going back several months. A CT scan was entirely normal. MRI scan showed signal change in the temporal neocortex, consistent with either a low grade glioma or a dysembryoplastic neuroepithelial tumor (Figure 8.1).

- MRI may miss acute hemorrhage or bony abnormalities: CT is the investigation of choice in acute trauma to evaluate hemorrhage or fractures.
- MRI requires the patient to lie still for longer and sedation or anesthesia may be required for those who are unable to do so – the acutely unwell, confused patient or young children.
- MRI is contraindicated in those who have pacemakers or other metal implants, which may be affected by the magnetic field.

THE TECHNIQUES OF MRI

- The head is placed in a strong, magnetic field with a rostro–caudal gradient. An electromagnetic pulse is generated perpendicular to the field that acts on tissue at a specific level of magnetization along the gradient and so excites a specific slice of the brain. The pulse of energy is absorbed by tissue in the slice and is then released when the electromagnetic pulse ceases. The energy released is detected and forms the basis of the magnetic resonance image. The pattern of energy release depends on which atoms have been excited and their chemical milieu.
- Protons in hydrogen are most commonly excited by MRI. These are very abundant and so generate a high resolution structural image. The quality of this image depends very much on parameters of the electromagnetic pulse that are beyond the scope of this book (and its author).

1. T_1 weighted images are best at identifying anatomical defects such as cortical developmental abnormalities and are used for volumetric imaging (below).

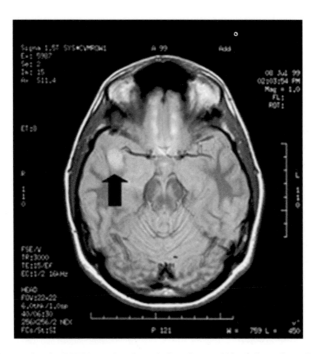

Figure 8.1. Proton density MRI scan showing a lesion that could be a dysembryoplastic neuro-epithelioma or a low grade glioma in a patient with temporal lobe epilepsy. An X-ray CT scan 2 weeks earlier had been normal.

2. T_2 weighted images are better at identifying foreign tissue lesions.
3. Proton density sequences have intermediate properties.

- A combination of sequences is sometimes needed to identify different tissue types, for example water is "bright" on T_2 and "dark" on T_1 sequences, whereas fat is "bright" on both.
- Specialized sequences include diffusion-weighted imaging usually looking for acute ischaemia and fluid attenuated inversion recovery (FLAIR) looking for inflammation and gliosis.

Standard Magnetic Resonance Imaging Applied to Epilepsy

- Major pathology such as infarction, tumors, vascular malformations and larger developmental abnormalities can be identified by standard MRI techniques.
- Subtle lesions such as mesial temporal sclerosis (MTS) or cortical developmental abnormalities are the commonest causes of refractory focal epilepsy and are much more difficult to detect with standard MRI techniques.

Volumetric Imaging

- Most MRI images sample slices at close intervals through the brain. Subtle lesions may lie between the slices sampled.
- In volumetric imaging, the slices are much thinner and are contiguous. This has several beneficial effects.

1. The whole brain is sampled, so that no structural abnormality is missed, which is within the resolution of the scanner.
2. A three dimensional reconstruction of the entire volume of the brain can be made. This enables accurate measurements of the volume of critical structures such as the hippocampi.
3. It allows one to reconstruct slices through the brain at unusual angles to highlight specific regions.
4. The three dimensional image can give an impression of the surface of the brain, which is of value to a surgeon as they embark on cortical resection.

Magnetic Resonance Spectroscopy in Epilepsy

- The chemical composition of the brain can be explored by magnetic resonance spectroscopy (MRS), which is tailored to excite atoms or molecules other than hydrogen. MRS can only be applied to a limited number of chemical species at the moment. Because their concentration is much lower than hydrogen, the scanner must excite a larger volume of brain with each pulse in order to generate a satisfactory image. This means that MRS has a low spatial resolution.

- *N*-acetyl aspartate (NAA) has been found to be useful in MRS. Its function is unknown but it is associated with viable neurons and is a marker of living neural tissue. The creatine/choline ratio (Cr/Cho) is a widespread tissue component and is used as a background marker. The NAA to Cr/Cho ratio can be compared between different regions to assess the amount of viable brain tissue. This has been applied particularly to comparisons between the two mesial temporal lobes.

MR Imaging of Mesial Temporal Sclerosis

- Mesial temporal sclerosis (MTS) is the commonest pathology for which surgery is considered. The hippocampi are small structures that are difficult to see on ordinary scans. A combination of techniques is often needed to categorize MTS.
- When there is hippocampal sclerosis, the internal structure of the hippocampus becomes disordered and the appearance may change on high resolution T_1 weighted imaging (Figure 8.2a).
- Increased signal on T_2 weighted images (Figure 8.2b), occurs in about 30 to 60 percent of MTS.
- The volumes of the amygdalae and hippocampi on each slice are measured by taking their cross-sectional area on each slice and multiplying by slice thickness. The hippocampi are remarkably symmetric in normal individuals. The volume is compared between the two sides to find relative differences. In unilateral disease, the abnormal hippocampus is smaller, anteriorly, diffusely or posteriorly but the difference in volumes may be as little as 10 percent.
- Bilateral disease may be missed with these relative measurements. To overcome this problem, the volume is also calculated as a ratio of the total volume of the hemisphere and compared against the mean of normal controls.
- MRS shows a reduction in NAA in hippocampi where there is also volume loss on MRI. NAA may also be reduced in the hippocampus ipsilateral to EEG evidence of seizure onset even when structural neuroimaging has not shown a clear abnormality. Surgery in these cases results in a remission rate of the epilepsy that is not as good as when there is demonstrable anatomical abnormality but better than in cases where MRS is also normal.
- T_2 relaxometry is a technique that measures rate of decay of the T_2 signal. Increased hippocampal T_2 relaxation time is a sensitive measure of hippocampal sclerosis, seen in 80 percent of patients with temporal lobe epilepsy (TLE) and can be found in patients with normal structural imaging. Since it does not rely on a ratio, it is also helpful in identifying patients with bilateral disease.

MR Imaging of Neocortical Epilepsy

- Developmental abnormalities of the cerebral cortex are the second commonest cause of refractory epilepsy after MTS. Figures 2.3 to 2.6, 5.5.
- Volumetric MRI allows scans to be reconstructed in unconventional planes to optimize regions of interest.

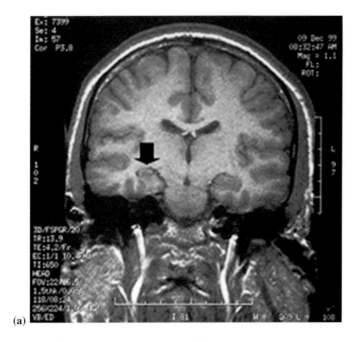

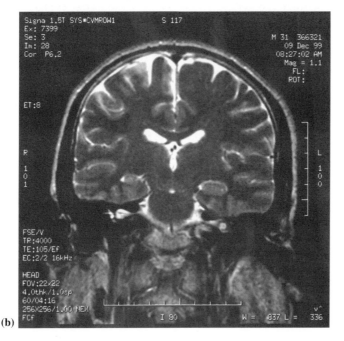

Figure 8.2. (a) T_1 weighted coronal MRI of mesial temporal sclerosis, showing loss of volume and internal architecture of the hippocampus. (b) T_2 weighted coronal MRI in the same patient showing increased signal representing gliosis within the hippocampus.

- Diffusion weighted imaging is a research tool that may occasionally detect abnormalities when other MRI techniques are normal.
- Statistical parametric mapping (SPM) is a research technique whereby a patient's scan is mapped onto a standard scan that is an average of a large number of controls. This can then be used to detect subtle anatomic differences in MRI, for example some abnormalities have been suggested in the frontal lobes in the idiopathic generalized epilepsies.

FUNCTIONAL NEUROIMAGING

- Functional neuroimaging (FNI) is mostly used clinically in planning epilepsy surgery.
- It can also be used to help with identifying the epileptogenic region. When a region of the brain generates a seizure, its regional blood flow, metabolic rate and glucose utilization increase. Immediately after the seizure there is a decline to below the level of other brain regions that may persist throughout the interictal period or may return towards normal. In some cases, FNI can help identify regions of seizure onset for example in lateralizing TLE, where structural imaging is normal or symmetric. Compared to structural imaging, FNI tends to overestimate the extent of epileptogenic cerebral cortex.
- FNI can be used to localize brain function. When a task activates a particular brain region, there is an increase in local cerebral blood flow and glucose utilization of up to 50 percent, which can be detected by neuroimaging. Much smaller increases occur in local blood volume and oxygen consumption (<10%). Experimental activation tasks can be designed to show an increase in blood flow compared to a control situation. For example, a simple finger-tapping test measures motor cortex activity and can be compared to a task of thinking about tapping the finger without actually doing it to subtract out background cortical activity. This can be related to the region of epilepsy onset to help determine if a specific critical function will be affected by focal cortical resection.

Table 8.2. Comparison of Different Forms of Functional Neuroimaging

	PET	**SPECT**	**fMRI**
Ictal imaging of epileptogenic zone	No, except by chance	Yes >90% sensitivity	No, except by chance
Interictal imaging of epileptogenic zone	Yes >80% sensitivity	Yes but <50% sensitivity and low specificity	No
Imaging activation procedures	Yes	No	Yes
Spatial resolution	<5 mm	5–10 mm	2 mm
Temporal resolution	Seconds to minutes	Seconds to minutes	<1 second
Availability	Specialized units only	Widely available	Increasingly available
Cost	High	Moderate	Moderate
Repeatability	No	No	Yes
Adverse effects	Exposure to radioactivity	Exposure to radioactivity	Probably none

Modes of Functional Neuroimaging

Positron Emission Tomography (PET)

- PET uses radio-isotopes, which decay rapidly to produce a pair of particles, an electron and a positron. These are emitted in opposite directions and are detected by banks of detectors around the patient's head. As these isotopes decay rapidly, they have to be produced on site just prior to the scan, which is expensive and it also means that scans are usually interictal as one cannot predict when a seizure will occur and produce the isotope at the right time.
- Cerebral glucose utilization is most commonly measured with 2-[^{18}F]fluoro-2-deoxyglucose (FDG), which is distributed in the brain in parallel with glucose.
- Blood flow and oxygen extraction can also be mapped.
- Specific neurotransmitter receptors may also be mapped, for example flumazenil (a benzodiazepine ligand) may be useful in identifying abnormal regions in patients whose structural scans are normal. Spatial resolution of PET is better than of single photon emission computerized tomography (SPECT) but lower than MRI.
- SPM may be applied to PET, to detect differences in activation, which may be helpful in epilepsy localization and in mapping during activation tasks.

Single Photon Emission Computerized Tomography (SPECT)

- SPECT also uses radio-isotopes that emit particles that can be detected outside the patient's head. The most commonly used isotope is Technetium^{99} in hexamethyl-propyleneamineoxime (^{99m}Tc-HMPAO). On injection it is distributed according to cerebral perfusion and is rapidly fixed into the brain, providing a snapshot of cerebral perfusion, that can be imaged sometime later. The isotope can be stored and injected during a seizure, then the scan is performed the following day, providing ictal blood flow SPECT images. This is compared to interictal SPECT and usually shows focal increased blood flow. SPECT has lower spatial resolution than PET but is widely available and is mostly helpful in lateralizing TLE.

Functional Magnetic Resonance Imaging (fMRI)

- There are several methods of functional magnetic resonance imaging. It provides an image of cerebral activation that has a high anatomical and temporal resolution, being able to detect changes over hundreds of milliseconds.
- Blood oxygen level-dependent (BOLD) contrast makes use of the changes in blood flow produced by cerebral activity. Since focal cerebral activity increases blood flow by up to 50 percent and oxygen utilisation by only 5 percent, oxygen extraction ratio is reduced and a higher proportion of hemoglobin in the capillaries and venous circulation remains oxygenated. Deoxyhemoglobin is paramagnetic and so influences the MRI characteristics of surrounding tissue, whereas oxyhemoglobin is not. This difference can form the basis of a subtraction image with an activation task.
- In bolus tracking fMRI, a bolus of contrast is injected intravenously, which causes a reduction in tissue signal intensity, proportional to the dose and local

cerebral blood volume. The change in signal can be compared before and after the cerebral activation procedure.

- Inflow imaging fMRI uses the difference in magnetization between moving blood and static tissue to generate an image that is proportional to blood flow and so can be used to compare activity during baseline and activation procedures.

COREGISTRATION OF INFORMATION

- The data gleaned from EEG, structural neuroimaging and functional neuro-imaging may be superimposed onto a single image, allowing simultaneous visualization of each type of information. This process of "coregistration" enables one to see the concordance of all the data regarding the region of onset of the epilepsy and how that region relates to the location of specific cerebral functions. This form of presentation is especially valuable in planning epilepsy surgery.
- To achieve coregistration, each investigation is related to markers on the patient's head. The more markers are used, the more accurately the image can be fixed in three dimensional space and the more reliable the coregistration process. The markers may be a frame attached to the patient's head or fixed bony anatomical landmarks on the surface of the head (frameless stereotaxy).

BIBLIOGRAPHY

Cascino GD, Trenerry MR, Jack CR *et al*. Electrocorticography and temporal lobe epilepsy: relationship to quantitative MRI and operative outcome. Epilepsia 1995;36:692–696.

Cook MJ, Fish DR, Shorvon SD, Straughan K, Stevens JM. Hippocampal volumetric and morphometric studies in frontal and temporal lobe epilepsy. Brain 1992;115:1001–1015.

Duncan R, Patterson J, Roberts R, Hadley DM, Bone I. Ictal/postictal SPECT in the presurgical localization of complex partial seizures. Acta Neurol Scand 1990;81:287–293.

Henry TR, Chugani HT. Positron emission tomography. In Engel J Jr, TA Pedley TA (eds). Epilepsy a Comprehensive Textbook. Philadelphia: Lippincott-Raven, 1997;947–968.

Henry TR, Duncan JS, Berkovic SF (eds). Advances in Neurology Volume 83: Functional Imaging in the Epilepsies. Philadelphia: Lipincott, Williams and Wilkins, 2000.

Jackson GD, Connelly A. New NMR measurements in epilepsy. T2 relaxometry and magnetic resonance spectroscopy. Adv Neurol 1999;79:931–937.

Knowlton RC, Wong STC, Woods RP, Mazziotta JC. Coregistration. In Engel J Jr, TA Pedley TA (eds). Epilepsy a Comprehensive Textbook. Philadelphia: Lippincott-Raven, 1997;1081–1097.

Li LM, Cendes F, Watson C, Andermann F, Fish DR, Dubeau F, Free S, Olivier A, Harkness W, Thomas DG, Duncan JS, Sander JW, Shorvon SD, Cook MJ, Arnold DL. Surgical treatment of patients with single and dual pathology: relevance of lesion and of hippocampal atrophy to seizure outcome. Neurology 1997;48:437-444.

Raymond AA, Fish DR, Sisodiya SM, Alsanjari N, Stevens JM, Shorvon SD. Abnormalities of gyration, heterotopias, tuberous sclerosis, focal cortical dysplasia, microdysgenesis, dysembryoplastic neuroepithelial tumour and dysgenesis of the archicortex in epilepsy. Clinical, EEG and neuroimaging features in 100 adult patients. Brain 1995;118:629–660.

Woermann FG, Sisodiya SM, Free SL, Duncan JS. Quantitative MRI in patients with idiopathic generalized epilepsy. Evidence of widespread cerebral structural changes. Brain 1998;121:1661–1667.

SECTION 3
Treatment

9

General Principles of Treatment

IMMEDIATE MANAGEMENT OF A FIRST SEIZURE

- First aid principles apply to the management of any seizure (Box 9.1).
- A first seizure may be the first manifestation of unprovoked epilepsy or the presentation of an acute illness (acute symptomatic or provoked seizure, Chapter 13).
- Patients with seizures not due to an acute cause generally recover to normal awareness within 2 hours. It is useful to take blood samples and urine for toxicology at this stage as this cannot be done later but other investigations can be undertaken as an outpatient.
- After an acute symptomatic seizure, the patient may remain drowsy and unwell. Other clinical clues are recurrent seizures, high fever or other systemic features, neck stiffness or focal neurological signs. These patients require urgent inpatient investigation and treatment of their seizures and the underlying cause (Box 9.2).

WHEN TO GIVE MEDICATION TO PREVENT SEIZURE RECURRENCE

- Acute symptomatic seizures have the lowest risk of long-term recurrence. Medication may be required to stop seizures in the acute phase but may be withdrawn early with a low risk of seizure recurrence (Case 1).
- The patient must be involved in any decision regarding longer-term medication and needs to be committed to treatment in order to be compliant and for treatment to be effective. Once anti-epileptic drug treatment is started, it is likely to be continued for a number of years.

Case History 1
A 65-year-old woman was admitted to hospital for surgical resection of adenocarcinoma of the rectum. Five days after the surgery she suffered a series of tonic–clonic seizures that were controlled with a loading dose of phenytoin. There was no recurrence of her seizures but she felt sleepy and unsteady with phenytoin levels in the

---

Box 9.1. Principles of First Aid for Convulsive Seizures

1) Convulsive Phase
Ensure the patient cannot injure themselves. Remove sharp objects, rest their head on a
  pillow. Nurse on the ground or in a bed with cot-sides.
Do not interfere with mouth or airway during the convulsive phase, but ensure they cannot
  suffocate.
If the convulsions last more than five minutes, call for help or give buccal, rectal or parenteral
  benzodiazepine.
2) Postictal Phase
Put drowsy patients into the recovery position and allow them to recover
  naturally. Call for help if the patient has a further seizure or patient remains drowsy and
  unresponsive more than two hours, or their breathing appears impaired.
Remove sharp objects on which the patient may injure themselves.
If the patient is confused, agitated or wandering, guide them gently away from danger. Use
  minimal interference, and avoid confrontation, which may be resisted violently.

Box 9.2. Guidelines for Management of a First Seizure in Adults

1) Criteria for admission to hospital. The purpose of admission to hospital is to diagnose and treat acute causes of seizures and to treat recurrent seizures in order to prevent status epilepticus

   Fever or signs and symptoms compatible with infection/meningitis

   Prolonged convulsion (>5 minutes of convulsive activity)

   Recurrent seizures: 2 tonic–clonic seizures or 3 focal seizures in 24 hours.

   Incomplete recovery after a seizure or prolonged drowsiness (>2 hours) after a seizure

   Focal neurological deficit after a first seizure

2) Outpatient investigations after a first seizure. A structural cause e.g. tumor or previous trauma are moderately common causes of epilepsy in adults

   Neuroimaging is mandatory

   An EEG is most helpful in the classification of seizures in children and young adults. Under-recognized causes are seizures related to alcohol or illicit drugs. Other metabolic disturbances are uncommon in previously healthy individuals

   Routine biochemistry, calcium, glucose, blood count

   Urine for toxicology

   Brain scan

   EEG

   Others as indicated for example CSF if features suggesting intracranial infection

3) Criteria for urgent neuroimaging. Urgent neuroimaging should be undertaken if there is clinical evidence of acute pathology underlying the seizure

   Criteria are as 1 above

4) Treatment of a first seizure

   Do not treat a single seizure

   A cluster of seizures over 24 hours that is self-limiting has the same prognosis as a single seizure. Acute treatment is indicated under certain circumstances:

   If the patient remains drowsy between attacks The attacks are prolonged

   There are more than two attacks in 24 hours

   Clinical features or investigations suggest a serious underlying cause

5) If acute treatment is required

   Use treatment that may be titrated rapidly e.g. phenytoin, phenobarbital or valproate (see Chapter 14)

6) Tell the patient

   They must not drive and must inform the licensing authority and their vehicle insurance company

   They must not operate dangerous machinery and must take care with swimming or other at risk hobbies

7) Arrange

   Neuroimaging and EEG if patient discharged from in Accident and Emergency

   Specialist referral

---

therapeutic range. Medication was withdrawn after three months and her symptoms improved. There had been no recurrence of seizures at one year.

Acute symptomatic seizures often do not develop into long-term epilepsy. Medication in the elderly is even more likely to cause adverse effects at standard doses and early drug withdrawal may be the best treatment.

Factors in the Decision Whether to Give Medication

- The risk of seizure recurrence is a major factor in determining treatment (Figure 9.1) and depends on the epilepsy syndrome, which may be difficult to diagnose

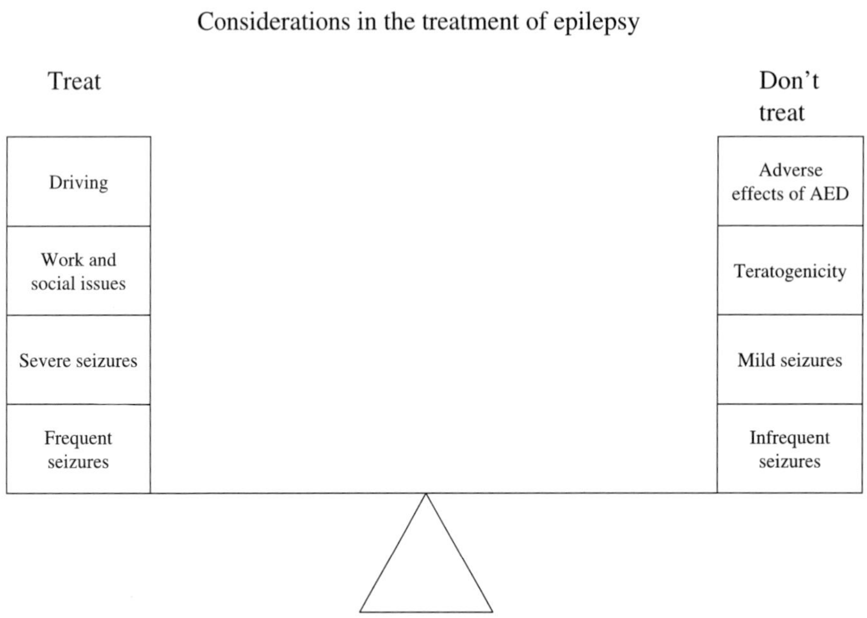

Considerations in the treatment of epilepsy

Figure 9.1. Factors in deciding on whether to treat epilepsy (see text).

after only a single seizure. In practice, treatment is usually only considered once seizures have recurred.

- The patient's age influences the diagnosis, the recurrence risk and the hazards of seizures. A child with a self-limiting, benign focal epilepsy syndrome may suffer more from anti-epileptic drugs (AEDs) than from occasional seizures. Focal epilepsy in the elderly usually recurs and the morbidity of falls due to seizures is likely to be much higher than in younger age groups, but so is the morbidity from medication.
- Patients whose occupations are very public, may find even a small recurrence risk intolerable, for example musicians, lawyers, teachers or other public speakers. Conversely, even very minor cognitive effects mean that some patients find themselves unable to work quite as well when taking medication and would prefer the occasional seizure. Often, but not always, a more satisfactory medication can be found for them.

Factors Weighing Against Medication

- Very mild seizures such as auras with no evidence of functional impairment may be left untreated. In some patients the seizures may evolve into a more severe form, in which case the decision may be revised. (Case 2, Chapter 5).
- Very infrequent seizures pose a difficult problem. The longer the interval between seizures, the longer it takes to know if treatment is having any impact. A threshold for treatment of more than one seizure per year is reasonable for many patients.
- The teratogenicity of many anti-epileptic drugs may make some women decline treatment if they are planning a family.

• Adverse effects or concern over potential adverse effects may cause some patients to decline treatment.

Factors in Favor of Long-Term Medication

• Severe seizures, prolonged seizures, seizures with severe injury or a history of status epilepticus, weigh heavily in favor of treatment.
• Frequent seizures usually require treatment unless they are very mild.
• Sudden death in epilepsy (SUDEP) is most commonly associated with severe epilepsy, but most specialists have experience of young patients with well controlled epilepsy, who have been found dead in bed (Chapter 4). Concern about this complication may increase the imperative to treat.
• Driving is such a major issue for some people that they would wish to receive treatment even if they fall into a low risk category for seizure recurrence.

Case History 2

A 32-year-old female office-worker had suffered about 10 convulsive seizures in her teens, which then remitted for many years. At the age of 32 she experienced another convulsive seizure the day after a hen night. In retrospect she realized she had suffered mild morning myoclonus regularly over the years that had never come to medical attention. Her original EEG had been typical of juvenile myoclonic epilepsy. She was taking the oral contraceptive pill and had completed her family. When she had first developed seizures she had decided she did not want to learn to drive and had been able to structure her life without driving. She decided against AED therapy, opting to try and control her seizures by managing her lifestyle and accepting continuing myoclonus.

   This woman's story illustrates the interplay of factors in making a decision about long-term treatment. She suffered very occasional seizures as part of juvenile myoclonic epilepsy (JME) that does not usually remit. Her most recent seizure was triggered by sleep deprivation and alcohol withdrawal. She hoped to prevent further seizures by avoiding these triggers. She had completed her family and was taking secure contraception so teratogenicity of AEDs was not an issue for her. She had no intention of learning to drive and worked in an environment where myoclonus or seizures would not have put her at physical risk and she accepted that myoclonus would continue, with a small risk of more serious seizures.

LIFESTYLE FACTORS IN THE TREATMENT OF EPILEPSY

• Sleep deprivation is a potent trigger for seizures, especially in idiopathic generalized epilepsy (Case 2).
• Alcohol withdrawal may also trigger seizures and this is often combined with sleep deprivation on the day after a "good night out."
• Some illicit drugs such as cocaine may trigger seizures directly or cause cerebrovascular disease that predisposes to epilepsy (Chapter 13).
• Dietary changes do not help patients who already have a normal diet. A ketogenic diet has been used in the treatment of epilepsy in very severely affected patients, mostly children (below).

- Herbal remedies are sometimes used to treat epilepsy but some herbs may cause seizures, even in the concentrations used for aromatherapy.
- Photosensitivity. Some patients suffer seizures triggered only at times of exposure to television or video-games. Control of exposure (Chapters 1 and 7) may prevent seizures and obviate the need for medication. Indeed, AEDs may be unsuccessful in this situation anyway.
- Psychological or emotional stress may cause an exacerbation of epileptic seizures. Stress can be addressed by increasing support, stress management and occasionally biofeedback strategies.

WHICH MEDICATION TO TREAT THE EPILEPSY?

General Principles

- Seizure-freedom can be achieved for 60 to 70 percent of patients with the first medication tried. Selection of AEDs is currently based on incomplete evidence but a multicenter study in the UK is currently comparing different drugs in newly diagnosed epilepsy.
- Syndromic diagnosis gives the best chance of finding an effective medication. The first stage is to distinguish between focal and generalized epilepsy (Chapter 6) as there are differences in AED efficacy between these types. Most trials of medication address seizure types rather than epilepsy syndromes, often lumping together all patients with convulsive seizures, masking differences between those due to focal or generalized epilepsies.
- Rarer syndromes, usually arising in childhood may need specific AED.
- Within epilepsy syndromes, some drugs are effective only for specific seizure types, and these need to be categorized for each patient.
- Adverse effect profile may be the key factor in the choice of AED in situations where there is no clear evidence of differences in efficacy between drugs.
- Gender influences drug choice: interactions with oral contraception and teratogenicity are specific to women.
- Cost is also an issue in some countries, ranging from less than £10 per year (phenobarbital) to more than £1000 per year for some new medications.

Spectrum of AED Efficacy (Table 9.1 and Appendices)

- Broad spectrum drugs have some efficacy across a broad range of focal and generalized epilepsy syndromes. They include valproate, lamotrigine, topiramate, possibly levetiracetam and felbamate (not available in the UK).
- Focal epilepsy drugs are primarily useful in focal epilepsy and may be helpful for tonic–clonic seizures of idiopathic generalized epilepsy (IGE) but often make IGE absences or myoclonus worse. These drugs include carbamazepine, phenytoin, oxcarbazepine, vigabatrin, gabapentin and tiagabine.
- Drugs for specific seizure types in IGE include ethosuximide for absences and piracetam for myoclonus. Clonazepam is also most useful for myoclonus but is often used more widely.

Table 9.1. Indications for Different AEDs

	Monotherapy	IGE Tonic–Clonic Seizures	IGE Myoclonus	IGE Absences	Focal Epilepsy
Acetazolamide	-	+?	+?	+	+
Carbamazepine	+	+	—	—	+
Clobazam	-	+	+	+	+[1]
Clonazepam	-	+	+	+	+[1]
Ethosuximide	+ (IGE absences)	-	-	+	-
Felbamate	-	+	+	+	+
Gabapentin	+	?	—	—[2]	+
Lamotrigine	+	+	+	+	+
Levetiracetam	-	+?	+?	?	+
Oxcarbazepine	+	+	—	—	+
Phenobarbital	+	+	?	?	+
Phenytoin	+	+	-	—	+
Piracetam	-	-	+	-	-
Tiagabine	-	?	?	—[2]	+
Topiramate	?	+	+?	+	+
Valproate	+	+	+	+	+
Vigabatrin	-	?	—	—[2]	+
Zonisamide	-	+	+?	+?	+

— Contraindicated
- Not indicated
? Unknown
+? Some evidence of benefit
+ Indication
[1]Effect often habituates
[2]May induce absence status

Proposed schemes for the treatment of focal and generalized epilepsy are shown in Figures 9.2 and 9.3. These are a synthesis of evidence, anecdote and personal experience.

Spectrum of AED Adverse Effects (Table 9.2 and Appendices)

Neurotoxic Effects

- Neurotoxic effects may occur with most drugs and are generally dose-related. They are often seen early in the course of treatment during the period of dose titration, which should usually be slow. This is especially important with carbamazepine, as it induces its own metabolism. Mild symptoms often settle if the titration rate is slowed or after the dose titration period. If the patient is forewarned they can be encouraged to persevere.
- Sedation and mild mood change are common with many AEDs but sometimes severe depression, confusion or psychosis occurs. It can be difficult to know if these severe mental symptoms are attributable to the drug or some other facet of the epilepsy (Chapter 17). Barbiturates, vigabatrin, benzodiazepines and topiramate may be particular culprits.

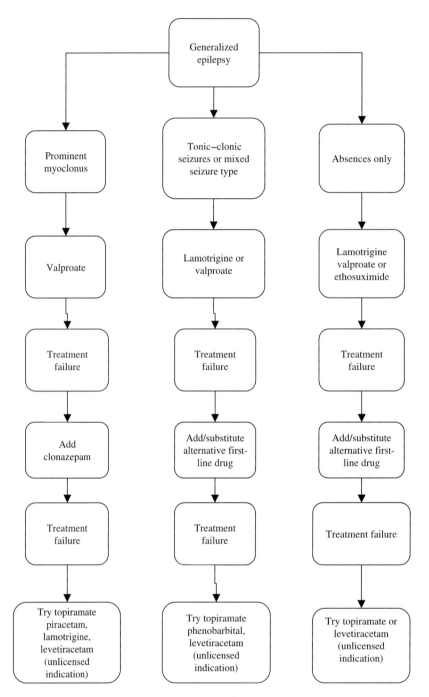

Figure 9.2. An example of a scheme for the treatment of generalized epilepsies (see text).

- Ataxia and diplopia are dose-related properties mainly of drugs that act on sodium channels: phenytoin, carbamazepine and lamotrigine.
- Speech disturbance is an unusual focal cognitive adverse effect, seen with topiramate.

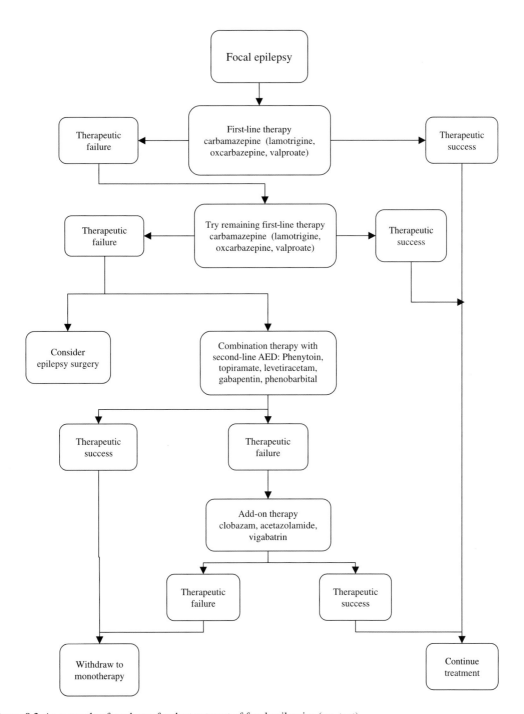

Figure 9.3. An example of a scheme for the treatment of focal epilepsies (see text).

Idiosyncratic Reactions

- Reported rates of allergic skin rash are around 1 to 3 percent with phenytoin, carbamazepine, lamotrigine and phenobarbital. Skin rash is less common with most other drugs. The risk of developing a rash with carbamazepine or

Table 9.2. Adverse Effects of AEDs

	Sedation	Mood Change	Allergy	Weight Change	Diplopia/ Ataxia	Other
Acetazolamide	+	+	+	Loss occasionally	-	Tingling extremities very common, occasional renal stones
Carbamazepine	+ (especially early in treatment)	+/- (also used as a mood stabilizer)	+	Loss or gain occasionally	+	Hyponatraemia common but not usually symptomatic. Lupus-like reaction
Clobazam	++	+	-	-	-	Occasional psychotic/severe depressive symptoms
Clonazepam	++	+	-	-	-	
Ethosuximide	+	+	+	Loss	+	Lupus-like reaction
Felbamate	+	-	++ (may be fatal)	Loss	+	Oesophageal burning
Gabapentin	+	+	-	Gain may be marked	-	
Lamotrigine	+/-	+/- (sometimes mood elevation)	+	-	+ (occasional)	Headache common at higher doses Sometimes insomnia
Levetiracetam	+	+/-	+	-	+	
Oxcarbazepine	+	-	+	-	+/-	GI disturbance, hyponatremia
Phenobarbital	++	++	+	Gain	+ (mostly ataxia)	Paradoxical agitation in children. Osteomalacia
Phenytoin	+	+/-	+	-	+ (mostly ataxia)	Facial coarsening, acne, gum hypertrophy, persistent ataxia, cognitive change and peripheral neuropathy. Osteomalacia, pseudo-lymphoma
Tiagabine	+	+	-	Gain	-	
Topiramate	+	++	+/-	Loss may be marked	-	Renal stones, cognitive effects especially dysphasia
Valproate	+	+/- (also used as mood stabilizer)	+/- (rare but severe pancreatitis or hepatitis)	Gain may be marked	-	Tremor common. Possible association with polycystic ovary syndrome. Rare metabolic encephalopathy. Lupus-like reaction rarely
Vigabatrin	+	+ psychosis reported	-	Gain may be marked	-	Progressive, irreversible visual field defects in up to 30%
Zonisamide	+	+	+	Loss	+/-	Renal stones

+, adverse effect moderately common; ++, adverse effect common or severe; -, adverse effect very unlikely; +/-, adverse effect possible but uncommon.

lamotrigine is significantly lower if the rate of dose titration is slow. More severe rashes, such as Stevens-Johnson syndrome are usually seen in the early stages of treatment when dose titration has been rapid. A severe rash necessitates immediate withdrawal of medication. Skin irritation without a visible rash also occurs. In this situation, the symptom may be transient and treatable with emollients. In occasional cases, patients have been restarted more slowly on the same drug and have not suffered a recurrence of their allergic reaction.

- The rate of cross-reactivity of skin rash is high between these drugs, up to 25 percent.
- Other immune-mediated reactions may be seen with the same group of drugs, including hepatitis, pancreatitis and bone marow suppression, which may rarely be lethal. The use of felbamate has been restricted in the US because of these problems and it is unlikely to be licensed in the UK.
- Hepatotoxicity with valproate may be due to a different mechanism, probably by interference with metabolic processes in the liver. This affects especially children under the age of two years with inherited metabolic disease, which may go unrecognized until valproate is administered.
- Blood indices are often affected by AEDs, for example a mild leucopenia or thrombocytopenia. These are reversible on stopping the medication but if the depression of the marrow is too great, or there are symptoms to suggest defective function such as infection or purpura then the drug needs to be withdrawn.
- Hyponatraemia is common with carbamazepine or oxcarbazepine. It is usually mild but may be severe (<125 mmol/l), especially with concomitant diuretics. It may cause drowsiness or worsening seizures.

Case History 4

A 65-year-old woman was admitted to hospital with focal motor seizures affecting the right leg associated with a left hemisphere subdural effusion. In hospital the seizures evolved into tonic–clonic convulsions. She was treated with intravenous phenytoin but developed a skin rash after one week and this was withdrawn. Sodium valproate was started and within five days she developed severe jaundice. The seizures had largely settled apart from occasional jerks of the right leg and her treatment was changed to clonazepam alone. A liver biopsy showed periportal inflammatory changes. Clonazepam was withdrawn successfully after four weeks, without seizure recurrence.

This case illustrates an immune-mediated reaction involving both skin and liver. The likely culprit for both is phenytoin, since valproate-induced hepatotoxicity is not usually immune-mediated but until the liver biopsy was available, the safest course of action was to stop the valproate and use a benzodiazepine in the short term, which is highly unlikely to cause allergic reactions.

Case History 5

A 35-year-old man had suffered poorly controlled epilepsy since the age of 10, including tonic–clonic seizures and myoclonic jerks. Previous treatment had been with phenobarbital, phenytoin and carbamazepine. Despite these he had had repeated admissions to hospital with clusters of tonic–clonic seizures. During one of these admissions his EEGs were reviewed. They showed a consistent pattern of frequent bursts of generalized spike and wave. He was thought to suffer juvenile myoclonic epilepsy and he started treatment with valproate. He had no further seizures and was discharged home. Two weeks later he was readmitted, drowsy but with no overt seizures. An EEG showed no epileptiform activity but the background activity was markedly slower than previously. Valproate was withdrawn and he started to improve. Blood ammonia and a urinary test for orotic acid showed elevated levels.

A deterioration in mental state soon after starting valproate may be due to hyper-ammonemia. This rare complication is most commonly seen in patients who have a pre-existing metabolic deficiency affecting nitrogen metabolism, such as ornithine transcarbamylase deficiency. The condition is lethal if valproate is not withdrawn promptly. Drowsiness or deteriorating seizure control are pointers to this rare complication.

- Osteomalacia may severely affect patients who have taken enzyme-inducing AED for many years, especially phenytoin. There is no agreed protocol for anticipating or dealing with this problem.

AEDs for Idiopathic Generalized Epilepsy (Figure 9.2)

- Valproate has traditionally been the drug of choice for most IGE although clear evidence is lacking. It is active against all seizure types in IGE probably rendering 80 percent of patients seizure-free. In mild cases, seizures may melt away with tiny doses of the drug, sometimes as little as 200 milligrams per day. More commonly doses of 600 to 1500 milligrams per day are required.
- Lamotrigine is useful for treating IGE. Absences and tonic–clonic seizures are often well controlled but myoclonus may respond less well. The dose required for adults may be as little as 100 milligrams per day but is sometimes 150 to 400 milligrams. It is easy to use in monotherapy but is profoundly influenced by concomitant enzyme-inducing or enzyme-inhibiting drugs.
- Topiramate may also have an increasing role treating IGE absences and tonic–clonic seizures.
- Phenobarbital is an effective drug in IGE but has more sedative adverse effects than most newer drugs. In combination with valproate, these can be severe.
- Levetiracetam is a new drug that may be helpful in IGE including myoclonus, but is not currently licensed for that indication in the UK.
- Focal epilepsy drugs may help tonic–clonic seizures of IGE, but they may unmask myoclonus or absence seizures.
- Myoclonus may respond to piracetam or benzodiazepines such as clonazepam and for this seizure type the effect does not appear to habituate.
- Ethosuximide has a specific effect on the absences of IGE and rarely helps other seizure types.

This combination of drug properties means that where a single drug is not fully effective, one can combine drugs in rational regimens.

Case History 6
A 17-year-old girl presented with three tonic–clonic seizures over two months. Each seizure was preceded by a cluster of myoclonic jerks. In retrospect she described having had myoclonic jerks most mornings for the previous 18 months. An EEG confirmed the diagnosis of juvenile myoclonic epilepsy. She was treated with

sodium valproate 1000 milligrams daily and there were no further tonic–clonic seizures, and myoclonic jerks were reduced but continued at a lower frequency. Further increases in sodium valproate did not eliminate myoclonus. Valproate was reduced to 600 milligrams per day and clonazepam was added at 0.5 milligrams nocte. Her myoclonus ceased.

This case illustrates targeting a second, seizure-specific drug at myoclonus or absences when first-line therapy has achieved control of tonic–clonic seizures.

AEDs for Focal Epilepsies (Figure 9.3)

There is even less information to guide choice of medication in the treatment of focal epilepsies. There are no studies that have addressed differential efficacy in different types of focal epilepsy, for example in frontal versus temporal lobe epilepsy or in epilepsy due to different etiologies. The overall success of treatment of focal epilepsy is less than for generalized epilepsy. Patients probably have no better than a 50 percent chance of achieving seizure-freedom, except children with benign focal epilepsies of childhood.

First-Line Drugs in the Treatment of Focal Epilepsy

- No consistent differences in efficacy as monotherapy have been proven between carbamazepine, valproate, phenytoin, phenobarbital and lamotrigine.
- Add-on trials cannot be used as a guide to monotherapy usage. For example, vigabatrin is a highly effective drug in add-on trials but compared poorly with carbamazepine in a monotherapy trial. A pragmatic study comparing carbamazepine, gabapentin, lamotrigine, oxcarbazepine and topiramate in monotherapy is under way in the UK.
- Carbamazepine is the standard medication for treating focal epilepsy in the UK. This is best introduced gradually and given as the slow-release preparation that is less associated with post-dose side effects such as transient blurred vision. A standard regime starts at 100 milligrams at night, increasing to 200 milligrams daily after a week and to 600 milligrams daily in 4 to 6 weeks.
- Oxcarbazepine is closely related to carbamazepine but has much less enzyme-inducing tendency. It is favored to carbamazepine in some parts of Europe but has only recently become available in the UK.
- Phenytoin is used widely as a first-line treatment for epilepsy, especially in the USA. It has a similar mechanism and spectrum of action but has some advantages over carbamazepine. It can be introduced rapidly: an oral loading dose can be given to rapidly achieve therapeutic blood levels. The dose is quite standard, usually between 250 and 400 milligrams per day and it is given just once. It is also cheap. A disadvantage is its zero order kinetics. In a drug with a narrow therapeutic window and a large number of drug interactions, this readily leads to toxicity or therapeutic failure. In addition there are large number of potential long-term side effects such as ataxia, osteomalacia, neuropathy, cosmetic changes, gum hypertrophy and possibly cognitive changes.
- Valproate compares well in clinical trials although many clinicians feel carbamazepine is more effective. Valproate may have advantages in some situations for example for the elderly as it is less prone to cause ataxia or hyponatremia.

- Lamotrigine has been compared directly to carbamazepine and was found to have similar efficacy with slightly fewer adverse effects. It is gaining in popularity as a broad spectrum first-line treatment.
- Phenobarbital is effective and very cheap. It remains the standard drug in countries with more limited health care budgets. It carries a higher risk of sedation and cognitive side effects than other standard, first-line drugs. In children there may be paradoxical hyperactivity and withdrawal seizures are also common.

ASSESSING THE RESPONSE TO TREATMENT

- Seizure-freedom is the goal of most epilepsy treatment. Quality of life studies show that it is only complete freedom from seizures that confers maximal psychosocial benefit.
- Seizure-reduction is a measure used in research studies to establish drug efficacy. A 50 percent reduction in seizures is considered a good pharmacological response, but it is a very poor second best to seizure-freedom: the patient still lives in fear of the next attack, cannot drive and may have difficulty finding work.
- Seizure-severity scales have been devised and correlated with psychosocial outcomes. For example, seizures with falls or incontinence of urine are more severe than seizures without these complications. The major impact of such scales is to help the clinician feel they are doing some good, even though the patient still has seizures.
- Seizure diaries are ingrained into many clinicians and patients. A diary may show a recurring pattern of seizures, which allows intermittent intervention, for example in catamenial epilepsy. Diaries help patients with very infrequent seizures to take a very long view of their epilepsy and may provide evidence that small changes in seizure frequency are part of the natural fluctuation of the patient's disease and are nothing to do with treatment changes. However, if a patient with refractory epilepsy needs to look at a diary to know if a treatment has reduced their seizures, then the impact is marginal.
- Under-reporting of seizures occurs with absences, seizures associated with amnesia or seizures in sleep; independent evidence is needed.

WHAT TO DO WHEN FIRST-LINE TREATMENT FAILS

There are two options available to the clinician: try a new first-line drug or add a second-line drug in combination therapy. Most clinicians would not give up an attempt for monotherapy after just a single drug, but how they approach changing drugs varies.

Trying a New First-Line Drug

1. Add in another first-line drug and if this is successful in treating the epilepsy, withdraw the first medication to assess the new drug in monotherapy. The advantages of this method are that the patient is never left with levels of medication that

are subtherapeutic and only one drug is changed at a time making it easier to determine the culprit if there is a problem. A disadvantage of the add-on method is that patients are more likely to end up on polytherapy.

2. Withdraw the old drug and introduce the new one at the same time. The advantages of this strategy are a lower risk of adverse effects of combination therapy and the pharmacokinetics of drug interactions are less likely to play a significant role. This crossover method must be planned carefully to avoid a vulnerable period of subtherapeutic doses of both drugs.

Adding a Second-Line Drug

- Failure of first-line AED leads to consideration of second-line drugs. All first-line drugs can be used in a second-line role but drugs that are exclusively second-line are of unproven value in monotherapy.
- Second-line drugs are added to existing therapy. Clear targets should be set for benefit in terms of seizures and adverse effects.
- Ineffective drugs should be withdrawn before another drug is added to avoid ever-increasing polypharmacy.
- Withdrawal to monotherapy. Occasionally, if a second-line drug is very valuable, other medication may be withdrawn, leaving the patient on monotherapy on the understanding that this may be unlicensed treatment.
- More than two AEDs concurrently rarely improves treatment efficacy and more than three is virtually never helpful. Severe epilepsy poorly controlled by one drug is better than severe epilepsy poorly controlled by four drugs with additive adverse effects (Chapter 12, Case 3).

HOW TO COMBINE AEDs

The number of potential combinations of AEDs is enormous and there is neither evidence on which to base a decision as to how to combine different AEDs nor any real prospect that this evidence will be available in the future. Rational polytherapy tries to apply pharmacological principles of pharmacodynamic and pharmacokinetic properties of different AEDs in deciding on treatment combinations. It is most easily applied to treating different seizure types in IGE but some aspects can be extrapolated into polytherapy of focal epilepsy. Table 9.3 summarizes drug combinations. (See also Table 9.4.)

- Combinations of enzyme-inducing drugs often lead to erratic blood levels and it may be difficult to achieve satisfactory levels of both drugs. For example the combination of carbamazepine and phenytoin often causes fluctuating phenytoin levels and subtherapeutic carbamazepine levels.
- Combining drugs with similar mechanisms of action may be expected to give additive adverse effects with little therapeutic benefit. For example the combination of vigabatrin and tiagabine, both of which have a specific GABAergic effect is unlikely to be helpful but may increase sedation and weight gain.
- Adding an enzyme-inhibiting drug such as valproate may inhibit the metabolism of other drugs, rendering them toxic. Under these circumstances, adverse effects are due to the old drugs, not the new one. Anticipatory changes in drug

Table 9.3. Rational Drug Combination

Shaded combinations are not recommended

	Clobazam	Ethosuximide	Gabapentin	Lamotrigine	Levetiracetam	Oxcarbazepine	Phenobarbital	Phenytoin	Piracetam	Tiagabine	Topiramate	Valproate	Vigabatrin
Carbamazepine	4	2	4	1,2,3	4	2,3*	1,4	1,2,3	2	1,4	1,4	1,4	4
	Clobazam	5	4	6	6	4	3	4	7	3	6	6	3
		Ethosuximide	2	5	5	2	2	2	7	2	5	1,5	2
			Gabapentin	4	4	4	2,3	4	2	2,3	4	4	2,3
				Lamotrigine	5	1,2,3	1,4	1,2,3	7	4	4	1,4	4
					Levetiracetam	4	6	4	2	4	6	6	4
						Oxcarbazepine	1,4	1,2,3	2	4	4	4	4
							Phenobarbital	1,4	7	1,3	1,4	1,3	3
								Phenytoin	2	1,4	1,4	1,4	4
									Piracetam	2	7	7	2
										Tiagabine	4	4	2,3
											Topiramate	1,6	4
												Valproate	4
													Vigabatrin

1 Pharmacokinetic interaction

2 Illogical combination

3 Additive adverse effects likely

4 Rational combination in focal epilepsy only

5 Rational combination in generalized epilepsy only

6 Broad spectrum combination

7 Rational combination in myoclonic epilepsy

* Despite this being an apparently illogical combination, one study has shown benefit from this combination

Table 9.4. Mode of Elimination of Different Anti-Epileptic Drugs

Renally Excreted	Hepatically Metabolized	Mixed Elimination
Gabapentin	Benzodiazepines	Topiramate[2]
Levetiracetam	Carbamazepine[2]	
Piracetam	Ethosuximide[1]	
Vigabatrin	Lamotrigine	
	Oxcarbazepine[2] (mild)	
	Phenobarbital[2]	
	Phenytoin[2]	
	Tiagabine	
	Valproate[1]	

[1] = hepatic enzyme inhibitor, [2] = hepatic enzyme inducer.

dosages and AED blood levels before and after making the change may be helpful.

- Adding an enzyme-inducing drug may reduce the efficacy of existing medication, leading to worsening of seizures. Here it is the drop in the old AED, not the new AED that is causing the problem.
- Pharmacodynamic interactions may cause adverse effects without any major change in blood levels. Many AEDs may cause adverse effects that can be reduced by a small reduction of concomitant medication during initial dose titration.
- Lamotrigine treatment is heavily dependent on concomitant therapy. In monotherapy its half-life is around 20 hours and therapeutic doses are usually 150 to 400 milligrams daily. With concomitant valproate its half-life is around 60 hours and therapeutic doses are usually 100 to 300 milligrams per day. With concomitant enzyme-inducing drugs, its half-life is around 10 to 15 hours and therapeutic doses are usually 300 to 800 milligrams per day. Lamotrigine needs to be introduced slowly to reduce idiosyncratic reactions and the titration rate also depends on concomitant therapy. Adding valproate to lamotrigine will cause a sudden rise in levels and may precipitate toxicity. Adding an enzyme inducer may cause a drop in levels and therapeutic failure.
- Felbamate is used in the USA for refractory epilepsy and has complex pharmacokinetic interactions. It reduces carbamazepine levels by 20 percent, but increases levels of the epoxide metabolite that is responsible for many adverse effects. Felbamate also increases blood levels of phenytoin, phenobarbital and valproate. Conversely carbamazepine and phenytoin reduce felbamate levels by 20 to 30 percent.
- Informing the patient enhances compliance. Without prior warning they reasonably blame the new medication for any problem and stop it rather than modifying previous medications.

USING NEW DRUGS

- New AEDs are marketed after trials showing efficacy and safety as add-on therapy. The limitations of such trials mean that these medications have a restricted role when they are first marketed and this role is gradually re-defined with post-marketing experience.

- Add-on therapy is the indication for new AED. Later experience and monotherapy trials may show benefit (lamotrigine) or lack of benefit (vigabatrin) in monotherapy.
- Focal epilepsy is the usual indication for new AED as this is the main group in refractory epilepsy studies. Later experience may suggest the drug is useful for generalized epilepsy (lamotrigine, topiramate) or may make it worse (gabapentin, vigabatrin).
- Teratogenicity of new drugs is only known in animal studies. Women who may become pregnant are excluded from studies so there is no information in this important patient group prior to marketing. Clinicians use new AEDs in this situation at their own risk and patients must be counseled.
- Pre-marketing usage is a few thousand patients. Serious adverse effects may emerge that are uncommon but not excessively rare (felbamate and bone marrow suppression) or common but difficult to detect (vigabatrin and visual disturbance).
- Recommended rate of dose titration may be modified (usually slowed down) after the drug is marketed. It is often wise to titrate more slowly from the outset.
- Effective doses in post-marketing populations may be lower (topiramate) or higher (gabapentin) than those used to achieve the artificial endpoints of pre-marketing studies.

WHEN TO STOP ANTI-EPILEPTIC DRUG THERAPY (TABLES 9.5 AND 9.6)

- The factors in the decision to stop AEDs mirror those in the decision to start therapy in the first place and have been evaluated in the Medical Research Council (MRC) study.
- Risk of seizure recurrence is the primary consideration including the medical and social consequences of recurrence. Set against this is the risk of continuing therapy, which is usually low, for a patient who has been seizure-free for a long time on stable medication.
- No investigation can predict seizure recurrence. There is no time when drug withdrawal can be said to carry no risk, seizures may occasionally recur on drug withdrawal after decades of seizure-freedom.

Table 9.5. Factors in Determining the Risk of Seizure Recurrence After AED Withdrawal

Factor	Consideration
Epilepsy syndrome	For example juvenile myoclonic epilepsy usually recurs, childhood absence epilepsy much less frequently
Duration of seizure-freedom prior to AED withdrawal (all cases combined)	2 years seizure freedom: 40% recurrence over next 2 years 10 years seizure-freedom, 10% recurrence over next 2 years
Duration of treatment	Longer duration prior to seizure freedom confers higher risk
Duration of epilepsy prior to treatment	Probably no effect
EEG	Important in syndromic diagnosis and slow waves have minor independent adverse effect on recurrence in children

Table 9.6. Risk of Withdrawal Seizures With Different Medications

High risk	Barbiturates, benzodiazepines, carbamazepine, vigabatrin
Moderate risk	Phenytoin
Low risk	Valproate
Unknown risk	Lamotrigine, topiramate, tiagabine, gabapentin, oxcarbazepine

- Driving is a central issue for many patients. Since a clinician cannot promise seizure-freedom, many patients opt to stay on therapy indefinitely. In addition in the UK, a patient withdrawing medication is required by law not to drive for 6 months after the completion of withdrawal.
- Employment may also be jeopardized by recurrent seizures.
- Teratogenic effects of AEDs may sway a woman to discontinue AEDs early if she wishes to conceive.
- In children, the social consequences of a seizure may be of less concern than the sedative effects of medication and treatment is often withdrawn earlier than in adults.

HOW TO WITHDRAW A DRUG

Withdrawal Because of Acute Complications

- Severe complications, for example a severe behavioral or allergic reaction, merit rapid withdrawal of the AED.
- Withdrawal seizures are a risk. The patient needs to be stabilized on another anti-epileptic drug. A benzodiazepine, such as clobazam 10 to 20 milligrams daily can be used to minimize seizures during the crossover period. In high risk cases with severe epilepsy the patient may need to be admitted to hospital.
- Minor complications can be dealt with as an outpatient by tapering medication over weeks to months whilst another is started.

Elective Drug Withdrawal

- Withdrawal seizures usually occur towards the end of the withdrawal phase or after the drug has been stopped. They are related more to low levels of medication than to the rate of withdrawal.
- A 6-week schedule is sufficiently slow for most drugs although patients may be more comfortable with a slower process.
- Barbiturates and benzodiazepines are more prone to withdrawal seizures than many other drugs. They are often withdrawn much more slowly, over months.

Case History 7
A 58-year-old man suffered severe focal epilepsy partly controlled on combination therapy including vigabatrin. The vigabatrin had not proved of long-term benefit and because of concerns regarding visual symptoms, a decision was made to withdraw the drug, reducing the daily dose by 500 milligrams per month. Five days after reducing the daily dose from 1000 milligrams to 500 milligrams he was admitted to hospital with a severe cluster of seizures – something he had not experienced

before. He was treated with clobazam 20 milligrams daily and remained seizure-free for the next 3 weeks. The final 500 milligrams of vigabatrin was withdrawn uneventfully.

Withdrawal seizures may occur with even very slow dose reduction. Benzodiazepines may help prevent withdrawal seizures in the short-term, but it may be necessary to reintroduce the withdrawn drug to reverse the imbalance that has triggered the seizures.

JUDGING DOSAGE AND ANTI-EPILEPTIC DRUG LEVELS IN TREATMENT (TABLE 9.7)

- AED dosage is a balance between therapeutic and adverse effects. In monotherapy, AED blood levels have very limited use as the clinical decision-making process only comprises four possibilities.

  1. The patient is seizure-free and has no side effects – continue current therapy.
  2. The patient is not seizure-free and has no side effects – increase treatment until seizure-free or side effects occur.
  3. The patient is not seizure-free and has side effects – change therapy.
  4. The patient is seizure-free but has side effects – reduce dose until adverse effects disappear or seizures recur.

Dose-Limiting Toxicity

- Sedation and mental slowing are dose-related effects common to many drugs that can be used in judging when maximum tolerated dose has been achieved. In polytherapy it may be difficult to judge which drug is responsible.
- Carbamazepine causes blurred vision, diplopia and sometimes ataxia, which first occur post-dose, reflecting toxicity at peak blood levels. These adverse effects are a reliable sign of developing toxicity that can be used to judge dosage. They are reduced by using the sustained release preparation.
- Lamotrigine may cause similar problems to carbamazepine but to a lesser degree.

Table 9.7. Value of Blood Levels for Different AEDs

	AED	Comments
Highest value	Phenytoin	Blood levels bear a strong relation to therapeutic and toxic effects Zero order kinetics mean that the therapeutic window is narrow A subgroup of patients (fast acetylators) require higher doses of phenytoin and are more difficult to manage
Intermediate value	Phenobarbital carbamazepine lamotrigine	Therapeutic and toxic effects bear a weaker relation to blood level
Low value	Vigabatrin valproate gabapentin topiramate benzodiazepines	For example, vigabatrin binds irreversibly to CNS target, blood levels bear no relation to its CNS effect. Levels of these AEDs not routinely available

- Phenytoin toxicity usually causes ataxia with less visual disturbance than carbamazepine.
- Valproate causes dose-related postural tremor. This can be treated with propranolol and is not necessarily limiting for the patient.
- Topiramate causes tingling extremities that is also quite drug-specific but may not be the dose-limiting adverse effect. It also causes an unusual speech disturbance.

Uses of AED Blood Levels in Monotherapy

- To monitor phenytoin monotherapy.
- To measure compliance.
- To ensure a reasonable carbamazepine level in patients with very infrequent seizures where a therapeutic effect will take a long time to assess.
- In women at the start of pregnancy to provide measurements against which to assess any later problems.

Case History 8

A 27-year-old woman achieved only incomplete seizure control with carbamazepine monotherapy. Her clinician decided to add sodium valproate. After two weeks she was admitted to hospital with severe nausea, vomiting, ataxia and nystagmus. A carbamazepine blood level was minimally elevated but its epoxide metabolite was grossly elevated. Her symptoms resolved when the carbamazepine dose was reduced.

This case illustrates a potential effect of valproate on the metabolic pathway of carbamazepine, triggering toxicity with only a slight effect on carbamazepine blood levels. Blood levels of carbamazepine are only loosely linked to adverse effects.

Anti-Epileptic Drug Levels in Polytherapy

- Changes in AED therapy can be monitored by blood levels before and after altering therapy and can help to attribute clinical effects to a particular drug. However, Case 8 shows that drug levels are not the whole story.
- Pharmacodynamic interactions occur that are not reflected in measurable changes in the blood. For example, adding topiramate to existing therapy may cause sedative adverse effects that can be eliminated by reducing concurrent therapy, without there having been any changes in blood levels.

PROPRIETARY *VERSUS* GENERIC ANTI-EPILEPTIC DRUGS

- Proprietary prescription is advisable for most AEDs as it is the only way of guaranteeing the same preparation each time.
- Bioavailability of generic drugs is within 20 percent of a standard, allowing up to 40 percent difference between different generic preparations. This fluctuation may influence efficacy and tolerability of preparations such as phenytoin with a narrow therapeutic window.
- Carbamazepine toxicity is closely related to blood levels and these can be smoothed out, with significantly improved tolerability by prescribing controlled release Tegretol™ (Novartis).

- Valproate is also available as a controlled release preparation, Epilim-Chrono™ (Sanofi-Synthelabo). This can be given as a once daily dose up to 1500 milligrams per day and may have slightly fewer adverse effects than generic valproate. Most newer AEDs are under patent and are necessarily proprietary.

SEIZURE CLUSTERS

- The timing of seizures is rarely truly random. Clustering of attacks is common and may be predictable or unpredictable. In the clearest cases, seizures occur at close intervals, sometimes separated by only minutes to hours but may then disappear until the next cluster is due, perhaps weeks later.
- Sometimes a seizure cluster may evolve into a more severe attack, for example flurries of morning myoclonus leading to a convulsive seizure or serial attacks evolving into status epilepticus. In this situation, if continuous treatment does not prevent attacks, intermittent treatment may be effective damage limitation.

Case History 9
A 37-year-old man suffered IGE. About once per month he would awake and develop serial absences over one to two hours culminating in a tonic–clonic seizure. Seizures were reduced but not eliminated by regular therapy with valproate and lamotrigine. He was provided with clobazam tablets, which he took on his bad mornings, reducing the duration of absences to a few minutes and preventing the tonic–clonic seizures altogether.

- A seizure diary can be used to try and identify causes for clustering such as life events, compliance problems, sleep deprivation or alcohol effects.
- Predictable clustering such as in women with catamenial epilepsy (Chapter 10) and regular menses, can be treated with clobazam. The drug is started the day before the cluster is due and continued at 10 to 20 milligrams daily until after the cluster is due to finish.
- Unpredictable clusters can also be treated with clobazam. The drug can be given after a first attack and for 2 to 3 days, in the hope of aborting the rest of the seizure cluster and preventing a more serious outcome.
- Clobazam may however simply convert seizures to a non-clustering pattern or simply move the seizures to after the short course of medication is finished, rather than stop them altogether.

CAN MEDICATION MAKE SEIZURES WORSE?

Anti-Epileptic Drugs

- Incorrect syndromic diagnosis may lead to inappropriate AED prescription and deterioration of seizures. The commonest example is carbamazepine given for juvenile myoclonic epilepsy.
- Toxic doses of AED, taken inadvertently or deliberately may make seizures worse.
- Enzyme-inducing AEDs may exacerbate seizures and encephalopathy in patients with acute intermittent porphyria.

- Valproate may exacerbate seizures and cause fatal encephalopathy in patients with defects of nitrogen metabolism such as ornithine transcarbamylase deficiency.
- Other cases of paradoxical increased seizures may not have a clear explanation. If a clinician is not aware of this possibility, they may attribute an increase in seizures to the patient's underlying condition, and further increase the dose of the offending medication.

Case History 10

A 33-year-old man suffered poorly controlled temporal lobe epilepsy. His neurologist started lamotrigine and he developed a new pattern of drop attacks. Concerned about the deterioration in his seizures, an increased dose was prescribed and the drop attacks worsened. Following withdrawal of lamotrigine the drop attacks ceased and he returned to his previous pattern of focal seizures.

Concomitant Medication

- Concomitant medication may have intrinsic pro-convulsive properties (Chapter 13).
- Medication may trigger epileptic seizures because of drug interactions with AEDs (below).
- Sometimes it is the intercurrent illness for which medication is prescribed that is the cause of seizures for example if the patient experiences a high fever that lowers the seizure threshold or diarrhea that reduces AED absorption.

Drug Interactions for Anti-Epileptic Drugs (Tables 9.8a–c)

- Interactions between AEDs are common.
- Interactions with other medications are common. These are often pharmacokinetic and may interfere with the action of the AED or with the other drug.
- Some pharmacodynamic group effects can be assumed to occur with most anti-epileptic drugs. These include enhanced neurotoxicity with other drugs acting on the CNS including antidepressants, neuroleptics and opioid analgesics. Patients taking these combinations should be warned particularly about sedation and their effects on driving or operating machinery etc.

Table 9.8a. Effects of Concomitant Medication on AED Therapy

Target AED	Interacting Drug(s)	Effect
Acetazolamide	Topiramate, Salicylates	Enhanced risk of metabolic acidosis
Carbamazepine	1. Erythromycin, isoniazid, verapamil, diltiazem, dextropropoxyphene, cimetidine, felbamate, lamotrigine, oxcarbazepine, valproate viloxazine, fluoxetine	1. Decrease hepatic metabolism and increase carbamazepine blood levels or may increase levels of the epoxide metabolite of carbamazepine, which is responsible for many of its neurotoxic adverse effects
	2. Phenobarbital, phenytoin, primidone, theophylline, clonazepam, retinoids	2. Decrease carbamazepine blood levels and reduced efficacy

Table 9.8a. *Continued*

Target AED	Interacting Drug(s)	Effect
Clobazam	1. Cyclo-oxygenase inhibitors e.g. cimetidine	1. Reduced metabolism and enhanced neurotoxicity
	2. Hepatic enzyme inducers e.g. phenytoin, phenobarbital or carbamazepine	2. Increased metabolism and reduced efficacy
Clonazepam	1. Cyclo-oxygenase inhibitors e.g. cimetidine	1. Reduced metabolism and enhanced neurotoxicity
	2. Hepatic enzyme inducers e.g. phenytoin, phenobarbital, carbamazepine	2. Increased metabolism and reduced efficacy
Ethosuximide	1. Valproate	1. May double ethosuximide half-life and increase toxicity
	2. Enzyme inducers: carbamazepine, phenytoin, rifampicin	2. Reduce blood levels by >50% and reduce efficacy
Felbamate	Enzyme inducers such as phenobarbital, phenytoin or carbamazepine	Reduce felbamate levels by 20–30%
Gabapentin	Magnesium containing antacids	Reduce gabapentin by up to 25%
Lamotrigine	1. Enzyme inducers e.g. phenytoin, phenobarbital, carbamazepine	1. Half life reduced to 12 hours, dose may need to be increased in the range 400-800 mg/day
	2. Hepatic enzyme inhibitors e.g. valproate	2. Half life increased to 70 hours. Low starting dose and maintenance reduced in the range 100–200mg/day
Levetiracetam	None known	
Oxcarbazepine	Enzyme-inducing drugs such as carbamazepine, phenytoin, phenobarbital	Increased metabolism, dose may need to be increased
Phenobarbital	1. Valproate	1. A potentially highly sedating pharmacodynamic interaction
	2. Valproate, phenytoin, dextropopoxyphene	2. Increased blood levels and toxicity
	3. Rifampicin	3. Reduced phenobarbital levels and efficacy
Phenytoin	1. Acetazolamide, amiodarone, antifungal agents, histamine H2 antagonists, diazepam, isoniazid, omeprazole, estrogens, oxcarbazepine salicylates, ethosuximide, tolbutamide, topiramate trazodone, viloxazine	1. Phenytoin levels increased and may precipitate toxicity. Regular monitoring advisable.
	2. Carbamazepine, reserpine, folic acid, vigabatrin	2. Phenytoin levels reduced and may impair seizure control. Regular monitoring advisable
	3. Phenobarbital, valproate, antineoplastic agents	3. Phenytoin levels may increase or decrease. Regular monitoring advisable.
Piracetam	None known	
Tiagabine	Enzyme inducers, phenytoin, phenobarbital, carbamazepine	Reduce tiagabine levels, efficacy may be reduced
Topiramate	Enzyme inducers: Phenytoin, carbamazepine, phenobarbital	Topiramate levels reduced, may impair efficacy
Valproate	1. Salicylates, naproxen, phenylbutazone	1. May displace valproate from binding sites, increasing blood levels
	2. Carbamazepine, phenytoin, barbiturates, mefloquine	2. Increased metabolism, dose may need to be increased
	3. Barbiturates	3. Enhanced sedation with this combination
	4. Clonazepam	4. Generally safe but rare reported cases of status epilepticus with this combination
	5. Cimetidine, erythromycin	5. Prolonged half-life, valproate dose may need reduction
Vigabatrin	None known	
Zonisamide	Phenytoin, carbamazepine, valproate	May decrease zonisamide levels and reduce efficacy

Table 9.8b. AED Effects on Concomitant Medication

AED	Drug Affected	Effect
Acetazolamide	1. Folic acid antagonists	1. May potentiate folate antagonism
	2. Hypoglycemic agents	2. May potentiate hypoglycemia
	3. Oral anticoagulants	3. May potentiate anticoagulation
	4. Salicylates, topiramate	4. May cause severe acidosis and CNS toxicity
	5. AED	5. Enhances tendency to osteomalacia
Carbamazepine	1. Warfarin, oral contraceptive pill, glucocorticoids, clobazam, clonazepam, ethosuximide, valproate, digoxin, doxycycline, haloperidol, imipramine, methadone, theophylline.	1. Increased metabolism, dose usually needs increasing. Use 50 µg estrogen pill but may still have suboptimal efficacy.
	2. Isoniazid	2. May increase isoniazid mediated hepatotoxicity
	3. Lithium	3. May increase lithium mediated neurotoxicity without increasing lithium blood levels
	4. Thiazide diuretics	4. May combine to cause severe hyponatremia
	5. Anesthetic muscle relaxants	5. Effect may be reduced, dose needs to be raised
Clobazam	Psychotropic medications such as other benzodiazepines, AEDs, antidepressants, neuroleptics and opioid analgesics	Enhanced sedation and neurotoxicity
Clonazepam	Psychotropic medications such as other benzodiazepines, antidepressants, AEDs, neuroleptics and opioid analgesics	Enhanced sedation and neurotoxicity
	Valproate	Rare reported cases of absence status epilepticus with this combination, uncertain significance
Ethosuximide	Phenytoin and valproate	Blood levels may rise
Felbamate	1. Carbamazepine	1. Reduced level by 20–30% but toxic epoxide metabolite levels rise
	2. Phenytoin, phenobarbital, valproate	2. Levels increase by 10–30%, dose reduction may be needed
Gabapentin	AED	Enhanced neurotoxicity
Lamotrigine	Carbamazepine, possibly other AED	Enhanced neurotoxicity and increased risk of diplopia or ataxia. Dose may require reduction
Levetiracetam	None known	
Oxcarbazepine	Oral contraceptive pill	Use 50 µg estrogen pill but oral contraceptive still may have suboptimal efficacy
Phenobarbital	1. Oral contraceptive pill	1. Use 50 µg estrogen pill but oral contraceptive still may have suboptimal efficacy
	2. Carbamazepine, clonazepam, clozapine diazepam, corticosteroids, warfarin, aminophylline	2. Enhanced metabolism reduces effect. Dose may need to be increased
	3. Phenytoin	3. Variable effect on phenytoin levels, which should be monitored
	4. Valproate	4. Combination may cause severe neurotoxicity and sedation
Phenytoin	1. Antifungal agents, antineoplastic agents, clozapine, corticosteroids, warfarin, digitoxin, frusemide, lamotrigine, theophylline, vitamin D	1. Enhanced hepatic metabolism reduces drug action
	2. Thyroxine	2. Thyroxine displaced from binding sites. Total and free concentrations reduced but TSH remains reliable
	3. Oral contraceptive pill	3. Use 50 µg estrogen pill but oral contraceptive still may have suboptimal efficacy

Table 9.8b. *Continued*

AED	Drug Affected	Effect
Piracetam	None known	
Tiagabine	None known	
Topiramate	1. Digoxin	1. Small reduction in digoxin levels
	2. Oral contraceptive pill	2. Use 50 µg estrogen pill but oral contraceptive still may have suboptimal efficacy
	3. Acetazolamide, salicylates	3. Increased risk of metabolic acidosis
	4. Drugs predisposing to nephrolithiasis	4. Increased risk of nephrolithiasis
Valproate	Warfarin	Protein binding reduced, probably minor but monitoring recommended
Vigabatrin	Phenytoin	Small reduction in phenytoin blood levels, not usually significant
Zonisamide	None known	

Case History 11

A 58-year old woman suffered her second convulsive seizure during which she bruised her hip and thigh, causing significant pain. Her physician started her on carbamazepine 400 milligrams daily combined with a paracetamol-dextropropoxyphene combination. One week later she was nauseated and vomiting with gross nystagmus. Her analgesic was changed and the dose of carbamazepine was reduced to 200 milligrams daily and then escalated gradually.

Carbamazepine induces its own metabolism over the first two weeks of therapy. Consequently the same dose of drug gives a higher blood level in the first week than later in treatment. The starting dose should be 1 to 200 milligrams per day. A high starting dose, combined with an enzyme-inhibiting drug (dextropropoxyphene) led to severe toxicity. Patients taking carbamazepine should avoid this analgesic altogether.

ALTERNATIVE THERAPIES IN EPILEPSY

- Alternative therapies are increasing in popularity among patients. Few have been evaluated in epilepsy and for most there are no systematic studies to prove benefit. They should never be used without consultation and traditional therapy should be continued.
- Pharmacologically neutral therapies are unlikely to be harmful. They include reflexology, massage, homeopathy, spiritual healing, meditation, qigong or biofeedback.
- Pharmacologically active therapies contain drugs at potentially therapeutic or toxic concentrations. Some practitioners postulate that many patients have a mild deficiency of a substance normally present in the body, such as calcium, that in gross deficiency triggers severe seizures. Treatment includes supplementation but over-supplementation in deficiency states can precipitate seizures and other complications. Other practitioners use foreign substances such as herbs in herbal medicine and aromatherapy and sometimes even heavy metals (Ayurvedic medicine).
- There is a small literature of case studies and small case series from which Table 9.9 is drawn. It includes those substances thought to be either beneficial or harmful to patients with epilepsy. There is some evidence of a mechanism of

Table 9.8c. Quick Guide to AED Pharmacokinetic Interactions

AED added	Existing AED													
	CBZ	CLB	CZP	ESM	GBP	LAM	LEV	PB	PHT	PRM	TGB	TPM	VGB	VPA
CBZ	AI	↓CLB	↓CZP	↓ESM	0	↓↓LAM	0	0	↑↑/↓↓PHT	↓PRM	↓↓TGB	↓↓TPM	0	↓↓VPA
CLB	↓CBZ	-	0	0	0	0	0	↑PB	↓/↑PHT	↓PRM	0	0	0	↑VPA
CZP	0	-	-	0	0	0	0	0	↓/↑PHT	0	0	0	0	0
ESM	0	0	0	-	0	0	0	0	↑PHT	0	0	0	0	↓↓VPA
GBP	0	0	0	0	-	0	0	0	0	0	0	0	0	0
LAM	↑CBZ-E	0	0	0	0	AI	0	0	0	0	?	?	0	0
LEV	0	0	0	0	0	0	-	-	0	0	0	0	0	0
PB	AI	↓↓CLB	↓CZP	↓ESM	0	↓↓LAM	0	-	↑↑/↓↓PHT	NCP	↓↓TGB	↓↓TPM	0	↓↓VPA
PHT	↓↓CBZ	↓CLB	↓CZP	↓ESM	0	↓↓LAM	0	↑↑PB	AI	↓/↑PRM	↓↓TGB	↓↓TPM	0	↓↓VPA
PRM	↓↓CBZ	↓CLB	↓CZP	↓ESM	0	↓↓LAM	0	NCP	↑↑/↓↓PHT	?AI	↓↓TGB	↓↓TPM	0	↓↓VPA
TGB	0	0	0	?	0	?	0	0	0	0	?	?	?	↓VPA
TPM	0	0	0	?	0	?	0	0	↑PHT	0	0	-	?	↓↓VPA
VGB	0	0	0	0	0	↑↑LAM	0	↑PB	↓PHT	↑PRM	?	?	-	0
VPA	↑↑CBZ-E	0	0	↓/↑ESM	0	↑↑LAM	0	↑↑PB	↑↑/↓↓PHT	↑PRM	0	?	-	-

0, none anticipated; ↓, infrequently observed decrease in concentration; ↓ ↓, frequently observed decrease in concentration; ↑, infrequently observed increase in concentration; ↑ ↑, frequently observed increase in concentration; interaction not known or not investigated; AED, antiepileptic drug; AI, autoinduction; CBZ, carbamazepine; CBZ-E, carbamazepine epoxide; CLB, clobazam; CZP, clonazepam; ESM, ethosuximide; GBP, gabapentin; LAM, lamotrigine; LEV, levetiracetam; NCP, not commonly prescribed; PB, phenobarbital; PHT, phenytoin; PRM, primidone; TGB, tiagabine; TPM, topiramate; VGB, vigabatrin; VPA, valproate.
Reproduced from Patsalos (2000) with permission of Elsevier Science.

Table 9.9. Herbal Remedies Effect on Epilepsy

Natural Remedies Thought Beneficial in Epilepsy	Natural Remedies Thought Harmful in Epilepsy
Deficiency type: Magnesium, manganese, taurine and zinc.	Eucalyptus, fennel, hysop, pennyroyal, rosemary, sage, savin, tansy, thuja, turpentine, wormwood, heavy metals
Herbal type: Saiko-Keisho-To, Coleus forskoli (mint family), Dan Jien Ning	

action for some herbs. For example Saiko-Keishi-To (SK) has been shown to reduce pentylenetetrazol-induced seizure activity in snails. SK has several components including derivatives of Bupleuri radix (Hare's ear root), Scutellaria radix (Scullcap), paeony, cinnamon, liquorice, ginseng and ginger. Dan Jien Ning has compared favorably to phenobarbital in a clinical trial.

Ketogenic Diet Therapy

- A ketogenic diet has been used in children and more recently in some adults. Some rare defects of carbohydrate metabolism may be particularly responsive.
- Ketosis is induced by a ratio of fatty acids to glucose of greater than 2:1. The diet is difficult to administer to children under the age of one and is unpalatable to older children although more imaginative recipes may make it more acceptable. The foods usually include a large amount of cream and butter. The child's required calorie intake is calculated as 60 to 80 kilocalories per kilogram per day, 20 percent less than normal intake.
- The ketogenic diet has produced seizure control in 29 percent of children with refractory epilepsy in one series. Potential adverse effects include thirst, hunger, weight loss and altered pharmacokinetics of antiepileptic drugs, causing toxicity. In adults there may be potential cardiovascular complications of a high fat diet.

BIBLIOGRAPHY

Brodie MJ, Richens A, Yuen AW. Double-blind comparison of lamotrigine and carbamazepine in newly diagnosed epilepsy. UK Lamotrigine/Carbamazepine Monotherapy Trial Group [published erratum appears in Lancet (1995);345:662; see comments]. Lancet 1995;345:476–479.

Burkhard PR, Burkhardt K, Haenggeli CA, Landis T. Plant-induced seizures: reappearance of an old problem. J Neurol 1999;246:667–670.

Gilman JT, Duchowny M. Allergic hypersensitivity to antiepileptic drugs: past, present, and future. Epilepsia 1998;39 Suppl 7:S1–S2.

Hart YM, Sander JWAS, Johnson AL, Shorvon SD. National General Practice Study of Epilepsy: recurrence after a first seizure. Lancet 1990;336:1271–1274.

Kwan P, Brodie MJ. Epilepsy after the first drug fails: substitution or add-on? Seizure 2000;9:464–468.

Kwan P, Brodie M.J. Early identification of refractory epilepsy. New Engl J Med 2000;342:314–319.

Marson AG, Chadwick DW. New drug treatments for epilepsy. J Neurol Neurosurg Psychiatry 2000;70:143–148.

Medical Research Council Antiepileptic Drug Withdrawal Study Group. Randomised study of antiepileptic drug withdrawal in patients in remission. Lancet 1991;337:1175–1180.

Sirven J, Whedon B, Caplan D, Liporace J, Glosser D, Dwyer JO, Sperling MR. The ketogenic diet for intractable epilepsy in adults. Epilepsia 1999;40:1721–1726.

Zaccara G, Muscas GC, Messori A. Clinical features, pathogenesis and management of drug-induced seizures. Drug Safety 1990;5:109–151.

REFERENCE

1. Patsalos PN. Pharmacokinetic profile of levetiracetam: towards ideal characteristics. Pharmacology and Therapeutics 2000;85:77–85.

APPENDIX

Acetazolamide

History	First used in epilepsy in 1952
Preparations	Tablets, controlled release tablets, parenteral injection
Indications	IGE tonic–clonic seizures, absences and focal seizures. Catamenial epilepsy
Mechanism of action	Carbonic anhydrase inhibitor increases seizure threshold in animal models
Age range (UK)	All ages
Cautions	Renal and liver failure, acid–base balance disorders, sulphonamide allergy
Pharmacokinetics	Bound to carbonic anhydrase with half-life 2–4 days
Therapeutic dose	Adults 250–1000 mg/day. Children 8–30 mg/kg/day
Dose titration	Over days to weeks
Adverse effects	Tingling extremities is usual. Anorexia, GI disturbance and altered taste are common. Drowsiness and confusion occasional. Sulphonamide-type reactions with toxic epidermal necrolysis or bone marrow suppression are rare. Occasional renal stones
Interactions	Increases phenytoin levels. May increase AED-induced osteomalacia. Antagonizes folate and potentiates anticoagulants. Aspirin in combination with acetazolamide may precipitate CNS toxicity
Teratogenicity	Teratogenic in animal models but not clear in humans
Lactation	Probably at too low a concentration to be significant
Summary	Acetazolamide is an occasional player with greatest efficacy in IGE absences. It is mostly an add-on therapy and may be valuable in intermittent use for catamenial seizures. Patients must be warned about the tingling it often causes

Benzodiazepines (BZ): Clobazam, clonazepam, diazepam, lorazepam, midazolam

History	First developed in the 1950s
Preparations	Tablets, rectal (diazepam) parenteral preparations, nasal and buccal midazolam under evaluation
Mechanism of action	Benzodiazepines bind to a specific receptor associated with the $GABA_A$ receptor, augmenting its action

Indications	Acute treatment of status epilepticus, intermittent treatment for seizure clustering. Chronic treatment of generalized epilepsies. Clobazam may help focal epilepsies long-term
Age range (UK)	All ages
Cautions	Respiratory depression in acute use, especially parenteral preparation
Pharmacokinetics	BZs except lorazepam and clonazepam are metabolized and glucuronidated in the liver.
Therapeutic dose	According to preparation
Dose titration	Can be rapid providing sedation is not excessive
Adverse effects	Acute administration: respiratory and cardiovascular depression, localized thrombophlebitis from diazepam injection. Dose related: sedation, ataxia, visual blurring, confusion Idiosyncratic: hyperactivity, psychosis
Interactions	Pharmacodynamic interactions with increased adverse effects, with other drugs acting on GABA, especially barbiturates. Relatively minor pharmacokinetic interactions
Teratogenicity	Not known to be a major problem but may augment teratogenicity of other drugs
Lactation	Secreted significantly into milk and may cause sedation and withdrawal symptoms in the baby, including jitteriness and rarely seizures
Summary	Benzodiazepines, especially lorazepam are very effective in stopping seizures in status epilepticus. They can also be used intermittently (usually clobazam) to prevent seizure clusters. They are of value in chronic treatment of generalized epilepsies, clonazepam is effective for myoclonus. For focal epilepsy they may occasionally be effective but tolerance usually develops after a few weeks. Clobazam is the least prone to tolerance formation. They are often sedating and withdrawal may provoke rebound seizures, insomnia and agitation; withdrawal should be slow

Carbamazepine

History	Introduced 1964, long experience
Mechanism of action	Predominantly blockade of sodium channels
Preparations	Tablets, chewable tablet, liquid, controlled release tablet (85% bioavailable), rectal preparation (75% bioavailable)
Indications	Focal epilepsy and TCS of IGE
Age range (UK)	All ages
Cautions	May worsen IGE absences and myoclonus. Major adverse effects rare. May depress cardiac conduction
Pharmacokinetics	Half-life 36 hours for single dose, falls to 16 hours with repeated dosing, "autoinduction." Metabolised by CYP 3A4 isoform of cytochrome P450. Epoxide metabolite causes many side effects
Therapeutic dose	Adults, 400–1600 mg; <1yr, 100–200 mg; 1–5 yrs 200–400 mg; 5–10 yr, 400–600 mg; 10–15 yrs 600–1000 mg
Dose titration	1–200 mg per week in adults
Adverse effects	Common: Diplopia, visual blurring, ataxia, sedation, skin rash, mild hyponatremia, mild elevation liver enzymes, mild depression of blood indices Uncommon: Psychiatric reactions, severe liver reactions or blood dyscrasias. Severe hyponatremia (with concomitant diuretics)
Interactions	Reduces half life of many hepatically metabolized drugs, including other AEDs, contraceptive pill, warfarin, cyclosporin. CBZ levels increased by macrolide antibiotics, dextropropoxyphene, fluoxetine, cimetidine. CBZ levels decreased by other enzyme-inducing AEDs. Valproate, lamotrigine and felbamate increase conversion to toxic epoxide

Teratogenicity	Rates reported of 0.5–2% including spina bifida. Vitamin K supplementation recommended in last trimester and to neonate
Lactation	No major risk
Summary	CBZ remains a benchmark drug in focal epilepsy. Dose escalation must be slow, side effects during this period often settle after 6–10 weeks. At higher doses, the development of visual blurring or sedation suggest that the maximum dose has been reached. The controlled release preparation is usually the best tolerated, especially at higher doses. Blood levels are of some limited value. Drug interactions are often significant with other AEDs and concomitant medication quite commonly triggers CBZ toxicity. CBZ reduces the effect of the contraceptive pill, even when higher dose pills are used and patients must be warned. CBZ is of value in patients with associated psychiatric disturbances as it has mood stabilizing properties. Withdrawal seizures are quite common, even after just one or two missed doses

Ethosuximide

History	Available since 1958
Mechanism of action	Specific action on thalamic T-type calcium channels
Preparations	Tablets and liquid
Indications	IGE absences and rarely other seizure types
Age range (UK)	Any age
Cautions	Abnormal liver or renal function
Pharmacokinetics	Low protein binding and 80% metabolized in the liver. Half-life 40–60 hours
Therapeutic dose	Over 6 years, 500–2000 mg daily. Under 6 years 15–20 mg/kg/day
Dose titration	Start at 250 mg/day and increase by 125–250 mg every few days. Given twice or three times daily to avoid GI adverse effects
Adverse effects	GI upset, somnolence, behavioral and cognitive disturbances including psychosis. Rare serious abnormal liver function or blood dyscrasias reported
Interactions	Affected by enzyme inducers such as carbamazepine and inhibitors such as valproate
Teratogenicity	May be teratogenic but no clear data
Lactation	Milk levels similar to blood so a potential for adverse effects in breast-fed babies
Summary	Ethosuximide is highly effective against IGE absences but usually not against other seizure types. Consequently it is often used as adjunctive therapy as many patients with IGE absences also have tonic–clonic seizures. It is generally well tolerated. It is easy to use with easy dose titration and relatively minor drug interactions

Felbamate

History	Licensed in the USA in the 1980s, this drug was found to have a relatively high risk of severe hepatotoxicity and bone marrow aplasia. It remains licensed for patients where it has been successful and other drugs have failed but use is limited
Mechanism of action	It blocks NMDA currents and may be a glycine antagonist. It may also augment $GABA_A$ inhibitory activity
Preparations	Tablets and suspension
Indications	Refractory epilepsies
Age range (UK)	Not available
Cautions	Fatal hepatotoxicity or bone marrow suppression is usually in the first

	year of treatment and is more likely in patients with a history of allergic reactions or immunological disease such as lupus. Blood tests recommended weekly
Pharmacokinetics	Metabolised by P_{450} system, its half-life is 12–24 h but is influenced by concomitant medication. Protein binding is minor
Therapeutic dose	Usually 1200–3600 mg/day in adults
Dose titration	Start at up to 1200 mg/day and increase by 4–600 mg each 2 weeks
Adverse effects	Nausea, vomiting, esophageal burning, blurred vision, ataxia, insomnia and weight loss. Rare fatal reactions as above
Interactions	Carbamazepine levels reduced but toxic epoxide metabolite increased. Phenytoin, valproate and phenobarbital levels increased. Enzyme inducers reduce felbamate levels by 20–30%
Teratogenicity	Unknown
Lactation	Unknown but not recommended
Summary	Felbamate is an effective broad spectrum AED but the incidence of severe toxicity has relegated it to the most refractory cases. It is unlikely to be licensed in countries where it is not yet available. It has complex drug interactions

Gabapentin

History	Gabapentin (GBP) has been licensed for the treatment of focal epilepsy since the early 1990s
Mechanism of action	Unknown, may be related to GABA metabolism
Preparations	Capsules, dosing is usually twice daily
Indications	Focal epilepsy, as monotherapy or add-on
Age range (UK)	12 years and over
Cautions	GBP is affected by renal impairment. It may exacerbate generalized epilepsies and has been reported to precipitate IGE absence status
Pharmacokinetics	Half-life is 5–7 hours. GBP is excreted unchanged in the urine and dosing can be predicted from the creatinine clearance
Therapeutic dose	Usually 1200–2400 mg, but up to 4800 mg daily in some cases
Dose titration	Initial dose of 300 mg/day can usually be increased by 300 mg every 3 days
Adverse effects	Drowsiness, sedation, weight gain and occasional mood change
Interactions	Magnesium containing antacids may reduce GBP levels
Teratogenicity	Unknown
Lactation	Probably safe
Summary	Gabapentin has been shown to be effective in partial epilepsy but doses may need to be very high. It is generally well tolerated and easy to use with no major interactions. It is often wise to titrate the dose more slowly than the manufacturer's recommendation

Lamotrigine

History	The observation that many older AEDs affect folate metabolism led to a search for a drug that affects folate and is an effective AED. Lamotrigine was discovered but it emerged that although it is an effective AED, it has minimal affect on folate. It was in development for many years and has been marketed for around a decade
Mechanism of action	Sodium channel blockade and calcium antagonist
Preparations	Tablets and dispersible tablets
Indications	Focal and generalized epilepsies, including symptomatic generalized epilepsies, monotherapy and add-on
Age range (UK)	Monotherapy over 12 years, add-on over 2 years
Cautions	None

Pharmacokinetics	Half-life around 20 hours in monotherapy. Metabolized in the liver, Not significantly protein-bound
Therapeutic dose	In monotherapy 150–400 mg per day, with valproate 100–300 mg/day, with enzyme inducers, 200–800 mg/day
Dose titration	Starting dose 25 mg daily in monotherapy, 25 mg alternate days with valproate, 50 mg daily with enzyme inducers. Very slow titration, with fortnightly increments minimizes risk of allergy
Adverse effects	Rash, nausea, headache, insomnia, drowsiness, dizziness, diplopia
Interactions	Half-life is increased to 70 h by enzyme inhibitors e.g. valproate and reduced to 11 hours by enzyme inducers e.g. carbamazepine
Teratogenicity	Unknown, safe in animal studies, presumed unsafe in humans
Lactation	Probably safe
Summary	Lamotrigine has been shown in studies to have comparable efficacy to older drugs. It has a broad spectrum of action and is useful as the first alternative to valproate in IGE. It is generally well tolerated and neurotoxicity may be less than for some older drugs but allergic reactions occur moderately frequently. It is becoming a first-line drug. Drug interactions need to be considered in titrating the drug and deciding the final dose but are relatively predictable. Dose titration should be very slow, especially in children in order to avoid rash

Levetiracetam

History	Licensed in the UK in 2000, this drug is a derivative of piracetam
Mechanism of action	May affect N-type calcium channels
Preparations	Tablets
Indications	Add-on therapy for focal epilepsy. It is also proving of value in IGE
Age range (UK)	Over 16
Cautions	Dose needs adjustment in renal impairment
Pharmacokinetics	Rapidly and completely absorbed. Half-life 7 hours and virtually entirely renally excreted unchanged
Therapeutic dose	1000–3000 mg daily
Dose titration	Manufacturer's starting dose 500 mg BD and increasing by 500 mg every few days. Experience from other AED suggests going more slowly
Adverse effects	Somnolence and asthenia.
Interactions	None
Teratogenicity	Unknown presumed unsafe
Lactation	Unknown presumed unsafe
Summary	Levetiracetam is a new drug with a high rate of response of refractory epilepsy in trials and few adverse effects. It is easy to use and appears a very promising addition. It is also proving of value in IGE

Oxcarbazepine

History	Developed from carbamazepine and licensed in some countries in 1980s. Only available in UK from 2000
Preparations	Tablets
Mechanism of action	Sodium channel antagonist
Indications	Focal epilepsy, monotherapy or add-on
Age range (UK)	Above 6 years of age (occasionally down to 2 years)
Cautions	Dose unchanged in mild to moderate liver failure but may need reduction in moderate renal failure
Pharmacokinetics	Rapidly metabolized to active 10 monohydroxy metabolite. 38% protein bound. Eliminated by glucuronidation and renal excretion. Minor

	induction of liver enzymes. Dose reduction in severe renal impairment. Half life 8–10 h
Therapeutic dose	600–2400 mg daily in three doses. Usually 900–1200 mg
Dose titration	In adults start with 150–300 mg daily and increase by 300 mg every few days
Adverse effects	Rash up to 10%, hyponatremia especially with other drugs e.g. diuretics. (avoid large fluid volumes). Occasional sedation.
Interactions	Contraceptive pill has reduced efficacy. Phenytoin levels may be increased. Enzyme-inducing drugs reduce levels of oxcarbazepine
Teratogenicity	Unknown presumed unsafe
Lactation	Probably safe
Summary	Oxcarbazepine has similar chemistry and mechanism of action to carbamazepine. Oxcarbazepine 250 mg is equivalent to carbamazepine 200 mg. It is of value in focal epilepsies and may be easier to use than carbamazepine as it can be introduced more quickly and has fewer interactions. It has been used for a long time in some countries, has proven efficacy and is well tolerated

Phenobarbital

History	The oldest effective AED, available since 1912. It is orders of magnitude cheaper than newer drugs, making it the treatment of choice in many developing countries
Mechanism of action	Its main effect is probably to open the chloride channel in the region of the $GABA_A$ receptor, augmenting hyperpolarization
Preparations	Tablets, liquid and intravenous injection
Indications	Neonatal seizures, focal onset seizures, IGE (second-line drug), emergency treatment of status epilepticus
Age range (UK)	Any age
Cautions	May trigger attacks in acute intermittent porphyria. Withdrawal seizures are common
Pharmacokinetics	75% metabolized in the liver, 25% excreted unchanged. Urinary excretion is increased if urine is alkaline. Very long half life (3–5 days in adults, 1.5 days in children)
Therapeutic dose	Under age 4 years, 3 mg/kg; age 4–14, 2.3 mg/kg; age 15–40, 1.75 mg/kg; age >40 years, 0.9 mg/kg
Dose titration	Increments every 2–3 weeks achieving target dose after three increments.
Adverse effects	Allergic reactions. Sedation may be severe (paradoxical hyperactivity in children)
Interactions	Potent enzyme inducer, it affects many drugs metabolized in the liver, including other AEDs warfarin and the contraceptive pill
Teratogenicity	Causes fetal malformations and hemorrhagic disease of the newborn through vitamin K deficiency. Vitamin K supplementation recommended
Lactation	May accumulate in the baby and cause sedation, jitteriness or withdrawal seizures
Summary	Phenobarbital is an effective AED for focal epilepsy with some activity in IGE. It causes more sedation than newer drugs, which has led to decreasing usage in developed countries but it remains widely used. It is extremely effective against status epilepticus. It has significant drug interactions

Phenytoin

History	Developed in 1952. Standard AED for many years
Preparations	Tablets, capsules, liquid, intravenous injection

Indications	Focal epilepsy, tonic clonic seizures of IGE and status epilepticus
Mechanism of action	Predominantly use-dependent sodium channel blockade. Some effects on calmodulin
Age range (UK)	Any age
Cautions	Severe allergic reactions may occur
Pharmacokinetics	Metabolism of phenytoin is non-linear. Small changes in dose cause major changes concentration and the therapeutic window is narrow. Phenytoin is highly protein bound. Total concentration changes in parallel with albumin concentration and clinically relevant concentration is of free phenytoin. Metabolism is age-dependent: fastest in young children and slowest in neonates and the elderly. Genetic variations in P_{450} CYP2C9 isoenzyme significantly affect metabolism. In liver disease, metabolism is slowed. In renal disease, half life is shortened. With standard blood levels (40–80 mmol/l) half-life is 24–40 h
Therapeutic dose	Children around 5 mg/kg/day. Adults usually 250–400 mg/day
Dose titration	In emergencies, a loading dose of 15–20 mg/kg, followed by standard dose (300 mg/day) in adults. Otherwise, 300 mg/day from outset and check blood levels after 2 weeks
Adverse effects	Dose-related toxicity. Sedation, ataxia, confusion, movement disorders, seizures, encephalopathy
	Allergic. Skin rash, hepatitis, serum sickness, lupus-like syndrome, blood dyscrasias, renal failure
	Chronic toxicity. Osteomalacia, gingival hypertrophy, facial coarsening, neuropathy, ataxia and possibly cognitive change
	On IV use. Cardiac depression, distal ischemia "purple-glove syndrome"
Interactions	Drugs metabolized by cytochrome P_{450} isoform CYP2C9 may increase phenytoin concentrations, including cimetidine, chloramphenicol, isoniazid, fluconazole, diltiazem, progabide, clobazam felbamate and carbamazepine. Phenytoin concentration may be temporarily increased by valproate, salicylates, tolbutamide that displace it from protein binding. Phenytoin lowers the concentration of carbamazepine, lamotrigine, valproate, zonisamide, warfarin, folic acid, digitoxin, theophylline
Teratogenicity	A fetal phenytoin syndrome similar to fetal alcohol syndrome has been described. Defects include craniofacial abnormalities, limb anomalies and cardiac abnormalities. The risk is probably 4–6%. Vitamin K supplements recommended in the last month of pregnancy and to neonate
Lactation	Phenytoin levels in breast milk are only 20% of maternal plasma levels so are unlikely to be important
Summary	Phenytoin has a long track record in the treatment of focal epilepsy and is as effective as other first line drugs but may cause more sedation. It has complex pharmacokinetics, but many patients require a standard dose with little monitoring. Caution must be exercised with concomitant medication and blood level monitoring may be needed. Of concern are the long term and possibly irreversible neurological side effects that have relegated it to second-line use in the UK, although it remains a first-line in the USA. It remains valuable in emergency treatment of status epilepticus, although is being superseded by fosphenytoin (Chapter 14)

Piracetam

History	Piracetam was developed in 1967 and used for memory enhancment. In 1978 it was found to be useful in post-anoxic myoclonus

Mechanism of action	Unknown
Preparations	Tablets or liquid
Indications	Add-on therapy for myoclonus
Age range (UK)	Over 16
Cautions	Contraindicated in severe renal impairment
Pharmacokinetics	100% oral bio-availability, half life 5 h, renally excreted with no metabolites
Therapeutic dose	7.2–24 g daily
Dose titration	Initially 7.2 g daily then increasing by 4.8 g, no faster than every 3 days. Twice or three times daily dosage
Adverse effects	Very well tolerated. No major adverse effects reported but it may cause some drowsiness and dizziness
Interactions	None
Teratogenicity	Safe in animals, unknown in humans, presumed unsafe
Lactation	Crosses into breast milk, presumed unsafe
Summary	Piracetam may be extremely effective adjunctive therapy in myoclonus. It has remarkably few side-effects. The main problem is the large number (often >10/day) of tablets required

Tiagabine

History	Licensed in the late 1990s in Europe, USA and Australia
Mechanism of action	Inhibition of GABA reuptake at GABAergic synapses
Preparations	Tablets
Indications	Add-on therapy for focal epilepsy
Age range (UK)	Over 12 years
Cautions	IGE absence epilepsy and myoclonus may be exacerbated
Pharmacokinetics	Hepatic metabolism with plasma half-life 7–9 h. Dose needs to be decreased in liver failure
Therapeutic dose	30–60 mg
Dose titration	Start at 5 mg twice daily and increase total daily dose by 5 mg per week
Adverse effects	Dizziness, somnolence, possible mood change, weight increase, flu-like symptoms, ataxia
Interactions	Enzyme inducers such as phenytoin carbamazepine and phenobarbital lower the concentration of tiagabine
Teratogenicity	Unknown, presumed unsafe
Lactation	Unknown, presumed unsafe
Summary	Tiagabine is an effective add-on in the treatment of focal seizures. It is a new arrival and serious adverse effects have not been encountered but sedation is a problem. There is no evidence that it affects vision, unlike vigabatrin which augments GABA by a different mechanism. It should be easy to use

Topiramate

History	Topiramate was licensed in early to mid 1990s as add-on therapy for focal epilepsy but it appears to have a broad spectrum of action
Mechanism of action	Several actions including sodium channel inhibition, carbonic anhydrase inhibition, $GABA_A$ augmentation via a unique mechanism and kainate inhibition
Preparations	Tablets
Indications	Add-on for most kinds of seizures and epilepsies. Under study as first-line
Age range (UK)	Over 2 years
Cautions	Renal stones, usually in patients with previous nephrolithiasis.

Pharmacokinetics	Topiramate is 20% hepatically metabolized in monotherapy but the proportion may increase to 50% in patients taking enzyme-inducing drugs. The half-life is normally 21 h, longer in renal failure
Therapeutic dose	Usual effective dose is 100–400 mg/day in adults. In children the dose is 5–9 mg/kg/day
Dose titration	Starting dose in adults is 25 mg/day and increments need to be slow in order to minimise toxicity – increasing by 25–50 mg each fortnight
Adverse effects	Common: paresthesia, weight loss, sedation, mild mood or speech disturbance. Uncommon: diplopia, ataxia, confusion, mood disorders severe speech disorders, renal stones
Interactions	Phenytoin and carbamazepine reduce topiramate levels. Topiramate may reduce the efficacy of the oral contraceptive pill, digoxin and warfarin
Teratogenicity	Topiramate is teratogenic in animal studies. Human data is not available, presumed unsafe
Lactation	Unknown, presumed unsafe
Summary	Topiramate is a potent AED for focal epilepsy but may have additional roles including IGE, Lennox-Gastaut and West syndromes. Preclinical studies as add-on showed more seizure-free patients than in similar studies for most other new drugs. It may cause significant CNS adverse effects that may be minimized by slow dose titration and by minor reductions in concomitant therapy during the dose escalation phase

Valproate

History	Valproate has been used in Europe since before 1970 and in the USA since 1978
Mechanism of action	Unknown but valproate is thought to affect sodium channels and a variety of excitatory and inhibitory neurotransmitters
Preparations	Tablets, controlled-release tablets, syrup, intravenous injection
Indications	Focal and generalized epilepsies including Lennox-Gastaut syndrome
Age range (UK)	Any, but caution below 2 years
Cautions	In patients with active liver disease or metabolic disturbance, valproate may precipitate metabolic coma. Hepatic failure occurs most frequently in children under 2 years old, with mental retardation, on polytherapy and in the first 3 months of therapy
Pharmacokinetics	Half-life is 8–16 h. It is eliminated by via hepatic metabolism and some metabolites are active. It is influenced by enzyme-inducing drugs
Therapeutic dose	Effective adult dose is usually 500–2000 mg daily. Childhood dose is usually 20–35 mg/kg/day
Dose titration	Dose titration can be quite rapid, starting with 500 mg/day in adults and rising by 250 mg every few days
Adverse effects	Common: dose-related postural tremor (responds to propranolol), weight increase, commonest in young women, reversible hair loss. Endocrine disturbances including polycystic ovaries are a suggested association. Rare: pancreatitis, thrombocytopenia, pancytopenia and hepatitis
Interactions	Valproate is affected by a number of drugs but these are not usually clinically significant. Valproate inhibits liver enzymes Concentrations of other hepatically metabolized AED are increased: phenobarbital, phenytoin, carbamazepine, lamotrigine. Other drug groups also affected
Teratogenicity	Neural tube defects reported in 2–4%, most if dose is above 1000 mg daily. Fetal valproate syndrome is also described and may cause severe mental retardation. Subtle cognitive effects have been suggested

Lactation	Valproic acid levels in breast milk are low but may occasionally cause idiosyncratic reactions
Summary	Valproate is a benchmark broad-spectrum AED with a low incidence of major toxicity. Most patients with IGE are rendered seizure-free with valproate monotherapy. Weight increase may be a problem and concerns over teratogenicity and more recently over fertility of women on this drug have led to more cautious use in women of reproductive age

Vigabatrin

History	Vigabatrin was the first of the new AEDs in the UK in the last decade. It was very effective in add-on studies of focal epilepsy but a monotherapy trial showed it to be less effective than carbamazepine. In the last few years, increasing concerns of visual disturbances due to the drug have relegated it to occasional use
Mechanism of action	Inhibition of GABA breakdown by GABA transaminase
Preparations	Tablets and sachets
Indications	Add-on for focal epilepsy and monotherapy in West syndrome.
Age range (UK)	All ages
Cautions	Previous psychosis. Vigabatrin may exacerbate IGE absences and myoclonus
Pharmacokinetics	Plasma half-life is 5–8 h but as vigabatrin binds irreversibly to its CNS target, this bears little relationship to its clinical effect. Vigabatrin is excreted unchanged in the urine
Therapeutic dose	Usually 2000–4000 mg daily in adults, 80–100 mg/kg per day in children. Much higher doses have been used
Dose titration	Adults start with 500–1000 mg daily and increase daily dose by 500 mg per week. Children start with 40 mg/kg per day and increase by 10–20 mg/kg/day per week
Adverse effects	Drowsiness, fatigue, weight increase and mild mood change. Irreversible visual field defects reported in up to one third of patients. This may start 1 month to years after starting treatment, typically with a binasal defect that progresses to a concentric defect. It is asymptomatic in the early stages. Visual field assessments by an ophthalmologist are recommended before treatment and 6 monthly during treatment. Psychosis reported in up to 3%
Interactions	Minor reduction in phenytoin levels, probably not clinically significant
Teratogenicity	None in animals, unknown in humans, presumed unsafe.
Lactation	Unknown, presumed unsafe
Summary	Although highly effective in preclinical studies and in early use, vigabatrin is now reserved for the most refractory patients or children with West syndrome. Withdrawal seizures may be a problem

Zonisamide

History	Zonisamide is a sulphonamide analog, originally developed in Japan in the 1970s. It has been available there for some time but concerns over nephrolithiasis prevented its release in many other countries for many years
Mechanism of action	Zonisamide increases the time to recovery from inactivation of sodium channels and like phenytoin, causes inhibition of sodium channels which increases with increased rate of firing. Zonisamide also inhibits T-type calcium channels
Preparations	Tablets
Indications	Focal and generalized seizures

Age range (UK)	Not available in UK
Cautions	Previous history of nephrolithiasis or renal tract surgery. Allergy to sulphonamides
Pharmacokinetics	Half-life of single dose is 50–68 h. Metabolism is by acetylation then urinary excretion
Therapeutic dose	200–600 mg daily in adults, 4–12 mg/kg per day in children
Dose titration	Initially 100–200 mg/day in adults and 2–4 mg/kg/day in children, increasing every 1–2 weeks
Adverse effects	Somnolence, loss of appetite, GI symptoms, nephrolithiasis, allergic reactions including Stevens-Johnson syndrome
Interactions	Enzyme inducers such as phenytoin or carbamazepine reduce the half-life to around 30 hours.
Teratogenicity	Zonisamide is a known teratogen in animal studies
Lactation	Unknown
Summary	Zonisamide appears to be a broad spectrum AED, although its value in generalized epilepsies remains to be clarified. It is relatively well tolerated. It will probably become available in the UK in due course. It is relatively free of drug interactions but may be teratogenic

10

Epilepsy in Special Groups: Women

Managing epilepsy in women requires understanding of the effects of epilepsy on sexuality, the menstrual cycle and fertility and of the influence of the menstrual cycle and reproduction on epilepsy. There are also some differences in the epidemiology of epilepsy between males and females (Table 10.1).

Table 10.1. Some Sex Differences in the Epilepsies

Commoner in Females	Commoner in Males
Childhood absence epilepsy	Benign epilepsy with centrotemporal
Eyelid myoclonias and epilepsy	spikes
Juvenile absence epilepsy	Post-traumatic epilepsy
Juvenile myoclonic epilepsy	Most malignant epilepsies of childhood
Benign epilepsy with occipital paroxysms	

THE HORMONAL INFLUENCE ON EPILEPSY

The Effect of Female Sex Hormones on Epilepsy

Key effects that have been identified are:

- Estradiol increases brain excitability and lowers seizure threshold in animals
- Progesterone lowers brain excitability and increases seizure threshold in animals.

The Effect of the Menarche on Epilepsy

- The onset of some syndromes is around puberty in boys and girls, for example juvenile myoclonic and juvenile absence epilepsies.
- Psychogenic non-epileptic seizures commonly arise in adolescence and the diagnosis may need to be reviewed.
- Behavioral problems and compliance difficulties may affect adolescents with epilepsy who find the diagnosis particularly hard to accept.

The Effect of the Menstrual Cycle on Epilepsy

- A few women suffer seizures predominantly or exclusively at specific times of their menstrual cycle "catamenial epilepsy." Many more have a weaker tendency to more seizures at particular phases of the cycle.
- A seizure diary kept for 3 to 6 months is necessary to reliably establish a catamenial epilepsy pattern.
- A possible mechanism for this relationship has been suggested on the basis of changes in relative concentrations of epileptogenic estradiol and anti-epileptic progesterone concentrations, tending to favor estradiol.
- Ovulatory menstrual cycles are associated with two patterns of catamenial epilepsy (Figure 10.1), premenstrual exacerbation and ovulatory exacerbation. In the premenstrual phase there is a fall in protective progesterone levels that outstrips the fall in estradiol and at ovulation there is a rise in both hormones, with estradiol preceding progesterone.
- Anovulatory cycles are associated with an increase in seizures during the entire second half of the cycle. These cycles are characterized by deficient progesterone secretion throughout the second half.
- Treatments have been suggested but not fully evaluated:
  - Intermittent clobazam 10 milligrams daily over the risk period
  - Acetazolamide 250 to 1000 milligrams daily over the risk period
  - Endocrine manipulations been evaluated in very small numbers of patients and some have been shown to give a modest reduction in seizures.

  1. Medroxyprogesterone in doses sufficient to produce amenorrhea but it has significant adverse effects
  2. Progesterone supplementation over the at-risk period (premenstrual or luteal according to seizure pattern)
  3. Depot progestogens.

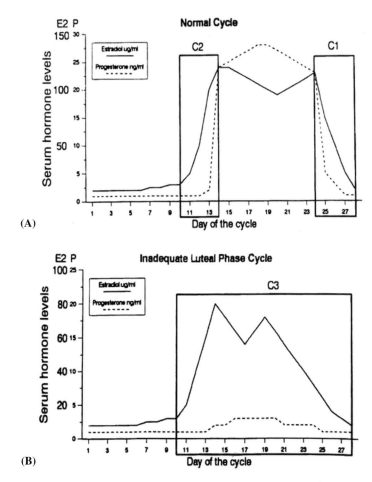

Figure 10.1. Patterns of seizure exacerbation in catamenial epilepsies, in relation to progesterone and oestrogen concentrations. A: Ovulatory cycles with pre-ovulatory and premenstrual exacerbations. B: Anovulatory cycles with exacerbation throughout the second half of the cycle. Reproduced with permission from Herzog *et al.* 1997.

The Effect of the Menopause on Epilepsy

- The hormonal effects of the reproductive years protect against cerebrovascular disease. With the menopause, this protection is removed and there is increased incidence of cerebrovascular disease and its complications, including epilepsy.
- The effect of the menopause on pre-existing epilepsy is unpredictable for most patients with epilepsy. Patients with catamenial epilepsy, may experience a reduction in seizures with cessation of menses but attacks may just become less predictable.

EPILEPSY AND FERTILITY IN WOMEN

- Fertility may be reduced for various reasons by as much as one third in women with epilepsy.

- Epilepsy syndrome: temporal lobe epilepsy (TLE) may have a greater effect on fertility than idiopathic generalized epilepsy (IGE).
- Psychosexual effects should be investigated in all women with epilepsy. Up to one-third report reduced sexual arousal and dissatisfaction with sexual intercourse for various reasons including social and psychological reasons, for example fear of seizures during intercourse and anti-epileptic drug (AED) effects.
- Social effects: Marriage rates are lower and divorce rates are higher than in the general population. Some women may opt not to have children, often for fear of not being able to look after a child. Some clinicians in the past advised women with epilepsy against becoming parents.
- Menstrual disorders may be commoner in women with epilepsy. Polycystic ovaries (PCO) may affect up to 20 percent of women with epilepsy although the incidence of full polycystic ovary syndrome is much less clear. This may be due to the effects of epileptic discharges on the release of gonadotrophins and prolactin.
- AEDs may also have an effect on fertility. It has been claimed that PCO may particularly affect women taking valproate.

EPILEPSY AND CONTRACEPTION

- All women of reproductive ability with epilepsy need counseling regarding contraception, particularly because of the teratogenicity of AEDs. Women with epilepsy are best advised to plan their pregnancies.
- Hormonal contraception is advisable for most women. Alternatives are a contraceptive coil or surgical sterilization, if a woman has completed her family.
- Non-enzyme-inducing AEDs maximize the efficacy of hormonal contraception if a woman does not wish to have children.
- Enzyme-inducing AEDs increase the rate of metabolism of hormonal contraceptives (Table 10.2). The dose of the hormonal contraceptive may need to be doubled or tripled with these medications. Intermenstrual bleeding whilst taking the combined oral contraceptive pill (OCP) is evidence of contraceptive failure. However, even with good cycle control, effective contraception is not ensured. The starting dose of estrogen is 50 micrograms in women taking the enzyme-inducing AED, sometimes increasing to 80 to 100 micrograms. This may need to be combined with a barrier contraceptive method. If depot

Table 10.2. Hormonal Contraception Requirements with Different AEDs

Drugs Requiring High Dose Contraception	Drugs Requiring Regular Dose Contraception
Carbamazepine	Benzodiazepines
Oxcarbazepine (slight effect)	Ethosuximide
Phenobarbital	Gabapentin
Phenytoin	Lamotrigine
Primidone	Levetiracetam
Topiramate	Tiagabine
	Valproate
	Vigabatrin

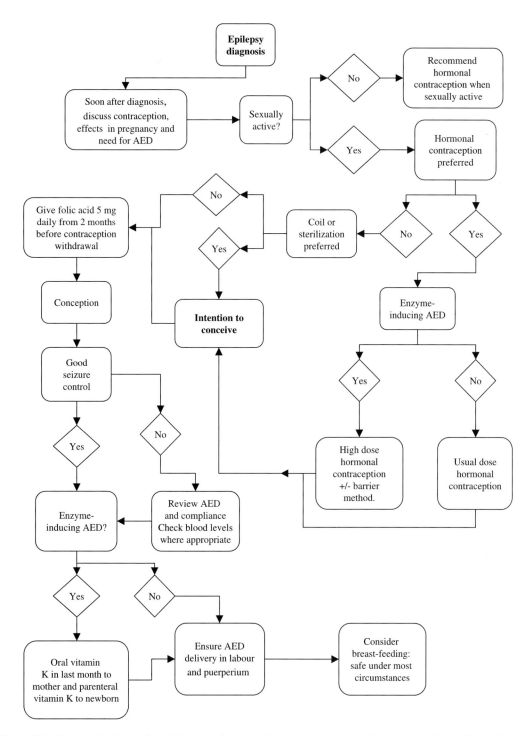

Figure 10.2. Suggested scheme of consideration of reproductive factors in women who develop epilepsy during the reproductive years.

> **Box 10.1.** Planning AED therapy in Pregnancy
>
> Epilepsy severity: Mild may need no treatment, severe needs
>   treatment
> Epilepsy syndrome: The best AED for the job
> Minimizing fetal risk:
> Avoid polytherapy
> Comparative teratogenicity of AED, review latest data
> Change successful AED only with a clear indication
> Minimize doses, especially valproate
> Preconceptual folic acid
> Vitamin K in last trimester if enzyme-inducing drugs

hormonal contraception is used, the interval between injections may need to be reduced to 8–10 weeks.

EPILEPSY AND PREGNANCY

The Effect of Pregnancy on Epilepsy

- Epilepsy severity remains unchanged on average during pregnancy. Roughly a quarter of women may experience an improvement and another quarter an exacerbation of their epilepsy.
- Deteriorating seizure control is more likely for women with focal epilepsy than generalized epilepsy and for women whose seizure control is already poor.
- Contributory factors include sleep deprivation and poor compliance with AED for fear of teratogenic effects.
- Counseling patients has been shown to increase compliance and improves epilepsy control in pregnancy.

The Effect of Pregnancy on Anti-Epileptic Drugs

- A number of factors influence blood levels of AED in pregnancy, including expansion of plasma volume, decreased serum albumin and increased hepatic activity. Some of these work in opposite directions and for many drugs no specific action is required but for others more regular monitoring may be recommended (Table 10.3).
- Reduced intake from fear of the teratogenic effects of AED is the commonest cause of a fall in AED blood levels.
- If blood levels fall and compliance is satisfactory, the clinician may need to alter AED dosage. In favor of a change are a deterioration in seizures, a history of a deterioration of seizures with small changes in blood levels, a decline in phenytoin levels to below the accepted therapeutic range, and previous freedom from seizures which is crucial to the patient. Factors against altering drug dosage are a history of only minor seizures, a small fall in levels within the accepted therapeutic range, and a change in the first trimester when the teratogenic risks of AEDs are greatest.

Table 10.3. Effects of Pregnancy on Different AEDs

Drug	Probable Effect of Pregnancy on AED Blood Levels
Carbamazepine	Blood levels often fall (2nd–3rd trimester)
Clonazepam	No major change
Ethosuximide	Highly variable – monitoring recommended
Lamotrigine	Variable but usually fall >50%. Consider if seizures recur
Phenobarbital	Blood levels often fall (1st trimester)
Phenytoin	Blood levels often fall (1st trimester)
Valproate	No major change

- If blood levels rise no action is usually required unless the patient is symptomatic.

The Effect of Epilepsy on Pregnancy and the Fetus

- Obstetric complications such as placental abruption, antepartum hemorrhage, pre-eclampsia, low birth weight and premature labor are all increased to a similar degree in some but not all studies of women with epilepsy.
- Convulsive status epilepticus carries a high risk of ischemic damage for the fetus from its systemic effects.
- Brief tonic–clonic seizures cause some degree of acidosis and affect fetal heart rate but probably cause little risk to the fetus.
- Falls during seizures may very rarely affect the fetus.
- Non-convulsive seizures are unlikely to have any major effects on the fetus.
- Cognitive disturbances may be commoner in the offspring of mothers with both convulsive and non-convulsive seizures. The effects of AEDs or a relationship to the epilepsy other than asphyxia, for example genetic factors, are likely to be the cause.
- The overall mortality of the baby in the first week after birth is increased up to three times in the offspring of women with epilepsy in some but not all studies.

Effects of Anti-Epileptic Drugs on the Fetus

- AEDs are the major determinant of fetal abnormality in the offspring of women with epilepsy. All older AEDs are teratogenic in humans. Some newer drugs are safe in animal studies. However, their risks to humans remain unknown at this stage and this needs to be balanced against the known but definite risks attached to older drugs. No AED can reliably be considered safe.
- Methodology is flawed in studies of this issue. Many studies are small or retrospective with wide margins of error. They consider live outcomes and there is little information about the risk of spontaneous fetal abortion. There is referral bias: these patients are often taking more than one drug, there is relatively less information regarding patients taking monotherapy, which makes it more difficult to tease out the teratogenic effects of individual drugs (Tables 10.4, 10.5). Pregnancy registers have been set up in recent years, which should improve the quality of information.

Table 10.4. Rate of Major Malformation According to Number of Maternal AEDs

Maternal Condition	Rate of Fetal Malformation
Normal population	2%
Epilepsy on no medication	2–3%
Epilepsy on one AED	4–7%
Epilepsy on two AEDs	5–10%
Epilepsy on three AEDs	10–50%

Table 10.5. Effects of *in utero* Exposure to Different AEDs

Drug	Abnormality	Possible Mechanism
Barbiturates	Craniofacial abnormalities and congenital heart defects.	Unknown
Benzodiazepines	Probably little effect themselves but may worsen valproate-associated defects.	Unknown
Carbamazepine	Spina bifida (0.5–1%). Also congenital heart disease, congenital dislocation of the hip, hypospadias	Unknown
Ethosuximide	Rarely used in monotherapy but an association with facial clefts suggested	Possible effect on endogenous retinoids
Hydantoins	Major deficits include facial clefts, congenital heart defects and urogenital abnormalities. Distal phalangeal hypoplasia in up to 11%. Fetal hydantoin syndrome comprises hypertelorism digital hypoplasia, growth delay, microcephaly and developmental delay.	Possibly due to hypoxia caused by suppression of the fetal heart during a sensitive phase of cardiac development. Folate antagonism may contribute
Valproate	Neural tube defects in 1–3%. Other abnormalities are radial ray aplasia, rib and vertebral abnormalities. Fetal valproate syndrome includes, microstomy, microcephaly thin lips, rotated ears and development delay, which may be severe.	Possible effect on folate metabolism or on endogenous retinoids important in fetal development. Effects possibly dose-related with highest risk over 1000 mg daily

Case History 1

A 35-year-old journalist had a history of infrequent convulsive seizures over the previous 8 years. She had been treated with valproate in various doses and was seeking advice as she wished to start a family. When her seizure diary was examined carefully, it was clear that there was no relationship between her treatment and the longer periods of seizure freedom. As her work was not jeopardized by occasional seizures she elected to stop medication until after she had completed her family and to accept occasional seizures during that time. The value of AED therapy needs to be established objectively for each woman and weighed against the risks if she wishes to become pregnant.

- Severe abnormalities have been found recently in roughly 6 percent of patients, whatever their medication regime and in none of 25 patients with epilepsy but who were not taking medication.
- Mild malformations occur with rates of up to 7 percent in monotherapy patients and 10 percent or more in patients on dual or triple therapy. In one study the rate of severe defects was greatest for valproate (13.6%) and carbamazepine (6.2%) with a high proportion of neural tube defects.

- Subtle cognitive deficits are poorly studied but may affect the offspring of women with epilepsy. They may not be apparent early on and require testing into adolescence. Suggested risk factors are drug therapy and the type of maternal epilepsy but not seizure number in pregnancy. Maternal polytherapy seems more consistently associated with cognitive abnormalities than monotherapy. Studies have suggested particular problems in offspring of mothers taking valproate or primidone.
- Common malformations are craniofacial abnormalities such as cleft lip and palate, congenital heart defects and spina bifida. A common more minor anomaly is distal digital hypoplasia.
- Drug-specific syndromes occur such as fetal valproate syndrome or fetal hydantoin syndrome. These combine a specific facial appearance with low IQ and other abnormalities (Table 10.5).
- Neural tube defects (NTD) are a common, severe consequence of AED therapy.
- Valproate appears to carry a higher risk than other AEDs of malformations and possibly of subtle cognitive deficits. NTD are increased tenfold to 2.5 percent. There may be a dose relationship, with lower risks at doses below 1000 milligrams daily.
- Folic acid supplementation may reduce the risk of NTD in non-epileptic patients at high risk by 75 percent. The supplement is taken from before conception to the end of the first trimester. The case remains unproven in relation to AEDs and the pattern of spina bifida is slightly different from that seen in sporadic cases. Many clinicians recommend 5 milligrams daily supplementation of folic acid for women taking AEDs who plan to become pregnant or who are sexually active without secure contraception.
- Enzyme-inducing AEDs reduce vitamin K levels in the fetus and may predispose to hemorrhagic disease of the newborn. Vitamin K supplementation (10 milligrams per day for the last month of pregnancy) and vitamin K injection for the newborn baby may help prevent this complication.
- Respiratory depression may be caused by sedative AEDs, for example barbiturates or benzodiazepines and increase the need for neonatal respiratory support.

Seizures Occurring During Pregnancy

- Eclampsia is the commonest cause of a first seizure occurring in the second half of pregnancy. The risk may extend a week (occasionally longer) into the puerperium.
- Other pregnancy-related acute symptomatic seizures need to be considered, including intracranial venous thrombosis and amniotic fluid embolus.
- Other causes for example tumors need to be considered as in the non-pregnant patient.

Pre-Eclampsia and Eclampsia

- Eclampsia complicates approximately 0.05 percent of deliveries in Western countries and carries a maternal mortality of 2 to 5 percent.
- Pre-eclampsia and eclampsia occur in the second half of pregnancy, most commonly in a first pregnancy. Eclampsia is defined as the occurrence of one or

more convulsions in association with the syndrome of pre-eclampsia. Pre-eclampsia is a multisystem disorder usually associated with proteinuria and hypertension and often with low albumin, hemoconcentration, and abnormal clotting or liver function.

- Seizures are usually convulsive but may have focal features and the ictal EEG shows generalized abnormalities. Neuroimaging may show cerebral edema and pathological examination of the brain reveals multiple petechial hemorrhages.
- Urgent delivery of the fetus can prevent pre-eclampsia from evolving into eclampsia but 44 percent of seizures occur post-partum.
- Magnesium sulphate (parenteral) is the treatment of choice for eclamptic seizures. It reduces the incidence of further seizures and decreases maternal mortality. Magnesium sulphate halves the chance of pre-eclampsia evolving into eclampsia and reduces maternal and fetal mortality. Its mechanism of action may relate to its antagonistic effect at N-methyl-D-aspartate (NMDA) receptors (Chapter 1).

Deterioration of Epilepsy in Pregnancy

A minor deterioration of epilepsy in pregnancy affects about one quarter of patients and is unlikely to affect the fetus.

- Coincidental eclampsia should be excluded.
- Check AED blood levels where relevant. The possibility of non-compliance and the woman's fears regarding medication should be explored.
- Mild deterioration. Consider weathering the storm or making a minor increase in AED dose, providing there are no adverse effects.
- Severe deterioration. Increase the dose of existing medication or if dose is maximal, add another drug. In this situation, controlling the mother's epilepsy is paramount and choice of drug should be tailored to her epilepsy syndrome.

Seizures around the Time of Delivery

- Peripartum seizure risk is 2 to 4 percent in patients with epilepsy. This risk is nearly tenfold higher than at other times during pregnancy.
- Acute symptomatic seizures including eclampsia need to be considered.
- For patients with established epilepsy, ensure continuation of AED therapy during delivery, especially of those that are prone to withdrawal seizures. Some AEDs can be given parenterally, others may be given by nasogastric tube.
- If a seizure occurs, then a benzodiazepine such as lorazepam 4 milligrams, may prevent further seizures. This may cause maternal sedation and increases the likelihood of requiring an instrumental delivery but a single seizure is not in itself an indication for Cesarian section. The drug may cause neonatal sedation and precautions should be taken to anticipate a possible need for ventilatory support in the first hours of the infant's life.

Anti-Epileptic Drugs and Lactation

- Breast-feeding confers significant health advantages for most infants. The decision whether to breast-feed needs to take this into account as well as the effects of AEDs.
- No currently available AED is contraindicated during lactation but the risks vary between drugs.
- The likelihood of an effect of an AED on the newborn baby depends on the proportion of the drug entering the breast milk, the bioavailability from breast milk to the baby and the baby's rate of metabolism of the drug (Table 10.6).
- Bottle-feeding causes rapid withdrawal of AEDs to which the baby has been exposed for an extended period *in utero*, which may in itself confer health risks on the baby.
- Sleep deprivation is a common trigger for seizures and bottle-feeding the baby allows both partners to participate in feeding, potentially having a beneficial effect on maternal epilepsy.

Epilepsy and the Puerperium

- Seizures affect about one percent of epilepsy sufferers during the puerperium. This may extend into the first few months of the baby's life, because of maternal sleep deprivation. It is probably best to leave medication unchanged unless the increase in seizures is severe or sustained. Increases in medication at this stage are likely to exacerbate sedation, fatigue and sleep deprivation.
- Pharmacokinetics change rapidly to the non-pregnant state. If medication has been increased, then it should be changed back, usually over six to eight weeks, during the puerperium to avoid drug toxicity.

Table 10.6. Different AEDs in Breast Milk

Drug	Breast Milk : Plasma Concentration Ratio	Comments
Carbamazepine	0.4–0.6	Usually safe and at low levels in the baby. Rare hepatic toxic effects in the baby
Clonazepam	0.3–0.4	May cause sedation or respiratory depression.
Ethosuximide	>0.8	May accumulate and cause sedation. May cause irritability on withdrawal
Lamotrigine	0.61	Nursed infants blood levels 25–50% of maternal levels. Probably safe
Oxcarbazepine	0.5	Presumed safe
Phenobarbital	0.4–0.6	Slow accumulation in the baby may cause sedation. Rapid withdrawal may cause jitteriness and seizures
Phenytoin	0.1–0.5	Safe
Primidone	0.7–0.9	Similar effects to phenobarbital but milder
Valproate	0.01–0.1	Generally safe but very rare idiosyncratic reactions to valproate in infants may occur

Case History 2

A 29-year-old woman had suffered refractory focal motor epilepsy since childhood. She was treated with carbamazepine 600 milligrams daily when she became pregnant. During the pregnancy, her seizures increased and her blood carbamazepine levels fell. Her dose of carbamazepine was increased to 1600 milligrams daily during the course of the pregnancy. Three days after delivery she became drowsy and ataxic with marked nystagmus in all directions of gaze. The level of carbamazepine in her blood was grossly elevated and reduction of the dose allowed her to return to normal.

CARE OF CHILDREN

- Fear of dropping, drowning or smothering their baby in a seizure is common. Such events are in fact rare and mothers can be reassured.
- Simple precautions:

    1. Changing the baby on the floor, rather than on a raised surface
    2. Washing the baby with someone else or else wiping them down rather than bathing them
    3. Pushing rather than carrying the baby
    4. Avoiding hot drinks, which may scald the baby.

BIBLIOGRAPHY

Adab N, Jacoby A, Smith D, Chadwick D. Additional educational needs in children born to mothers with epilepsy. J Neurol Neurosurg Psychiatry 2001;70:15–21.

Canger R. Malformations of women with epilepsy: a prospective study. Epilepsia 1999;39:1231–1236.

Chien PF, Khan KS, Arnott N. Magnesium sulphate in the treatment of eclampsia and pre-eclampsia: an overview of the evidence from randomised trials. Br J Obstet Gynaecol 1996;103:1085–1091.

Crawford P, Appleton R, Betts T, Duncan J, Guthrie E, Morrow J. The Women with Epilepsy Guidelines Development Group. Best practice guidelines for the management of women with epilepsy. Seizure 1999;8:201–217.

DeToledo JC, Lowe MR, Puig A. Nonepileptic seizures in pregnancy. Neurology 2000;55:120–121.

Goetting MG, Davidson BN, Status epilepticus during labor. A case report. J Reprod Med 1987;32:313–314.

Herzog AG, Klein P, Ransil BJ. Three patterns of catamenial epilepsy. Epilepsia 1997;38:1082–1088.

Holmes LB, Harvey EA, Coull BA, Huntington KB, Khoshbin S, Hayes AM, Ryan LM. The teratogenicity of anticonvulsant drugs. New Engl J Med 2001;344:1132–1138.

Koch S. Long-term neuropsychological consequences of maternal epilepsy and anticonvulsant treatment during pregnancy for school-age children and adolescents. Epilepsia 1999;40:1237–1243.

Licht EA, Sankar R. Status epilepticus during pregnancy. A case report. J Reprod Med 1999;44:370–372.

Morrell M.J. Guidelines for the care of women with epilepsy. Neurology 1998;51:S21–27.

Penovich PE. The effects of epilepsy and its treatment on sexual and reproductive function. Epilepsia 1999;41(Suppl. 2):S53–61.

The Eclampsia Trial Collaborative Group: Which anticonvulsant for women with eclampsia? Evidence from the Collaborative Eclampsia Trial. Lancet 1995;345:1455–1463.

The Magpie Trial Collaborative Group: Do women with pre-eclampsia and their babies benefit from magnesium sulphate? The Magpie Trial: a randomized placebo-controlled trial. Lancet 2002;359: 1877-1890.

REFERENCE

1. Herzog AG, Klein P, Ransil BJ. Three patterns of catamenial epilepsy. Epilepsia 1997;38:1082–1088.

11

Epilepsy in Special Groups: Children and Adolescents

Epilepsy in children presents specific problems. The differences from adult epilepsy extend across the whole spectrum of technical issues, including differential diagnosis, clinical seizure expression, pathophysiology, and drug treatment. The clinical situation also requires a different approach. Not only the child but the whole family must be managed. Parents who care for their child balance their own needs against the other demands of the family and cope with their own as well as the child's anxieties. Children with epilepsy can become fully integrated adults, even if seizure control is suboptimal. However, children with epilepsy often have more psychosocial handicaps than patients with other physical conditions causing equivalent disability.

DIAGNOSIS OF EPILEPSY

Up to one quarter of all children under the age of two years have at least one paroxysmal event that may resemble an epileptic seizure and they may suffer a number of paroxysmal conditions not seen in adults, consequently the differential diagnosis is different (Table 11.1).

INVESTIGATION OF EPILEPSY

- Different investigations are required for some of the conditions in Table 11.1.
- EEG can be performed in children of all ages. Its interpretation is strongly age-dependent and is more difficult than in adults. The EEG is central to the diagnosis of many pediatric epilepsy syndromes.
- MRI is undertaken in up to 75 percent of children with epilepsy. Children under the age of eight may require sedation or anesthetic for the procedure. The yield is lower than in adults. Imaging is not usually required for benign focal epilepsies or idiopathic generalized epilepsy (IGE), but is mandatory in other focal epilepsies, symptomatic generalized epilepsies, epilepsy with

Table 11.1. Conditions Mimicking Epilepsy in Childhood

Diagnosis	Age Affected	Clinical Features
Benign myoclonus	3–9 months	Jerky movements affecting trunk more than limbs, especially around sleep. Spontaneous remission
Sandifer's syndrome	Infancy	The child stiffens but retains awareness. Attacks occur during or soon after feeding, probably due to gastro-oesphageal reflux
Neonatal hyperekplexia (rare)	Infancy	Rare: myoclonic or tonic attacks triggered by startle, that may cause hypoxia. Usually remits. Treatment clonazepam. Associated with infantile hypertonia
Breath-holding attacks (affect 5% of children).	7–18 months	Attacks are provoked by fear, pain or emotional stress. Cyanotic form: the child cries intensely for up to 60 seconds before holding their breath for 30 seconds. They go blue and rigid with some clonic movements and sometimes a tonic–clonic seizure. Pallid form: the child has a vasovagal episode, often triggered by a blow to the head. Crying is less prominent. Ocular compression may reproduce the attacks
Night terrors	Over 2 years	Affect 3% of children and some adults (Chapter 5)
Masturbatory episodes	From 2–3 months	Episodes of sudden stiffening associated with rhythmical movements, facial flushing and irregular breathing
Munchausen syndrome by proxy	Any age	Attacks induced by an adult, usually a parent. Clinical features vary, for example poisoning or suffocation. The parent often claims to be the only one to have seen the attacks
Cardiac arrhythmia	Any age	Sudden collapse with pallor and rapid recovery
Alternating hemiplegia (rare)	Onset 10 days to 1 year	Unilateral posturing with nystagmus. There is sometimes transient hemiparesis that switches sides and becomes more prolonged. There may be developmental delay and other neurological deficits
Psychogenic non-epileptic seizures	Usually over 10 years	They may reflect many problems including sexual abuse, bullying, or learning difficulty (Chapters 5, 17)

developmental delay or neurocutaneous syndromes. The commonest abnormalities are either developmental or evidence of prenatal or perinatal insults or mesial temporal sclerosis.
- An extensive screen may be needed for children with symptomatic generalized epilepsies, which are normally associated with developmental delay.

PATHOPHYSIOLOGY

- Febrile seizures are the commonest form of seizure in young children, affecting 3 to 5 percent. Young children are especially susceptible during fever, irrespective of its cause.
- Early-onset pathologies are more likely to present with seizures in childhood. These include most forms of cortical dysplasia, inherited metabolic or degenerative conditions, lesions acquired *in utero* such as rubella infection or perinatal trauma.
- Tonic–clonic seizures (TCS) cannot occur until after about 6 months-old because only after then is myelination completed, which is required for expression of this seizure type.
- Age-dependent seizure expression occurs in most childhood epilepsy syndromes and probably reflects different stages of brain maturation (Figure 11.1).
- A continuum of age-dependent syndromes may occur, for example in the malignant symptomatic epilepsies. There is a high risk that epilepsy in infants with Ohtahara's syndrome will develop West's syndrome and then Lennox-Gastaut syndrome (Figure 11.2).
- Developmental delay may be the main manifestation of many forms of epilepsy but some rare syndromes cause cognitive decline with few or no overt seizures. Some authors consider there is an overlap between these syndromes and autism.
- Electroclinical syndromes may be due to various causes. For example West syndrome may be due to tuberose sclerosis or to metabolic abnormalities.
- Status epilepticus is more common in children than in adults. The mesial temporal lobes of a child are particularly sensitive to the damaging effects of severe seizures and temporal lobe epilepsy (TLE) is more likely to arise after status epilepticus in children than in adults.

PSYCHOSOCIAL CONSEQUENCES OF EPILEPSY IN CHILDREN

Cognitive Development

The cognitive and emotional developments of a child are multifaceted processes that may be disrupted both by epilepsy itself and by a variety of associated factors (Chapter 16). About one-third of children with refractory epilepsy need some kind of learning support.

Key factors include:

- The etiology of the epilepsy may itself be associated with cognitive and emotional disturbance for example tuberose sclerosis. Mesial temporal sclerosis often causes more focal memory disturbance.

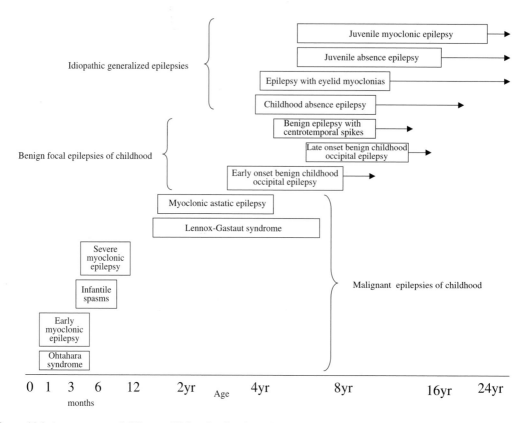

Figure 11.1. Age spectrum of different childhood epilepsies. The syndromic expression of epilepsy is strongly age-related. Boxes shows the common age range at presentation and arrows the persistence of the syndrome.

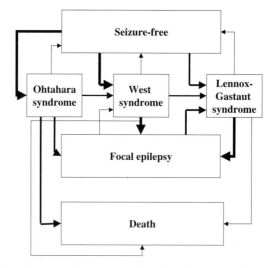

Figure 11.2. Evolution of malignant epilepsies. The effect of age-related expression is that malignant epilepsies often evolve through a distinct series of syndromes as children get older. In other children the epilepsy changes into a less specific focal or generalized epilepsy syndrome.

- Seizure activity temporarily interferes with normal mental activity, including ictal, postictal and interictal effects. IGE absences may have a profound effect because of their high frequency.
- Sleep disturbance from nocturnal seizures can have an effect.
- The social environment may contribute to cognitive difficulties. Worried carers may impose restrictions on children with epilepsy for fear they will have a seizure in public. They may not be allowed out to the shops, or to play with friends, inhibiting development and increasing dependency.
- Peer group rejection may lead to stigmatization and low self-esteem. The child may refuse to attend class or may be sent home by teachers if they suffer a seizure. This adds to isolation and time lost from education.
- All anti-epileptic drugs (AEDs) may slow the speed of mental processing. Some cause more specific effects such as paradoxical agitation with barbiturates, or speech disturbance with topiramate.
- Regression of existing skills may occur if the epilepsy is due to a degenerative condition such as progressive myoclonus epilepsy (Chapter 3). Some malignant epilepsy syndromes may manifest primarily with cognitive effects, for example Landau-Kleffner syndrome. In others such as Lennox-Gastaut syndrome, regression may be a consequence of severe epilepsy.

Emotional Development

- Amygdala lesions may be associated with emotional lability and severe behavioral disturbance. Orbitofrontal or frontopolar lesions may cause disinhibition and more mesial frontal lesions are associated with apathy and withdrawal.
- Seizures may cause emotional changes including irritability during the prodrome for hours to days, ictal agitation or postictal confusion, agitation or psychosis (Chapter 17).
- Interictal behavior disturbances may make children profoundly disruptive between seizures and may disappear on remission of seizures.
- Family dynamics may be disrupted if a child has epilepsy. The child may receive a disproportionate amount of attention from their parents, to the detriment of other children in the family and leading to jealousy. Divorce rates are higher in families with a child with epilepsy. Positive parenting attitudes and coping styles are associated with enhanced development in a child with epilepsy and are a greater determinant of emotional development than measures of seizure frequency or severity. The positive predictors for a successful environment are family esteem and communication, extended social support, family adaptation, financial well-being and low family stress.
- AEDs may affect mood, most often causing mild depression but elevated mood has also been claimed occasionally, independent of any AED effect on seizures. Cosmetic effects such as weight increase with some drugs and skin changes, especially with phenytoin may make children, who are already self conscious, even more reticent about social contact, increasing their isolation. This may have a particular effect on sexual development in adolescence.

Social Development

- The fear of seizures may lead to restrictions on a child's social activities. These restrictions may be imposed by carers or school afraid for the child's safety, by the child themselves who feels stigmatized by their epilepsy or by members of the child's peer group who are embarrassed by having to deal with the seizures.
- Associated learning disabilities may make it difficult to cope with the demands of adolescence and development of their own identity.

Case History 1

A 16-year-old girl suffered from learning disability and frontal lobe epilepsy due to cortical dysplasia. Her seizures manifested as drop attacks, absences and occasional tonic–clonic seizures. She left school at 16 with no formal qualifications and started a college course to acquire basic skills in literacy, numeracy and information technology. Three months into the course, she started to develop episodes of agitation. At first these were thought to be associated with seizures and she was admitted to hospital for evaluation. She presented as a shy and insecure girl who found it difficult to talk to any of the clinical staff. Her parents were caring and supportive. Numerous EEGs were normal and only occasional absences were observed during a long admission. She expressed fear over returning home and recommencing her course and refused to allow herself to be discharged from hospital. She was referred to an inpatient pediatric epilepsy and learning disability service.

This girl illustrates the difficulty that children with learning disability and epilepsy may have in coping with normal adolescent development. In her case it manifested with episodes that were initially incorrectly attributed to her epilepsy, which was in fact quite well controlled.

TREATMENT OF EPILEPSY IN CHILDREN

In the decision whether to initiate treatment, the key clinical principle of a balance of risks is the same in adults and in children but there may be a difference of emphasis. The decision involves the views of both parents and child.

Starting Treatment

- In favor of starting treatment are severe seizures, status epilepticus, cognitive decline and frequent seizure recurrence.
- Against treatment is a self-limiting, benign epilepsy syndrome, cognitive effects of AEDs and infrequent seizures. In the relatively protected environment of family and school, occasional seizures may be more acceptable than the cognitive effects of medication.

Stopping Treatment

- Just as the threshold to initiate treatment tends to be higher in children, withdrawal tends to be attempted sooner after remission than in adults.

- The prognosis for remission of epilepsy in children is affected by:

  1. The epilepsy syndrome
  2. The age of seizure onset (childhood onset is generally better than infantile or adolescent onset)
  3. A positive family history that confers a higher risk of recurrence
  4. Seizure frequency
  5. Seizure types: prognosis is adversely affected if there have been akinetic seizures or multiple tonic–clonic or focal seizures
  6. Continuing EEG abnormalities: this probably carry a greater adverse significance for most childhood epilepsy syndromes than for adults
  7. The seizure-free interval before discontinuation: this is important in children as it is in adults (Chapter 4).

TYPES OF TREATMENT

Although doses of medication differ, the day-to-day drug treatment of epilepsy is largely similar in children and in adults. Some important differences should be noted:

- New AEDs are developed in adults and studies in children only appear after the launch of the drug. Post-marketing studies in children are often inadequate. New drugs are not generally licensed for use in children and evidence of their value in children accumulates only slowly after release of the drug. However, all post-marketing studies in children over the age of four years suggest similar outcomes to adults.
- The large number of specific epilepsy syndromes affecting young children means that data concerning AED efficacy from trials in adults are often not directly comparable.
- Specific syndromes in childhood may respond to certain drugs and not to others, for example vigabatrin is very effective in West syndrome but not in Lennox-Gastaut syndrome.
- Pharmacokinetics in children are different to those in adults and doses may not be directly comparable.
- Adverse effects may occur more frequently in children than in adults, for example rash with lamotrigine, or may be different, for example phenobarbital causes hyperactivity in children and sedation in adults.
- Rare, idiosyncratic side effects may be different, for example fatal valproate-induced hepatotoxicity is largely limited to children under the age of 2 years. Valproate probably unmasks an inborn error of metabolism in these children.
- Dietary treatment (ketogenic diet) may be a more successful treatment for refractory childhood epilepsy than for adult epilepsy.
- Radical surgical treatment is life-saving in some severe epilepsies of childhood such as hemimeganencephaly. Curative resective surgery may be carried out in children with refractory focal epilepsy. There is increasing evidence that the earlier it is undertaken, the better the psychosocial development of the child, unhindered by continuing epilepsy. The issues have to be explored particularly carefully to secure the understanding of the child and the informed consent of their parents.

SEIZURE SYNDROMES IN CHILDHOOD

Neonatal Seizures

Clinical Features

- Major seizure types are tonic, myoclonic, automatisms and fragmentary jerks affecting localized body parts. There may be just slight deviation of the eyes, orofacial movements, rowing, pedalling or boxing movements.
- Pure autonomic seizures may occur, producing effects such as apnea or arrhythmia.
- Tonic–clonic seizures do not occur in the newborn.
- Ictal EEG changes may be absent or difficult to interpret.
- Differential diagnosis includes "jitteriness," benign neonatal sleep myoclonus and benign myoclonus of early infancy. The increased tone of hyperekplexia (startle disease) can mimic seizures in the first few months of life (Table 11.2).

Etiology

The causes and investigation of epileptic seizures in neonates reflect the wide variety of illnesses they may suffer that can affect the CNS (Tables 11.3 and 11.4).

Treatment of Seizures in the Neonate

- Neonatal intensive care is beyond the scope of this text.
- The cause of the seizures should be identified and treated rapidly.
- Pyridoxine 50 to 100 milligrams daily for 1 week in the absence of an identifiable cause.

Table 11.2. Differential Diagnosis of Neonatal Seizures (differentiating features are highlighted)

Clinical Feature	Neonatal Seizures	Jitteriness	Benign Neonatal Sleep Myoclonus	Benign Myoclonus of Early Infancy
Occurs awake	Yes	Yes	No	Yes
Occurs asleep	Yes	Yes	Yes	No
Tremulous movements	Yes	Yes	Yes	Yes
Tonic movements	Yes	No	No	Yes
Limb movements	Yes	Yes	Yes	No
Bilaterally synchronous movements	No	No	Yes	No
Stimulus sensitive movements	No	Very	No	No
Eye deviation	Yes	No	No	No
Autonomic changes	Yes	No	No	No
Automatisms	Yes	No	No	No
Abnormal EEG	Yes	No	No	No
Etiology	Various – see Table 11.3	Hypoxic-ischemic encephalopathy	None identified	None identified

Table 11.3. Causes of Seizures in Neonates

Cause of Seizures	Clinical Association
Cerebrovascular event	Infarction or hemorrhage
Hypoxic-ischemic encephalopathy	Respiratory distress syndrome, pneumonia, pneumothorax
Infection	Meningitis (especially Streptococcus, e-coli, Listeria), or encephalitis (Toxoplasma, Herpes simplex, Coxsackie B, Rubella or Cytomegalovirus, human immunodeficiency virus)
Cerebral malformations	Dysplasia, neurocutaneous disorders, chromosomal abnormalities
Pyridoxine-sensitive seizures	Start in the first hours of life with clonic episodes. The EEG is characterized by bilaterally synchronous 1–4 Hz EEG activity and the clinical and EEG response to pyridoxine is usually dramatic, occurring within minutes
Metabolic	Hypoglycemia, hypocalcemia, kernicterus, inborn errors of metabolism
Drugs	Drug withdrawal e.g. barbiturates or benzodiazepines taken by mother, drugs administered e.g. penicillins (Chapter 13)
Benign familial neonatal seizures	Present on day 2–3. Seizures are frequent but between them the child appears well. Attacks stop by age 6 months but there is a 10% risk of later seizures. Caused by a potassium channel mutation
Benign idiopathic neonatal seizures (fifth day seizures)	Occur from day 4–6 of life and manifest as clonic seizures, apnea and even status epilepticus. It usually remits by day 15. Cause unknown, low zinc levels implicated
Epileptic encephalopathies	See Table 11.5

- Phenobarbital 20 milligrams per kilogram is infused intravenously as first-line treatment and the dose may be increased to 40 milligrams per kilogram if there is no response.
- Phenytoin 20 mg/kg or lorazepam 0.05 to 0.1 milligrams per kilogram are alternative or second-line treatments.

In severe cases, therapy should be guided by EEG as clinical seizures may be difficult to identify in a heavily sedated neonate.

Prognosis of Neonatal Seizures

- Poor prognostic factors are prematurity, low birthweight, hypoxic ischemic damage abnormal background EEG. Only 10 percent with intraventricular

Table 11.4. Investigation of Neonatal Seizures

First-Line Investigations	Second-Line Investigations for Rare Causes
Metabolic screen: blood glucose, sodium, potassium, calcium, magnesium, urea and liver function	EEG
	Metabolic screen:
	Urine – organic acids
Blood count and clotting	Blood – ammonia, lactate, amino acids, transferrin isoelectric focusing
Blood cultures	
CSF analysis for meningitis, matched blood glucose	Maternal urine for drug toxicology CSF glycine, lactate, PCR for Herpes simplex
Cranial ultrasound for cerebral infarction or hemorrhage	Wood's light examination, eye examination

Table 11.5. Early Infantile Encephalopathies Causing Status Epilepticus

Syndrome/ Age of Onset	Etiology	Clinical Seizure Pattern	EEG Pattern	Treatment and Prognosis
Early infantile encephalopathy (Ohtahara's syndrome, very rare). Onset before 3 months	Asymmetric lesions on imaging e.g. malformations	Tonic spasms Focal motor and hemiconvulsions	Burst-suppression throughout waking and sleeping disappears by 6 months	ACTH is tried. Death or severe handicap common
Neonatal myoclonic encephalopathy	Congenital malformations and inborn errors of metabolism	Massive myoclonus Partial motor and tonic spasms. Family history common	Burst-suppression mainly during sleep and is persistent	None effective. Death or severe handicap common

hemorrhage will develop normally compared to nearly all those with appropriately treated, late onset hypocalcemia.

- Overall outcomes are: death, 20 percent; seizures, 15 to 20 percent (highest in very premature infants); neurological sequelae including mental retardation, 25 to 35 percent.

Epilepsy Syndromes in Infants and Young Children

Febrile Seizures

Epidemiology and Pathophysiology

- Five percent of all children in the age group 3 months to 5 years suffer febrile seizures (FS).
- They are seizures occurring in this age group during fever but without intracranial infection. In nearly 90 percent of cases the cause is a viral infection but in some it is a bacterial infection. The temperature is usually above 38 degrees Celsius before a seizure will occur. In about 10 to 25 percent there is a family history of FS or epilepsy and in a small proportion they may form part of the inherited syndrome "generalized epilepsy with febrile seizures plus" (GEFS+, Chapter 3).

Clinical Features and Diagnosis

- Febrile seizures may be a non-specific manifestation of fever in this age group but occasionally are due to primary CNS infection such as meningitis or encephalitis. Clinical indicators of possible CNS infection include:

    1. Signs of meningitis: headache or neck stiffness (which may be absent in very young children with meningitis) or meningococcal rash
    2. Absence of another obvious source of infection

3. Drowsiness or unresponsiveness prior to the seizure or beyond the normal recovery period from a seizure
4. Recurrent seizures: benign febrile seizures are single in over 90 percent.

- Differential diagnosis includes rigors, drug intoxications and syncope.
- A source of infection should be sought.
- EEG is generally unhelpful.

Treatment

- Acute treatment of febrile seizures:

  1. Antipyretic measures include adequate fluid intake and removal of excess clothing. Tepid sponging is ineffective and paracetamol (acetaminophen) gives symptomatic relief but has little effect on seizure recurrence.
  2. Benzodiazepines may be of value in terminating a prolonged febrile seizure or febrile status epilepticus but are otherwise unhelpful.
  3. Infections should be treated.
  4. AED prophylaxis, valproate and phenobarbital have been shown to reduce febrile seizure recurrence but are probably not worth the adverse effects.

Prognosis

- Epilepsy follows FS in 7 percent of patients by 25 years of age and is usually temporal lobe epilepsy due to mesial temporal sclerosis but may be GEFS+.
- Simple FS are brief, bilateral tonic–clonic or clonic seizures not followed by any neurological sequelae. They recur in subsequent illnesses in about one third of cases and 9 percent have three or more episodes. They are associated with later epilepsy in 2.4 percent compared with a population risk of 1.5 percent.
- FS associated with neurodevelopmental disorder or with complex features (below) substantially increase the risk of later developing epilepsy (see Chapter 4):

  1. Duration longer than 20 minutes
  2. Focal or unilateral features during the ictus
  3. Repeated seizures in one illness
  4. Neurological deficit following the ictus such as Todd's paresis.

West Syndrome (Infantile Spasms)

Epidemiology and Pathophysiology

- Incidence one in 3000 live births.
- Peak onset of spasms at 4 to 6 months old, 90 percent before 12 months.
- Commonest causes are tuberose sclerosis (TS) and other developmental abnormalities. Other causes: perinatal infection, ischemia or trauma and some

Table 11.6. Rare Epilepsies of Infancy and Early Childhood

Syndrome	Pathophysiology	Clinical Features and Diagnosis	EEG	Treatment and Prognosis
Benign myoclonic epilepsy of infants (rare) Onset 3 months to 4 years	Cause unknown. Children normal prior to onset. Family history of epilepsy or febrile seizures common	MS with falls. Several daily but not serial attacks. Differential: non-epileptic myoclonus (normal EEG), LGS or MAE (other seizure types and problems, below)	Generalized poly SW, more in sleep, sometimes photosensitive	Usually respond to valproate and remit within 2 years. Development usually normal
Severe myoclonic epilepsy of infancy. Incidence 1/40 000. 67% male. Onset before age 1	Family history of epilepsy in 25–64% suggests a genetic cause. Children normal prior to onset	Seizure often febrile at first. Focal or generalized myoclonic seizures (MS) are frequent, often clustered and triggered by movement. Also absences and PS in 40–50%. Developmental delay, ataxia and pyramidal signs develop	Initially SW when drowsy and during seizures. Later fast generalized SW with focal abnormalities	Very refractory seizures, severe mental retardation stabilizing by age 6 but all patients become dependent adults
Myoclonic astatic epilepsy (MAE) 1% of early childhood epilepsy. Onset before age 5	Close family history of epilepsy in 15% of siblings but myoclonic astatic epilepsy (MAE) in only 2%	Violent MS sometimes triggered by fright or light. Astatic seizures with head-nodding or knee-buckling. Absences (62%), TCS (75%), TS (30%). Myoclonic/ absence status epilepticus (36%)	May be normal at onset but develops 4 Hz occipital waves and 2–3 Hz SW with MS	Valproate may help but neurological decline common in early onset cases

inherited metabolic diseases such as non-ketotic hyperglycinemia or pyridoxine dependency. Relatively few patients with each of these conditions will develop West syndrome (WS), more will develop other forms of epilepsy. With MRI, the proportion of West syndrome due to unknown cause is 10 to 20 percent.

- The pons is proposed to be a fundamental site of abnormality unlike in other forms of epilepsy. However, TS is also associated with widespread cortical developmental abnormalities.
- Corticosteroids may profoundly influence WS and the hypothalamic–adreno-cortical axis may be important in the condition.

Clinical Features

- Spasms are the hallmark first described by Dr West in his own son in 1841. They last 1 to 2 seconds, longer than a myoclonic jerk but shorter than a tonic seizure.
- Flexor spasms are typical and consist of an abrupt flexion of the head, trunk and limbs. Extensor spasms may also occur, as may mixtures of the two. The spasms may be symmetric or asymmetric. Spasms often cluster with dozens occurring over a period of minutes, each separated by a few seconds. The spasms occur when waking or in non-REM sleep. Consciousness is lost briefly with the spasms, but this is rarely noticeable.
- Other seizure types: tonic, atonic seizures or partial seizures may occur.
- Specific pathology such as TS is suggested by extensor spasms, asymmetric spasms or other seizure types.

EEG in West Syndrome

The EEG is distinctive:

- There is no recognizable background rhythm.
- High amplitude slow waves and spikes are widespread, irregular, of variable amplitude and asynchronous between the two hemispheres. This chaotic pattern is termed hypsarrhythmia (Figure 11.3).
- During REM sleep the EEG may be nearly normal.
- Ictal recordings usually show an initial high amplitude slow wave and then fast activity or attenuation of the EEG. Hypsarrhythmia disappears between the spasms of an individual cluster and reappears at the end of the cluster.

Neuroimaging in West Syndrome

- Developmental abnormalities are often detectable on MRI but some are recognizable only on pathological examination.

Treatment of West Syndrome

- Vigabatrin up to 200 milligrams per kilogram may have a dramatic effect on spasms. In one study, a third of patients with symptomatic spasms became seizure-free, including those refractory to other therapies.
- Corticosteroids induce a remission of spasms within two weeks in 50 to 80 percent of patients. They recur in 30 percent but may respond to a second treatment. There have been no trials comparing vigabatrin and steroids.
- Valproate and pyridoxine in combination may also induce remission.

Prognosis of West Syndrome

- Mortality is 5 percent.
- Other epilepsy syndromes develop in half of those with West syndrome – refractory focal epilepsy or Lennox-Gastaut syndrome (Figure 11.2).
- Mental retardation develops in up to 90 percent of patients.

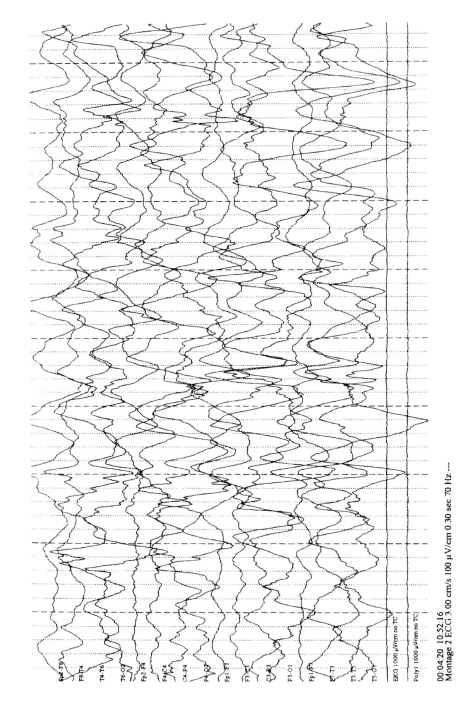

00:04:20 10:52:16
Montage 2 ECG 3.00 cm/s 100 μV/cm 0.30 sec 70 Hz ---

EKG 1000 μV/cm no TC

Poly1 1000 μV/cm no TC|

Figure 11.3. Hypsarrythmia typical of infantile spasms (West syndrome) showing the chaotic giant slow waves.

- Cryptogenic WS in neurologically normal children has the highest chance of a good outcome.

Lennox-Gastaut Syndrome

Definition

- Lennox-Gastaut syndrome (LGS) is a malignant epilepsy syndrome character-ized by three features:

  1. Specific seizure types, especially atypical absences, axial tonic and atonic seizures
  2. EEG abnormalities comprising slow spike and wave discharges on waking and 10 hertz fast rhythms in sleep
  3. Delayed mental development and behavioral disorders.

Epidemiology and Pathophysiology

- In specialist centers LGS may comprise 2 to 3 percent of early childhood epilepsy. It is somewhat commoner in boys.
- Peak onset is between ages 3 and 5 years and nearly all cases start before age 8.
- Symptomatic forms are due to neurodevelopmental disorders such as TS, perinatal insults, postnatal infection or radiotherapy for intracranial tumour.
- Pathological examination of brains with LGS has shown selective neuronal necrosis in a number of sites, including the neocortex, hippocampus, thalamus and cerebellum.
- Cryptogenic cases have an increased incidence of a family history of epilepsy.
- West syndrome precedes 20 percent of LGS. Focal epilepsy precedes some other cases.

Clinical Features

- Presentations vary but the syndrome evolves to a common pattern, with a high seizure frequency.
- Axial tonic seizures affect nearly all patients. The neck and body are suddenly flexed with posturing of the arms. The child falls and there may be autonomic features. If the seizure lasts more than 10 seconds, there may a tremor of the whole body "vibratory seizure."
- Atypical absences occur in nearly all cases. The seizures start and end gradually and consciousness is impaired rather than lost. The attack may be associated with irregular perioral and eyelid myoclonus.
- Massive myoclonus and atonic seizures also occur. All cause falls or drop attacks. Tonic–clonic and partial seizures also occur.
- Status epilepticus affects half or more of children with LGS and may last days to weeks, often with obtundation and serial tonic attacks.
- Development slows in LGS and there may be regression. Up to 90 percent develop mental retardation. During bouts of status, transient neurological signs

may appear and may become permanent if the bouts are too long or frequent.

EEG

- Waking interictal EEG usually shows slowing of the background rhythms with widespread or multifocal discharges of slow spike and wave (SSW) at 2 to 2.5 Hz.
- Sleeping interictal EEG typically shows 10 hertz spike discharges over the anterior regions in addition to SSW.
- EEG flattening is seen anteriorly prior to tonic seizures, which evolves during the seizure into fast bilateral bursts or generalized SSW.
- Ictal EEG may be relatively unchanged during atypical absences.

Neuroimaging

- Developmental abnormalities are the commonest finding in the symptomatic group.

Treatment

- Valuable AEDs include valproate, ethosuximide, benzodiazepines, barbiturates, lamotrigine and topiramate.
- Potentially adverse AEDs include phenytoin, carbamazepine and vigabatrin.

Prognosis

- Only 10 percent ever become seizure-free.
- LGS usually evolves into focal epilepsy before adulthood. Some cryptogenic cases persist into adulthood.
- Learning disability usually persists.

Landau-Kleffner Syndrome (LKS, Acquired Epileptic Aphasia) and Epilepsy with Continuous Spikes and Waves in Slow Wave Sleep (ECSWS)

- These two conditions may be part of the same spectrum of disorders.
- They are conceptually very important, although rare. In both cases, there is a very persistent electrographic 2 hertz spike and wave abnormality but relatively few overt seizures. Despite the paucity of seizures and absence of major structural pathology, these syndromes present with developmental delay or regression.
- Severely abnormal electrographic discharges may thus have a profound effect on normal development even without causing obvious seizures.

Epidemiology and Pathophysiology

- Onset is usually between the ages of 5 and 7 years and boys are affected twice as often as girls.
- Both conditions appear during the period when major functional connections are determined. In the neonate there is an overproduction of synapses and neuronal activity during normal use determines the selective pruning process. A

current hypothesis is that the almost continuous abnormal electrical activity in these conditions may prevent the formation of normal connections. In LKS, speech is primarily affected. In strictly unilateral lesions in this age group, such as trauma, speech often transfers to the contralateral hemisphere. In LKS, although the discharges are generated unilaterally, they propagate bilaterally, perhaps preventing transfer of speech to the non-dominant hemisphere.
- Some authors consider that LKS is in the same spectrum of disorders as the benign focal epilepsies of childhood.

Clinical Features of LKS and ECSWS

- LKS presents with acquired aphasia in a previously normal child, without an obvious structural cause but with marked EEG abnormalities. The onset may be subacute or more gradual. Understanding is affected first but soon speech is also affected, for example with paraphasias. In the most severe cases the child becomes mute and may also not react to non-speech sounds, such as the bark of a dog, implying some auditory agnosia as well as aphasia.
- ECSWS presents with more widespread cognitive decline.
- Seizures usually occur in both conditions but are relatively infrequent.

Treatment

- There are no clear guidelines as the condition is rare.
- AED therapy controls most seizures, except atypical absences and atonic seizures. Some patients are refractory.
- The EEG abnormality requires more aggressive treatment. This level of treatment is more difficult to achieve.
- Multiple subpial transection may be of benefit in preventing the cognitive decline (Chapter 15).

Prognosis

- Profound aphasia, preventing normal life affects half of those with LKS.
- ECSWS has an even worse prognosis.

The Benign Focal Epilepsies of Childhood

- These are characteristic clinical syndromes with a strong genetic component, which run a benign course. Some are common (below) and others are rare (Table 11.7).
- Different cortical regions are abnormally activated in different syndromes. They share similar electrographic phenomena, albeit in different parts of the brain with similar prognoses and responses to treatment.
- Occasional individuals develop more than one type of benign focal epilepsy.
- The gender predominance varies between syndromes.
- Different members of the same family may also suffer different benign focal epilepsies, which has led to the concept of a genetic seizure susceptibility syndrome with individual clinical expression influenced by other genetic or environmental factors.

Table 11.7. Rarer Benign Focal Epilepsies

Syndrome	Clinical Features	EEG	Treatment and Prognosis
Benign partial epilepsy with affective symptoms. Onset age 2–10. Family history common. Differential diagnosis, night terrors, behavioral disorder	Onset with fright or terror, screams, then chewing, autonomic features and loss of awareness. Duration 1–2 minutes. May have frequent seizures, asleep and awake	Fronto-temporal spikes similar morphology to BECTS, on either side and increase in sleep. Generalized S+W common. Ictal EEG focal or diffuse onset	Responds to monotherapy with carbamazepine or phenytoin and then remits in early teens
Benign partial epilepsy with parietal spikes. Onset 4–8 years. Commoner in boys. Febrile seizures common	Occasional, brief partial motor seizures with head version. May have recurrent seizures/focal status.	Sagittal and parasagittal spikes with giant somatosensory evoked potentials	Seizures usually persist for about 1 year and then settle. Too few patients to evaluate medication
Benign frontal epilepsy. Onset 4–8 years	Occasional daytime episodes including absences, tonic or atonic seizures. Commoner nocturnal convulsive seizures	Frontal EEG spikes move around the frontal lobe. They spread across the hemisphere and between frontal lobes in sleep	Seizures remit by age 9–11

Benign Epilepsy with Centrotemporal Spikes (BECTS)

Epidemiology

- BECTS is also known as Benign Rolandic Epilepsy.
- Up to 15 percent of childhood epilepsy is BECTS.
- Boys account for 60 percent of cases.
- Age at presentation is 7 to 10 years in 75 percent.
- There appears to be independent inheritance of the EEG trait and epilepsy tendency with possible linkage to chromosome 15.

Clinical Features

- Nocturnal seizures are commonest.
- A few attacks only before remission is the rule. Ten to 20 percent of patients only ever experience one seizure and only about 10 percent have frequent recurrent attacks.
- Seizures are stereotyped. They start with an odd sensation on one side of the mouth followed by drooling and twitching of the side of the mouth. Speech is affected and breathing may become difficult. Clonic jerks then spread down one side of the body. In most cases consciousness is retained but in some the seizure spreads to become a full tonic–clonic seizure with loss of consciousness.
- Normal cognition is usual. Some authors describe subtle changes reminiscent of those seen in LKS and suggest an overlap with this syndrome.

Investigations

- Sleep EEG recording is mandatory. Waking EEG is often normal.
- The characteristic abnormality is blunt, high voltage centrotemporal

spikes. These may occur on either side and on different sides in different recordings in the same individual and bears no relation to the side of the clinical seizure.
- Neuroimaging is normal in BECTS.

Treatment

- No treatment is usually needed.
- Seizures remit with most AEDs but low dose carbamazepine is generally favored.

Prognosis

- Remission is usual within two to 4 years of diagnosis and almost always by the age of 16.
- Generalized epilepsy develops in 2 percent later in life but BECTS does not relapse.

Benign Childhood Occipital Epilepsy (BCOE)

- Occipital seizures represent 4 to 5 percent of epilepsy in children. Girls are slightly more affected than boys.
- There are two types of BCOE, young onset and older onset.

Early Onset Benign Childhood Occipital Epilepsy (EOBCOE)

CLINICAL FEATURES

- EOBCOE accounts for about 17 percent of benign partial epilepsies of childhood. The median age of onset is 5 years, few present after age 8.
- The clinical pattern is unusual. Seizures are very infrequent but are prolonged, lasting 30 minutes or more. The child then usually sleeps and is well on awakening. The attacks are mostly nocturnal.
- Despite its name the features are more of autonomic than occipital involvement. In a typical episode the child feels unwell, often with a headache, becomes agitated and may retch or vomit after a few minutes. Other autonomic features are common, including pallor, flushing, mydriasis, meiosos and occasionally cardiorespiratory abnormalities. The child's eyes become tonically deviated to one side. Consciousness is usually affected during the course of the seizure. Classical occipital symptoms of ictal blindness or visual hallucinations are uncommon.
- Focal status epilepticus evolving to hemiclonic or tonic–clonic status affects some children.

INVESTIGATIONS

- EEG shows paroxysms, which are commonly occipital but may be more anterior, occurring whenever the eyes are closed. They may also occur with the eyes open but are abolished if the child actively fixes their gaze "fixation-off sensitivity." Centrotemporal spikes and giant somatosensory evoked potentials may also occur.

Treatment

- No regular treatment is usually required.
- Rectal diazepam may be indicated for occasional bouts of focal status epilepticus.

Prognosis

- Up to 30 percent of children have only one seizure. The median is three seizures.
- Remission is the rule but a few children may later develop BECTS.

Late Onset Benign Epilepsy with Occipital Paroxysms (LOBCOE)

Clinical Features

- LOBCOE accounts for 2 to7 percent of benign focal epilepsies.
- Median age of onset is 8 years, range of 3 to 16 years.
- Frequent seizures are found, often several per day.
- Patients have brief, waking seizures, lasting from seconds to three minutes. Typically they start with simple visual hallucinations or ictal blindness that leads on to a postictal headache. The visual loss may be quite prolonged. The visual hallucinations are often colored as distinct from migraine (black and white or silver). Other sensations may occur such as sensations of movement, illusions, ocular pain, tonic eye deviation or eyelid closure. They may evolve to hemiclonic or tonic–clonic seizures.

Investigations

- The EEG shows occipital paroxysms with fixation-off sensitivity.

Treatment

- AEDs are indicated because of the high seizure frequency.
- Carbamazepine is commonly used but may precipitate absences or myoclonus and many AEDs are effective.

Prognosis

- Remission occurs in 60 to 90 percent in the late teens. AEDs can usually be withdrawn 2 years later.
- Refractory cases may have subtle structural abnormalities, such as occipital cortical dysplasia and are therefore not truly LOBCOE.

Idiopathic Generalized Epilepsy

Idiopathic Generalized Absence Epilepsies

- Syndromes are childhood absence epilepsy (CAE), juvenile absence epilepsy (JAE) and eyelid myoclonias with absences (EMA), see Table 11.8.

Table 11.8. The Clinical Features of Distinct IGE Absence Epilepsy Syndromes

Feature	Childhood Absence Epilepsy	Juvenile Absence Epilepsy	Eyelid Myoclonias with Absences
Frequency	Common, 10% of childhood epilepsy	Common, 5% of epilepsy in adolescence	Uncommon
Age of onset	Peak 4–8, range 8–12	Peak 10–12, range 7–16	Peak age 6, usually first decade
Sex predominance	Strongly female	Slightly commoner in females	Almost all female
Genetics	Family history in 44%	Identical twins may both have JAE and family history of seizures quite common.	A strong genetic preponderance in some families
Duration of absences	Median 12 seconds	Median 16 seconds	Median 4 seconds
Frequency of absences	Many each day	Every few days or weeks	Hundreds of times daily
Automatisms	Involve hands and face and are common if absences last longer than 15 seconds	Perioral myoclonias	4–6 Hz jerking of eyelids and eyeballs, then head and shoulders may move up
Eyes	Usually open and staring, may blink at 3 Hz	Staring less common than CAE	Distinctive rapid fluttering
Consciousness	Usually complete loss of awareness and amnesia for events during the episode	Partial loss of awareness and may have partial recall	Loss of consciousness in longer discharges
Additional seizure types	Other seizure types uncommon. Tonic–clonic seizures in 10%, occasional myoclonus	Occasional tonic–clonic seizures in 90%, usually first thing in the morning. Some myoclonus. Absence status in 27–35%, occasional tonic–clonic status.	Tonic–clonic seizures develop in nearly all in adolescence or adult life
EEG	Normal background. Typical 3 Hz spike and wave discharge, frontally predominant. Almost always triggered by hyperventilation	Normal background. Symmetrical discharges at 3.5–4 Hz, sometimes 3–4 spikes preceding a slow wave. Reliably triggered by hyperventilation	Normal background. Frequent bursts of 3–6 Hz polyspike and wave. Triggered by eye closure except in darkness
Photosensitivity	Uncommon	20%	Marked in all. Some patients enjoy the sensation and seek photic stimulation, e.g. sitting close to the television
Prognosis	25% remit by age 16, 75% by age 30	Good response to treatment in >70% but spontaneous remission uncommon	Persists into adult life, absences difficult to treat, other seizures may respond

- Absence attacks are a key clinical feature.
- Absences differ a little between CAE and JAE, but it may require video-EEG-telemetry to make that distinction. The syndromes are distinguished more by epidemiology, age of onset, associated seizure types and prognosis.
- Subtle attacks, often without major motor manifestations, are often unrecognized as epileptic phenomena.
- Learning difficulties is a common presentation for children with CAE and frequent absences. They may be accused of daydreaming and their epilepsy can go unrecognized; this can severely affect educational development (Case 3, Chapter 16).

- A positive family history is common but the nature of the genetic abnormality is not clear (see Chapter 3).
- The EEG shows typical generalized spike and wave, which is at around 3 Hertz in classical CAE (Figure 11.4).
- Four sub-syndromes of CAE have been suggested and are the basis of further genetic analysis. Up to 60 percent are due to one subgroup of classical CAE or pyknolepsy.
- AEDs are similar for all syndromes: valproate, lamotrigine, ethosuximide, topiramate, acetazolamide and sometimes benzodiazepines or phenobarbital. Valproate and lamotrigine may be a particularly valuable combination. Ethosuximide can be used alone in CAE where absences are often the only seizure type, but other seizure types do not usually respond. Other AEDs may make seizures worse and may trigger absence status epilepticus, including phenytoin, carbamazepine, gabapentin, tiagabine and vigabatrin.

It is difficult to better Gowers' description of the attacks of CAE. "A patient suddenly stops for a moment in whatever he or she is doing, very often turns pale, may drop whatever is in the hand, and then is better. There may be no visible spasm or there may be a slight stoop forward, or a slight quivering of the eyelids. The patient may or may not fall. … The attack usually lasts only a few seconds. The return of consciousness may be sudden, and the patient, after the momentary lapse, may be in just the same state as before the attack, may even continue in a sentence or action which was commenced before it came on, and suspended during its occurrence. … When full consciousness is regained, although it had only been for a second or two completely lost, the patient may not know of the occurrence of the attack, and only become aware of it by finding that persons are looking at him with surprise."

Case History 2 (EMA)

A 17-year-old girl presented with a history of three seizures. On each occasion she had been watching television and went to insert a new video cassette into the video cassette recorder under the television. As she approached the television, she collapsed into a tonic–clonic seizure. During the course of the consultation there were numerous episodes of rapid flickering of her eyelids, lasting 1 to 2 seconds. The episodes were too brief to interfere with function. When asked about these, her mother said they had been going on for many years and she had attributed them to a habit. Her EEG showed frequent bursts of polyspike and wave and confirmed a photoparoxysmal response.

Juvenile Myoclonic Epilepsy (JME)

Epidemiology

- Commonest form of IGE; 3 to 12 percent of all epilepsy
- Genetic input is significant, but most cases are sporadic
- Subdivisions of JME have been proposed according to age of onset and presence of absences and may be of value in genetic analysis
- Female to male preponderance 3:2
- Misdiagnosis is common: the myoclonus may be subtle and is not reported by the patient and not sought by the clinician.

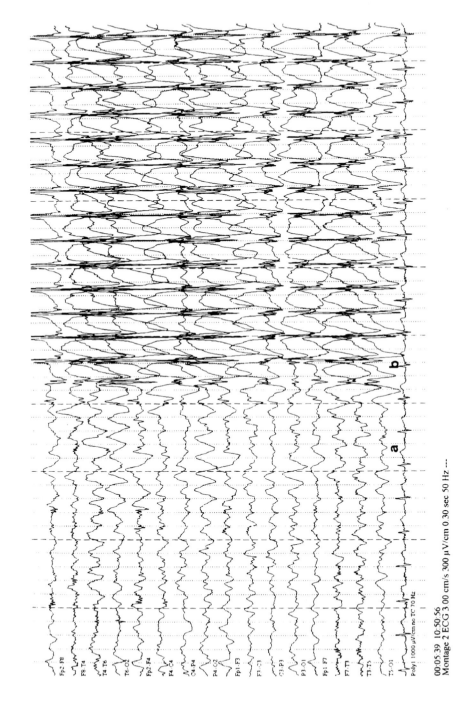

00:05 39 10:50 56
Montage 2 ECG 3.00 cm/s 300 μV/cm 0.30 sec 50 Hz ...

Figure 11.4. Three Hertz spike and wave of childhood absence epilepsy. The EEG shows symmetric slow waves (a) typical of hyperventilation, which triggers typical 3 Hz spike and wave of absence epilepsy (b).

Clinical Features

- Tonic–clonic seizures and myoclonus affect nearly all patients. The commonest presentation is with the first tonic–clonic seizure and prior myoclonus comes to light in the clinical assessment (Table 11.9).
- Absences occur in around 20 percent of patients and CAE may evolve into JME.
- Occasional patients have just myoclonus.
- The typical myoclonic jerk affects the proximal upper limb muscles, making the arms jerk upwards. The jerks may affect either side alone or both simultaneously. Occasionally the jerks may cause the patient to fall. Usually the patient retains awareness during the jerks but if they occur serially, with high frequency, awareness may be impaired.
- Waking (morning) myoclonus is typical. Jerks are worst within 30 minutes of waking. Tonic–clonic seizures are also most frequent soon after waking and often follow a flurry of myoclonus.

Case History 3

A 19-year-old boy gave a history of tonic–clonic seizures occurring every few months for 4 years. He did not volunteer any further seizure types but on direct questioning he admitted that most mornings he would experience two or three jerks of his limbs over about half an hour after waking. These jerks could affect any limbs without warning. He sat on the side of his bed for a few minutes before getting up so as to try and minimize the jerks and he had taken to sliding down the stairs on his bottom before breakfast as a jerk had once thrown him down the stairs. He drank cold coffee as his jerks had made him throw his drink across the room. His current treatment was with valproate and carbamazepine. Carbamazepine was withdrawn and lamotrigine was added. Myoclonus and tonic–clonic seizures ceased.

- Seizure triggers are very important in JME, especially sleep deprivation and alcohol withdrawal. These circumstances commonly combine in a normal teenager's social life and need to be sought in the history.
- Rarer seizure triggers include complex manual movements such as doing up buttons or brushing teeth, mental activities, such as making decisions, calculations and certain games such as chess. The combination of a complex mental task with a manual task such as using an abacus is especially likely to cause these "praxis-induced seizures." For some patients, emotional stress and the premenstrual syndrome may be triggers.

Table 11.9. The Age of Onset of JME

Manifestation	Age Range of Onset (Median)
Myoclonus	7–26 (15)
Absence	7–18
Tonic–clonic seizure	6–32 (16)

EEG

- The background EEG is normal.
- Repeated recordings may be needed to identify the typical abnormality of JME. Even with three recordings, it may be missed in 16 percent of cases.
- The typical interictal abnormality is of polyspike and wave complexes lasting 0.5 to 20 seconds (mean 7 seconds). The disturbance is characterized by 5 to 20 spikes at 12 to 15 Hz preceding the slow wave complex (Figure 11.5).
- Photosensitivity is present in 20 to 57 percent (mean 34 percent).

Catches in the Diagnosis of JME

The key errors in making the diagnosis are:

- Missing it altogether:

    1. The myoclonic jerks are not sought in the history.
    2. The patient gives a history of clumsiness rather than myoclonus (may be praxis-induced).

- The asymmetry of the presentation leads to an incorrect diagnosis of focal epilepsy:

    1. Myoclonic jerks are often asymmetric, affecting one limb, leading to an erroneous impression of focal seizures.
    2. Asymmetric features are common in the tonic–clonic seizures, for example with the patient's head turning to one side.
    3. The EEG discharges may show asymmetry, which often changes from side to side between recordings.

Treatment

- Valproate monotherapy fully controls up to 85 percent of patients. The dose required varies greatly according to the severity of the condition, from 200 milligrams daily to more than 2000 milligrams daily in adults.
- Other AEDs that are of value for all the seizure types in JME are lamotrigine, topiramate, phenobarbital and probably levetiracetam.
- Myoclonus may respond to clonazepam or piracetam.
- Absences may respond to ethosuximide or acetazolamide.
- Polytherapy may be of value in treating refractory JME (Chapter 9, Case 6).
- AED may exacerbate JME, especially carbamazepine, phenytoin, vigabatrin, tiagabine and gabapentin triggering myoclonus or absences.

Prognosis

- Seizure-freedom may be achieved in up to 90 percent of patients.
- Poorer prognosis is associated with learning disability, a history of major psychiatric problems and the presence of all three seizure types.
- Epilepsy persists for most patients. Only 10 percent can expect continued remission after drug withdrawal at any time in adult life.

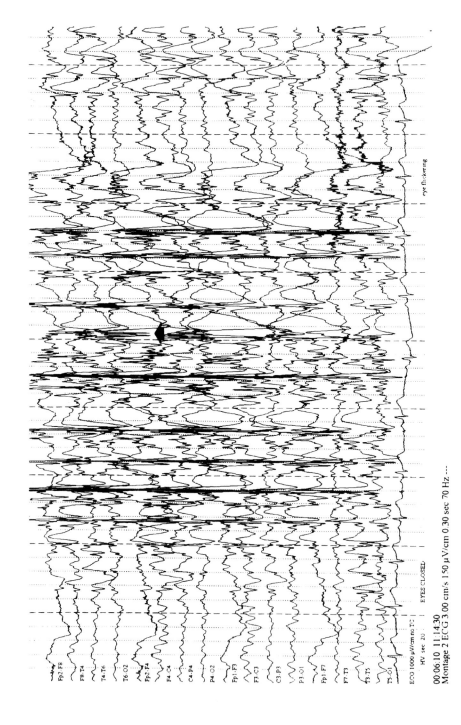

Figure 11.5. Typical polyspike discharge of juvenile myoclonic epilepsy. The polyspike discharge contrasts with the single spike of childhood absence epilepsy (Figure 11.4).

- Driving is prohibited in the UK by patients with any seizure type including myoclonus.

Primary Generalized Epilepsy with Tonic–Clonic Seizures on Awakening

- Differentiating epilepsy with TCS on wakening (ETCSA) from JME or absence epilepsy may be difficult. Patients with absence epilepsy or myoclonic epilepsy complicated by convulsions usually experience them soon after waking. A careful evaluation with video-EEG-telemetry may reveal myoclonic jerks prior to the TCS.
- Pure ETCSA is probably less common than the other IGE syndromes. A family history is seen in about 12.5 percent of cases, with 3.3 percent of first degree relatives affected, less than in other IGE syndromes.

Clinical Features

- By definition, a minimum of six seizures must occur within minutes of waking. The relationship is to the sleep–wake cycle rather than to a particular time of the day.
- Onset is usually in the second decade but may be from age 6 to age 35. It is about twice as common in males.
- Seizures triggered by fatigue and alcohol withdrawal are common.

EEG

- The background EEG may show some slow wave abnormalities.
- Spike and wave activity is seen in only 40 percent of patients.
- Sudden waking from sleep followed by hyperventilation substantially increases the yield of generalized epileptiform abnormalities.

Treatment

- The most effective drug has not been established but seizure-freedom is achieved in 59 to 85 percent.

Prognosis

- If drugs are withdrawn after only 2 years of seizure-freedom, 83 percent will relapse.

BIBLIOGRAPHY

Annegers JF, Hauser AW, Lee JR-J, Rocca WA. Factors prognostic of unprovoked seizures after febrile convulsions. N Engl J Med 1987;316:493–498.

Beaumanoir M. Continuous Spikes and Waves During Slow Sleep/Electrical Status Epilepticus During Slow Sleep. London: John Libbey 1995.

Delgado-Escueta AV, Medina MT, Serratosa JM, Castroviejo IP, Gee MN, Weissbecker K, Westling BW, Fong CY, Alonso ME, Cordova S, Shah P, Khan S, Sainz J, Rubio Donnadieu F,

Sparkes RS. Mapping and positional cloning of common idiopathic generalized epilepsies: juvenile myoclonus epilepsy and childhood absence epilepsy. Adv Neurol 1999;79:351–374.

Duncan JS, Panayiotopoulos CP (eds). Typical absences and related syndromes. Edinburgh: Churchill Livingstone, 1995.

Gowers WR. Epilepsy and other chronic convulsive diseases: their causes symptoms and treatment. London: J. and A. Churchill, 1981.

Hermann BP, Austin J. Psychosocial status of children with epilepsy and the effects of epilepsy surgery. In: Wyllie E (ed). The Treatment of Epilepsy: Principles and Practice. Philadelphia: Lea & Feibiger 1993: 1141–1148.

Ito M. Antiepileptic drug treatment of West syndrome. Epilepsia 1998;39 (Suppl. 5):38-41.

Panayiotopoulos CP. Benign Childhood Partial Seizures and Related Epilepsy Syndromes. London: John Libbey and Co., 1999.

Panayiotopoulos CP. Panayiotopoulos syndrome. A common and benign epilepsy syndrome. John Libbey & Co., 2002.

Roger J, Bureau M, Dravet Ch, Dreifuss FE, Perret A, Wolf P (eds). Epileptic syndromes in infancy, childhood and adolescence 2nd Edition. London: John Libbey and Co., 1992.

Schmitz B, Sander T (eds). Juvenile Myoclonic Epilepsy, the Janz Syndrome. Philadelphia: Wrightson Biomedical, 2000.

Shinnar S, Vining EP, Mellits ED, D'Souza BJ, Holden K, Baumgardner RA, Freeman JM. Discontinuing antiepileptic medication in children with epilepsy after two years without seizures. A prospective study. N Engl J Med 1985;313:976–980.

Volpe JJ. Neonatal seizures. In: Neurology of the Newborn. Philadelphia: WB Saunders, 1995;172–211.

12

Epilepsy in Special Groups: The Elderly and those with Learning Disability

EPILEPSY IN THE ELDERLY

Epidemiology

- Epilepsy arises more commonly in the elderly in Western populations, than in any other age group with an incidence of approximately 150 per 100, 000 and a prevalence of 12 per 1000 in the over 70s.
- The commonest causes are cerebrovascular disease, tumors or in association with dementias. Other causes include metabolic disturbances, including drug or alcohol-induced seizures, which are under-diagnosed in the elderly.
- Tonic–clonic status epilepticus is the presentation of epilepsy in 10 to 30 percent, usually as an acute symptomatic event complicating acute cerebral infarction.

Diagnosis

- The differential diagnosis of collapse is very broad in the elderly, including locomotor disturbances such as arthritis of the hip, ataxia, spinal spondylosis or peripheral neuropathy (Chapter 5). Loss of consciousness may be difficult to establish.
- Vascular conditions are common including cardiac arrhythmia and neurocardiogenic syncope. The typical prodromal symptoms of syncope are commonly absent.
- In the elderly, migraine commonly presents with focal neurological symptoms without headache, which may be mistaken for seizures or transient ischemic attacks (TIA). The aura is otherwise typical in terms of the nature and duration of symptoms.
- Transient global amnesia (TGA) is a condition of unknown etiology, sometimes associated with migraine that occurs above the age of 50. The condition is characterized by a failure of anterograde memory, which may mimic confusion with no associated physical deficits (Case 1, Chapter 5). TGA episodes usually last hours and recur infrequently. Brief, recurrent amnesic episodes are more likely to be epileptic.
- Transient ischemic attacks may present with positive motor phenomena but these are usually more prolonged than focal motor seizures, are not associated with altered awareness, and the motor manifestations have a less clear-cut evolution than those in a seizure.
- Parasomnias are common in the elderly, especially in association with neurodegenerative disease (Chapter 5, Case 7). They may manifest with prominent motor activity, mimicking seizures and a sleep laboratory may be needed to differentiate them.
- Acute confusion is a common presentation in the elderly, due to a wide variety of conditions. Non-convulsive status epilepticus is an uncommon cause, which should be considered if no other cause has been found (Chapter 14). Diagnosis is with EEG. Some patients have a history of epilepsy that may have been inactive since early adulthood but *de novo* presentation is also common.
- The EEG shows non-specific abnormalities in a high proportion of elderly patients. Some slowing of background rhythms is common and focal temporal slowing may be found in 30 to 40 percent of volunteers over the age of 60. This is usually secondary to cerebrovascular disease and should not be over-interpreted.
- Neuroimaging should be undertaken in elderly patients with new onset epilepsy, to exclude a tumor but other changes such as small vessel ischemia or atrophy are so common in asymptomatic patients they have little diagnostic value.

Epilepsy Syndromes in the Elderly

- Epilepsy syndromes in the elderly are usually focal.
- Generalized epilepsies rarely present in older age but a first presentation with absence status epilepticus is seen in this age group and needs to be considered in the differential diagnosis of confusional states.

Epilepsy and Stroke

- Stroke is responsible for about half of both acute symptomatic seizures and chronic epilepsy in the elderly. Five to 10 percent of cerebrovascular events are complicated by epilepsy. Intracerebral hemorrhage carries the greatest risk (15%) and lacunar infarction the lowest risk (2%). Embolic stroke carries a higher risk than thrombotic stroke.
- The pathophysiological basis of early post-stroke seizures may include lactic acidosis, cytotoxic edema with electrolyte imbalance, activation of NMDA receptors and downregulation of GABA. Factors in the mechanism of late seizures may include deposition of hemosiderin, which is highly epileptogenic, and reorganization of neural circuitry, predisposing to neural hyper-synchronization.
- Acute symptomatic seizures occur in 5 percent of strokes and may be the presenting feature. One tenth of these may be focal motor status epilepticus or sometimes generalized status epilepticus. Focal motor status after a stroke may last several days and usually resolves spontaneously, treatment usually has relatively little impact (Case 4, Chapter 14).
- Early seizures put the patient at 20 to 30 percent risk of later epilepsy but only a small minority of patients with stroke-related epilepsy have had early seizures.
- Fifty to 90 percent of epilepsy starts in the first year after a stroke and nearly all cases within 2 years.
- EEG is generally unhelpful in the diagnosis of post-stroke epilepsy.
- The prognosis of stroke-related epilepsy is usually good. Seizures are usually infrequent and about 90 percent are controlled by monotherapy.

Epilepsy and Dementia

- The incidence of seizures in dementias has been estimated from 2 to 16 percent. Seizures are usually tonic–clonic with no focal clinical features. They occur with low frequency and are usually easily controlled.
- Classical Creutzfeldt-Jakob disease is a rare, rapidly progressive dementia. It is complicated by prominent myoclonus in its final stages that may be very sensitive to startle stimuli.

Other Common Causes of Epilepsy in the Elderly

- Trauma is more likely to cause late epilepsy in the elderly than in any other age group.
- Medication usage is greatest in the elderly and may be responsible for up to 10 percent of acute symptomatic seizures (Chapter 13).
- Alcohol should not be forgotten as a cause of seizures in the elderly.
- Metabolic and systemic disturbances are responsible for up to 20 percent of acute symptomatic seizures, including hypoglycemia, hyperglycemia, hyponatremia, hypernatremia, hypercalcemia, hypoxia, hypotension, renal failure, hepatic failure or severe infection.

The Decision to Treat Epilepsy in the Elderly

- In favor of early treatment is that most late onset epilepsy is focal, and consequently has a very high risk of recurrence. Seizures may also have more severe consequences in the elderly. Falls lead to fractures that carry a significant morbidity and mortality. In Western cultures, many elderly patients live alone and have physical disability for example due to arthritis. They are often heavily dependent on their cars for shopping and social activity. Loss of their driving licence and the associated social withdrawal increase the pressure for early medical therapy of seizures.
- Against treatment are acute symptomatic seizures, which are common in the elderly. The elderly also suffer from an increased risk of adverse effects from medication, both because of increased sensitivity and from drug interactions with therapy for concomitant conditions.

Kinetics and Dynamics of Anti-Epileptic Drugs in the Elderly

- In the elderly, the kinetics of drugs may be altered by changes in absorption, distribution or elimination (Table 12.1).
- Reduced serum albumin in malnutrition or systemic disease such as renal disease, liver disease, rheumatoid arthritis or malignancy tends to cause a rise in unbound, active fractions of highly bound drugs such as phenytoin. Total phenytoin levels need to be adjusted in proportion to serum albumin.
- Renal clearance declines by 1 percent per year after age 40 and may reduce the required dosage for drugs, which are predominantly renally excreted such as gabapentin, levetiracetam or vigabatrin.
- Cytochrome P_{450} activity declines by 1 percent per year after age 40 and may reduce the required dosage for drugs metabolized through this system such as carbamazepine.
- Polypharmacy is most common in the elderly. This may cause pharmacokinetic and pharmacodynamic interactions (Chapter 9). For example, carbamazepine and oxcarbazepine often cause mild hyponatremia but when combined with a thiazide diuretic are more likely to precipitate symptomatic hyponatremia. The sensitivity of the aging brain to medications is increased and pharmacodynamic

Table 12.1. Age-Related Factors Affecting AED

Drug	Age-Related Factors	Recommendations
Carbamazepine	Reduced hepatic metabolism Increased tendency to ataxia	Slow dose titration and dosage reduction up to 40%
Gabapentin	Reduced renal function	Reduced dosage if impaired creatinine clearance
Lamotrigine	Increased tendency to ataxia	Dosage changes are minor
Phenobarbital	Increased sedative effect Reduced hepatic metabolism	Small dose reductions often necessary
Phenytoin	Reduced serum albumin Reduced metabolism	Initial dosage 3–4 mg/kg. Small dose increments. Total blood level proportionate to serum albumin
Valproate	Reduced serum albumin Reduced hepatic metabolism	Dosage may need to be reduced by 40%

interactions are enhanced. Nocturnal sedatives may exacerbate the cognitive adverse effects of AED.

Adverse Effects of Anti-Epileptic Drugs in the Elderly

- Altered pharmacokinetics and increased sensitivity to pharmacodynamic effects combine to increase the likelihood of adverse reactions in the elderly.
- Sedation and confusion are enhanced, especially if there is concomitant medication.
- Ataxia due to anti-epileptic drugs (AEDs), for example carbamazepine, phenobarbitone, phenytoin, and lamotrigine is enhanced, increasing the risk of falls.
- Osteoporosis may be exacerbated by phenytoin-induced osteomalacia, leading to more severe consequences from falls in seizures.
- Cardiac disturbance may be precipitated by drugs with sodium channel activity such as phenytoin and carbamazepine.
- Tremor and Parkinsonism may be exacerbated by valproate.

Choice of Medication in the Elderly

- There are no satisfactory comparative trials of AEDs in the elderly and medication should be guided in the first instance by epilepsy syndrome.
- Carbamazepine and phenytoin are somewhat less popular for elderly patients because of their adverse effect profile, especially their propensity to ataxia.
- Valproate has a broad spectrum of anti-epileptic efficacy, is often well tolerated and is available in a variety of forms, including liquid. It is indicated for patients with idiopathic generalized epilepsy (IGE) but may also have a broader role.
- Gabapentin and lamotrigine are also being used increasingly. Gabapentin has no major drug interactions and both drugs are reputed to have favorable adverse effect profiles in the elderly.

Case History 1

An 84-year-old man had suffered seizures as teenager and into his twenties, before they went into remission. Temporal lobe epilepsy (TLE) recurred in his seventies and was controlled with phenytoin, but he became unacceptably drowsy, despite "normal" phenytoin blood levels. His medication was changed to lamotrigine 150 milligrams daily, which rendered him seizure-free, without adverse effects.

Duration of Therapy in the Elderly

- Acute symptomatic seizures may require only brief therapy.
- Other causes of epilepsy, including dementia and cerebrovascular disease, tend to cause epilepsy that may be mild but persistent and recurs on drug withdrawal.
- Seizure freedom can be achieved in 70 percent of elderly patients. The morbidity of seizures is high in the elderly so that once a patient is established in a successful regime, lifelong treatment may be the safest course of action.

EPILEPSY AND LEARNING DISABILITY

- This section is concerned with the issues relating to the management of epilepsy in patients with pre-existing learning disability. The relationships between epilepsy and cognitive dysfunction are considered in more detail in Chapter 16.
- The prevalence of epilepsy among patients with severe learning disability (IQ < 70) is 20 to 30 percent and the lifetime prevalence may be over 50 percent. The more severe the developmental delay the higher the risk and the risk is also increased if there is associated cerebral palsy. Absence seizures are common and absence status epilepticus is seen much more frequently in the learning-disabled population.
- Epilepsy may be especially severe in this group of patients and most children with the malignant epilepsies of childhood (Chapter 11) have pre-existing developmental delay. These epilepsies lead to further cognitive decline and may compound retardation.
- Social aspects of epilepsy cause particular problems in this age group.

Etiology

- Many genetic disorders cause learning disability and seizures, common ones are Down syndrome, fragile X syndrome and neurocutaneous syndromes (Chapter 3). Tuberose sclerosis is especially likely to be associated with the severe epilepsies of childhood.
- Acquired intra-uterine causes include maternal infection, intra-uterine growth retardation, drugs and alcohol.
- Perinatal and postnatal causes include infections and intracranial vascular events.

Differential Diagnosis

- The diagnosis of seizures may be difficult in patients with severe learning disability. The patient may be unable to describe essential features such as subjective sensations, which a cognitively intact individual is able to report (Table 12.2).
- Stereotypic behaviors may mimic epilepsy and are common in patients with learning disability. For example staring into space, vocalizations or repeated movements, during which the individual may appear distracted or absent. These may represent a form of self-stimulation, on which the subject becomes emotionally dependent. Stereotopies are often more variable than seizures and may persist throughout much of the waking day. However, their clinical manifestations overlap with epilepsy and as both disorders are common in this patient group, video and EEG recordings may be needed to make a clear diagnosis.
- Dissociative reactions with violent motor activity mimicking a seizure are also common. Cognitive and personal limitations of the learning-disabled may make them feel more challenged by minor everyday stresses or changes in routine triggering these reactions.

Table 12.2. Aspects of Clinical Seizure Patterns Affecting Patients with Learning Disability

Seizure Pattern	Comments
Convulsive seizures	Common but often unclear whether focal or generalized onset
Atypical seizure symptoms	Common, including visceral symptoms, periodic headache, dizziness or paresthesiae
Absence status epilepticus	Commonest in this patient group
Recurrent tonic–clonic status epilepticus	Commonest in this patient group
Malignant epilepsies of childhood	Usually preceded by learning disability
Drop attacks	Commonest in learning disabled patients with severe epilepsy

Case History 2

A 38-year-old man had lived with his parents throughout his life. He had required special schooling and had never been in regular employment but attended a day centre with a workshop tailored to individuals with learning disability. Once a month he suffered brief tonic seizures affecting his right arm and sometimes leading to loss of consciousness. One year earlier his mother had died, following which he developed new episodes. These were characterized by vigorous shaking of the limbs and lasted up to 30 minutes. They occurred at times when he was asked to perform tasks such as dressing with which his mother would previously have helped him. He appeared initially unresponsive but when his father sat and talked gently to him, the movements would ease and eventually stop. Afterwards he was exhausted and slept. A home video confirmed the non-epileptic nature of the disorder.

This case illustrates the common co-existence of epileptic and non-epileptic disorders in patients with learning disability and the timing of the episodes to emotional stresses or changes in routine. The attacks are often rather longer than seizures and there may be evidence of responsiveness.

Electroencephalography

- The background EEG may be very abnormal in patients with severe learning disability. In some cases, the EEG may be so abnormal that it is difficult to discern a clear evolution of electrical discharges into the ictus. It is important to rely only on EEG abnormalities that have a high specificity for epilepsy in diagnosis of paroxysmal disorders.
- Video recording may be of most value in diagnosis.

Treatment

- The principles of treatment are the same for this group as for any other – the goal is seizure-freedom with no adverse effects.
- Seizure-freedom is probably more difficult to achieve than in any other patient group.
- Detecting adverse effects requires particular vigilance in the context of disability.

  1. Patients with motor deficits may be particularly prone to ataxia caused by phenytoin, carbamazepine or lamotrigine.

2. The cognitive effects of drugs are more difficult to detect when patients cannot give a history and the reports of carers are particularly important in detecting changes. A small improvement in seizures may not justify an impairment of cognition if the patient becomes more drowsy, less interactive or more difficult to care for (Case 3).
3. Behavioral disturbances are particularly likely in a group who may be unable to articulate their distress in any other way.

- Polypharmacy must be avoided in order to minimize adverse effects. Unhelpful AEDs should be discontinued.

Case History 3

A 21-year-old man had suffered severe perinatal problems and developed hydro-cephalus and developmental delay. He suffered severe epilepsy despite taking high doses of carbamazepine, topiramate and gabapentin. Gabapentin was withdrawn without a deterioration of his epilepsy but he became more alert and regained continence of feces and urine.

- Severe epilepsy may remain refractory and stopping medication may have other significant benefits.
- Frequent spike-wave discharges may interfere with cognitive function without necessarily causing frequent overt seizures.

Case History 4

An 18-year-old girl had a lifelong history of learning disability and seizures of unknown cause. Her seizures manifested as absences occurring several times each day, without aura but with manual and oro-alimentary automatisms. Between these she was quiet and passive, showing little interest in her surroundings. An EEG showed multifocal spike and wave discharges and neuroimaging was normal. She started treatment with lamotrigine and the frequency of overt absences decreased by about one-third. However she became brighter and started to look at magazines and develop hobbies such as cooking and caring for a pet rabbit. In some ways her parents found her more demanding as she was less passive but they felt greatly rewarded by her increased responsiveness. A repeat EEG showed that spike-wave discharges had reduced by more than 90 percent.

Even though overt seizures decreased only slightly there was a major change in behavior paralleled by a reduction in abnormal EEG activity. Carers can discover that a more alert patient may be more challenging to care for and other behavioral problems such as frustration can be unmasked.

Choice of Medication

Epilepsy syndrome determines the choice of drug in learning-disabled individuals as in any other patient. Although claims are made, there is no good evidence to suggest that one particular drug is indicated because it is being used in a disabled population. Malignant epilepsy syndromes are often associated with learning disability and may respond to a particular AED, for example vigabatrin in infantile spasms.

Absence seizures may be exacerbated by vigabatrin, gabapentin or tiagabine, which may even precipitate absence status epilepticus.

Social Aspects of Epilepsy and Learning Disability

- Developmental problems in numerous spheres may complicate learning disability, affecting education, personal and sexual development and employment.
- Individuals with severe epilepsy may become socially isolated. They are rejected by their peers and fail to develop normal friendships or sexual relationships.
- Support services may be unable to cope with severe epilepsy or bouts of status epilepticus. The patient may end up entirely dependent on family and carers.
- Aging parents reach a crisis point as they become unable to care for a severely disabled child. It may be difficult at this late stage to help the sufferer to a level of independent living and the only solution becomes some form of residential care.

Case History 5

A 44-year-old man had suffered with epilepsy and moderate learning disability. He had been cared for by devoted parents who had attended to his every need. His father died when he was 30 and his mother continued to look after him at home. He suffered seizures roughly once per week and attended a day centre but had no experience of independent living. His mother became ill and he was admitted to hospital as she was unable to continue caring for him. He remained in hospital for a long period and his medication was changed so that his seizures reduced to once per month. Many residential homes locally were unable to accommodate him and he was finally placed long-term into a residential centre specializing in epilepsy.

The supportive environment of his family had provided excellent care but had not nurtured the skills needed for any degree of independent living and as an adult these skills are harder to acquire.

BIBLIOGRAPHY

Proceedings of the Workshop on Epilepsy and Learning Disabilities. Troina, Italy, April 28–30, 2000. Epilepsia 2001;42 Suppl 1:1–61.

Besag FM, Wallace SJ, Dulac O, Alving J, Spencer SC, Hosking G. Lamotrigine for the treatment of epilepsy in childhood. J Pediatr 1995;127:991–997.

Cloyd JC, Lackner TE, Leppik IE. Anti-epileptics in the elderly: pharmacoepidemiology and pharmacokinetics. Arch Fam Med 1994;3:589–598.

Crawford P, Brown S, Kerr M. A randomized open-label study of gabapentin and lamotrigine in adults with learning disability and resistant epilepsy. Seizure 2001;10:107–115.

Dey AB, Stout NR, Kenny RA. Cardiovascular syncope is the most common cause of drop attacks in the elderly. Pacing Clin Electrophysiol 1997;20:818–819.

Everitt AD, Sander JW. Incidence of epilepsy is now higher in elderly people than children [letter; comment]. BMJ 1998;316:780.

Paul A (1997). Epilepsy or stereotypy? Diagnostic issues in learning disabilities. Seizure 1997; 6:111–120.

Rowan AJ, Ramsay RE. Seizures and Epilepsy in the Elderly. Boston: Butterworth-Heinemann 1997.

Siemes H, Brandl U, Spohr HL, Volger S, Weschke B. Long-term follow-up study of vigabatrin in pretreated children with West syndrome. Seizure 1998;7:293–297.

Stephen LJ, Brodie MJ. Epilepsy in elderly people. Lancet 2000;355:1441–1446.

SECTION 4
Special Situations

13

Acute Symptomatic Seizures

INTRODUCTION AND EPIDEMIOLOGY

- Acute symptomatic seizures (ASS, synonyms provoked seizures, situation related seizures) are seizures occurring in the context of acute illness. The illness may be a direct brain insult such as stroke or a secondary effect of a wide variety of metabolic and toxic conditions (Table 13.1).
- The lifetime risk of a symptomatic seizure is 3 to 5 percent.
- Acute symptomatic seizures represent about 40 percent of presentations with first seizures in community-based studies.
- Men suffer ASS nearly twice as commonly as women, because of higher rates of common causes such as head injury and alcoholism.
- ASS are commonest in the first year of life, relating to perinatal insults and then decline to a low level between age 10 and 40. After that age they increase steadily in parallel with the illnesses that trigger them.
- The prognosis of ASS is generally good, better than for unprovoked seizures, if the provoking illness is non-recurring. Some causes are recurring, for example alcoholism and some cause cerebral damage predisposing to later unprovoked epilepsy, for example stroke.

Table 13.1. Relative Frequency of Common Causes of Provoked Seizures

Cause	Percentage of Acute Symptomatic Seizures
Head trauma	15%
Infection	15%
Stroke	15–30% (strongly age-dependent)
Drugs and alcohol	15–30%
Metabolic	10%

GENERAL MANAGEMENT

- A wide variety of common conditions may cause seizures during the acute phase of illness.

  1. Intracranial causes: head injury, cerebral vascular events, intracranial infection (meningitis, cerebral abscess or encephalitis) and neurosurgical procedures
  2. Extracranial causes: alcohol withdrawal, drug intoxication or drug withdrawal, metabolic disturbance including liver disease, renal disease, cardiac or respiratory disease causing significant hypoxia, diabetic coma, especially hypoglycemia or hyperosmolar non-ketotic coma, electrolyte disturbances including sodium, potassium, calcium and magnesium and eclampsia, myxedema and Hashimoto's encephalopathy

- For a patient presenting with their first seizure, the clinician needs to differentiate between the first attack of unprovoked epilepsy and an acute symptomatic seizure.
- Clinical clues to the presence of an acute cause include:

  1. A history of any of the causes above
  2. A significant prodromal illness prior to the onset of seizures
  3. Fever (although this may occasionally be due to the seizure itself) or other signs of intracranial infection such as neck stiffness
  4. Focal neurological signs
  5. Delayed recovery after the seizure (longer than 2 hours)
  6. Recurrent seizures or status epilepticus.

- Investigation of seizures thought to be acute symptomatic seizures includes:

  1. Venous blood for urea, electrolytes, glucose, calcium, magnesium, liver function
  2. Arterial blood gases
  3. Toxicology in urine or blood where appropriate
  4. Urgent neuroimaging especially if there are focal neurological signs
  5. CSF analysis if there is fever or other signs of intracranial infection or prolonged unconsciousness, providing neuroimaging does not contraindicate lumbar puncture

- Management of these conditions comprises three aspects:

  1. Treatment of the underlying cause.
  2. Acute anti-epileptic treatment where seizures are life-threatening, prolonged or recurrent. The principles are the same as those for status epilepticus (Chapter 14). Firstly, stop the seizures for example with a benzodiazepine. Secondly, keep them away with a rapidly acting anti-epileptic drug (AED), for example phenytoin, fosphenytoin, phenobarbital or sometimes valproate.
  3. Long-term treatment is not always indicated as some conditions may be non-recurring and others such as alcohol withdrawal may be unaffected by long-term AEDs.

SPECIFIC CAUSES OF ACUTE SYMPTOMATIC SEIZURES

Seizures Following Head Injury

- Concussive seizures occurring within seconds of an impact to the head were first described on the sports field. The patient stiffens, collapses to the ground, convulses then recovers after 20 to 30 minutes. This is not associated with identifiable intracranial damage and no treatment is required. There is no increased risk of later epilepsy.
- Early post-traumatic seizures (within one week of injury) occur in patients with severe head injuries. Although some features of more severe injuries may be associated with the later development of epilepsy (Chapter 4), early post-traumatic seizures do not themselves confer any additional risk. A brief period of AED therapy may be needed to control early post-traumatic seizures, but this can be withdrawn early.
- Prophylactic AEDs after head injury do not prevent later epilepsy and treatment should wait until seizures occur.

Seizures Associated with Neurosurgery

- Neurosurgery is controlled brain injury and the same principles apply with respect to seizures. The risk of seizures following neurosurgery depends on the nature and location of the pathology for which surgery is being undertaken.
- Infratentorial lesions carry a low risk of peri-operative or post-operative seizures.
- Supratentorial lesions carry a higher risk of seizures. The highest risk are infectious (>25% risk), neoplastic (25% risk) or vascular malformations, within the brain substance.
- Extra-parenchymal lesions such as subdural hematomas less frequently cause seizures. Infectious lesions are an exception: epilepsy complicates one quarter of subdural empyemas, probably due to secondary vascular changes in adjacent brain substance.
- Hydrocephalus carries a low risk of seizures. Seizures follow ventriculo-peritoneal shunting in approximately 7 percent, probably partly attributable to surgery and partly to the shunt (a potentially epileptogenic foreign body) left *in situ*.

- Prophylactic AEDs do not affect the risk of developing later unprovoked seizures and AED therapy should be reserved until after seizures have developed.

METABOLIC AND TOXIC CAUSES OF ACUTE SYMPTOMATIC SEIZURES

- Metabolic or toxic causes of seizures are common. Over 10 percent of patients admitted to intensive care units for non-neurological reasons develop neurological complications and in 25 percent of these the problem includes seizures.
- With metabolic causes of seizures, the risk depends on the rate of change of the metabolic parameter as well as its absolute level.

Seizures Associated with Alcohol

Epidemiology

- Seizures occur in up to 10 to 35 percent of patients with high alcohol ingestion.
- The risk of alcohol-related seizures is strongly dose-related. A daily consumption, over 200 milligrams per day confers a high risk.
- The seizures are usually tonic–clonic, but focal seizures may occur in 10 percent of cases.
- Alcoholism may affect up to 15 percent of patients with pre-existing epilepsy.

Pathophysiology

- Alcohol-related seizures may result from a variety of mechanisms:

  1. Acute alcohol withdrawal in a binge drinker
  2. Delirium tremens: acute alcohol withdrawal in a chronically dependent drinker
  3. Pre-existing epilepsy exacerbated by alcohol withdrawal, especially idiopathic generalized epilepsy
  4. Acute Wernicke's encephalopathy in a chronic drinker. This syndrome is also characterized by reduce consciousness, confusion, ataxia and nystagmus. It occurs in malnourished drinkers and is due to thiamine deficiency
  5. Acute metabolic disturbances secondary to alcohol such as hypoglycemia, hepatic encephalopathy or hyponatremia
  6. Focal brain damage secondary to trauma from recurrent falls with head injury in chronic drinkers
  7. Cerebral atrophy from the chronic neurotoxic effects of alcohol

- Alcohol inhibits N-methyl-D-aspartate (NMDA)-induced calcium fluxes and enhances chloride fluxes. These anti-epileptic effects cause an upregulation of excitatory NMDA receptors and downregulation of chloride. Abrupt alcohol withdrawal unmasks these compensatory changes leaving a hyperexcitable state, predisposing to seizures. Alcohol withdrawal may also have a kindling-like effect on seizures.

Clinical Diagnosis

- About half of alcoholic patients deny their alcohol consumption. There are no reliable biochemical markers for excessive alcohol ingestion. The most sensitive is probably carbohydrate-depleted transferrin, but it is affected by AEDs, gender of the patient and body mass index. Studies have consistently shown that the best indicator of alcohol ingestion is clinical suspicion.
- Alcohol withdrawal is the commonest cause of seizures in alcoholics. Seizures usually occur 6 to 48 hours after cessation of alcohol ingestion.
- Other complications of alcohol or coincidental pathologies need to be considered, including hyponatremia, subdural hematoma, acute hepatic encephalopathy, intracranial tumor and bacterial meningitis including tuberculous meningitis. Six percent of alcoholics admitted with seizures may have another cause on investigation.
- Blood tests and brain imaging should be undertaken to exclude these causes at first presentation and CSF should be analyzed if the patient's recovery from the seizure is slow or there are other suspicious features such as focal seizures, seizures after 48 hours, fever or neck stiffness.

Management

- Thiamine should be prescribed both acutely and long-term to any patient with chronic alcoholism, to try and prevent Wernicke's encephalopathy and Korsakoff's psychosis.
- Acute alcohol withdrawal, may occur through choice or circumstance, for example when admitted to hospital with intercurrent illness. Seizures can be prevented by substituting a benzodiazepine or chlormethiazole and phasing drug withdrawal.
- If additional treatment is required acutely, a barbiturate should be used, such as phenobarbital. Phenytoin has no effect on alcohol-withdrawal seizures.
- Withdrawal seizures carry a high risk of evolving into delirium tremens, which has a significant mortality. Patients with seizures should be observed for 72 hours, until this complication can reasonably be excluded. A benzodiazepine should be given in tapering dosage during this time.
- Abstention is the only effective long-term treatment for alcohol-related seizures. Chronic AEDs carry numerous problems in this patient group and are of little proven benefit. Poor compliance leads to a cycle of drug ingestion and withdrawal with the potential for withdrawal seizures. Fluctuating liver function leads to unpredictable blood AED levels that may be subtherapeutic or toxic. AED treatment may be precipitate or worsen hepatic encephalopathy in patients with critical liver function.
- AED should probably be reserved for patients with severe or frequent seizures or those in whom there is good evidence that excessive alcohol consumption has ceased. Carbamazepine has been reported to be of some value in treatment of alcohol-related seizures but is prone to withdrawal seizures. Valproate may be a reasonable choice, but if liver function is severely impaired, it could theoretically precipitate hyperammonemic encephalopathy. Gabapentin is unproven but is a theoretical choice as the only purely renally excreted first line AED with low toxicity.

Other Drugs of Abuse – See Table 13.2

Liver Failure

- Depression of mental function is a hallmark of liver failure and in severe cases may lead to seizures, irrespective of the cause of liver failure. In many cases, the condition is due to alcohol and the combination of liver failure and acute alcohol withdrawal commonly causes seizures.
- Reye's syndrome should be considered in patients with liver failure and seizures. It is commonest in children and is associated with aspirin, but may affect adults.
- The diagnosis of hepatic encephalopathy is not always straightforward as standard test of liver function may be non-contributory. Hyperammonemia may be diagnostically helpful in some cases.
- The EEG may show characteristic triphasic waves in hepatic encephalopathy.
- The choice and dose of medication is influenced by its effect on liver disease, by its effect on mental function and by its pharmacokinetics.
- Benzodiazepines are effective in stopping seizures in patients with liver failure but must be used with caution as they may increase sedation and encephalopathy.
- Phenytoin and carbamazepine may be effective in controlling seizures but deteriorating liver function may cause unpredictable blood levels, which should be monitored very regularly in these patients.
- Valproate is a rare cause of hepatic failure in children. Many clinicians would be cautious about using it in this context.
- Gabapentin and levetiracetam are entirely renally excreted and may be a logical choice for patients with liver disease but there are no trials to support their use.

Renal Failure

- Ten percent of patients with severe renal failure suffer seizures.
- Seizures are caused through electrolyte disturbances or as a result of encephalopathy when renal failure becomes severe.
- Blood urea nitrogen is a poor predictor of seizures.
- The commonest clinical sequence is for the patient to develop asterixis evolving to multifocal myoclonus then to tonic–clonic seizures.
- Most drugs used in the treatment of epilepsy are predominantly metabolized in the liver. Nevertheless when glomerular filtration rate (GFR) falls below 10 milliliters per minute, blood levels of carbamazepine and phenytoin should be monitored, as they become less predictable.
- Gabapentin is renally excreted and dosage should be adjusted in proportion to the reduction of GFR.
- The proportion of a drug removed during dialysis depends on the proportion free in plasma. Those drugs highly bound to plasma proteins are preferred as they are least dialyzed and dosages are least likely to need adjustment (Table 13.2).

Table 13.2. Drugs Which Can Affect Epilepsy

Drug Group	Approximate Risk of Seizures	Best Drugs	Worst Drugs	Comments
Antidepressants	0.5–4%	Moclobemide Citalopram Nefazodone	Tricyclics Fluoxetine Paroxetine	Seizure risk is dose related and usually occurs early in treatment. Risk of seizures in overdose is 10%
Antipsychotics	0.5–1%	Butyrephenones Sulpiride Pimozide	Chlorpromazine (1.2–9%) Clozapine (4%) Lithium (in overdose)	Incidence of seizures is closely dose-related
Antihistamines	Uncertain		Ethylenedienes Ethanolamines e.g. diphenhydramine	Case reports of focal seizures triggered from existing focal lesions. Rare status epilepticus, children are particularly susceptible. Many of these drugs are available over the counter
Antimicrobials	Variable	Aminoglycosides	Quinolones (0.9–2.1%)	Quinolones enhance glutamate activity and have synergistic epileptogenicity with theophyllines
		Cephalosporins Tetracyclines	Penicillins (0.3%) Imipenem Metronidazole Isoniazid (1–3%)	Penicillins may cause focal seizures at sites of breaches blood brain barrier Isoniazid-induced seizures are reduced by prescribing pyridoxine
Analgesics	Low		Pethidine	Pethidine-induced seizures are commonest in renal impairment and in combination with monoamine oxidase inhibitors
Theophyllines	Seizures in 8.2% in overdose			Synergistic proconvulsive effect with quinolones. Probably act via adenosine receptor. Valproate or barbiturates are probably best treatment
Antimalarials		Proguanil Tetracyclines	Mefloquine	Risk of mefloquine is clearly greatest in patients with a history of seizures or psychiatric illness
Glucocorticoids				Confusional states, psychosis and seizures in occasional patients at normal doses
Anti-neoplastic and immunosuppressive agents	About 1%	Fluorouracil Busulphan Azathioprine Vinca Alkaloids Bleomycin Anthracyclines	Cyclosporin (1–3%) Tacrolimus Asparaginase Chlorambucil (5%)	Cyclosporin causes a reversible encephalopathy with abnormal neuroimaging, most commonly at high blood levels Asparaginase causes seizures through hemorrhagic or thrombotic cerebrovascular events Chlorambucil reproduces generalized spike-wave activity in rats
General anesthetics		Thiopentone Propofol	Enflurane Isoflurane	Although general anesthetics are used in the treatment of status epilepticus, low doses of thiopentone can enhance EEG signs of epilepsy and enflurane is proconvulsant at higher doses
Drugs of abuse		Cannabinoids	Alcohol – see text Cocaine Ecstasy	2.5% of hospital attendance in cocaine abusers relates to seizures: exacerbations of pre-existing epilepsy or acute symptomatic seizures Heroin causes occasional seizures as other opiates. Seizures are a common toxic effect of ecstasy Seizures are less common with amphetamine than with cocaine but risk is dose-related Cannabinoids have some anticonvulsant effect

Table 13.3. Dialysis of Different AEDs

Highly Dialyzed	Least Dialyzed
Ethosuximide	Carbamazepine
Gabapentin	Phenytoin
Lamotrigine	Valproate
Levetiracetam	Topiramate
Oxcarbazepine	
Phenobarbital	
Piracetam	
Primidone	

Hypoglycemia

- Acute symptomatic seizures may occur if the blood sugar drops below 2.2 millimoles per liter.
- Hypoglycemic treatment for diabetes mellitus is the main cause. Other drugs may cause hypoglycemia as an incidental effect, including quinine and pentamidine. Insulinoma is rare and often difficult to diagnose.
- Patients classically have a premonitory phase of minutes to hours of confusion, agitation and sympathetic activation followed by a tonic–clonic seizure.
- Hypoglycemic attacks may mimic nocturnal epilepsy. Nocturnal hypoglycemia is common and a sleeping patient is less aware of the premonitory symptoms.
- Atypical or focal attacks may occur. Patients who take beta-blockers or who have had repeated hypoglycemic attacks may not experience the premonitory phase as they have become habituated.

Hyperglycemia

- Hyperglycemic non-ketotic coma (HONC) is commonly associated with seizures (Case 8, Chapter 14). Hyperglycemia is intrinsically epileptogenic and levels of blood glucose triggering seizures may be as low as 15 to 20 millimoles per liter, if there is associated significant hyperosmolarity. Cerebrovascular disease is often present.
- Focal seizures are common including focal status epilepticus. The commonest pattern is focal motor status, which may last for days. Treatment is by correction of the metabolic abnormality and antiepileptic drugs have relatively little effect.
- Diabetic ketoacidosis is not particularly associated with seizures.

Thyroid Disease

- Myxedema coma is now rare but severe hypothyroidism causes seizures in 20 percent of cases.
- Hashimoto's encephalopathy is associated with autoimmune thyroid disease. It is a rare, relapsing, subacute encephalopathy. Patients present with behavioral disturbance and cognitive decline, evolving over days to weeks. They develop

myoclonus, tonic–clonic seizures and depressed consciousness with focal neurological signs. Investigations do not reveal another cause but antithyroid antibodies are usually at very high titers. Glucocorticoids reverse the condition within hours. AEDs have little effect.

Electrolyte Disturbances

- Numerous electrolyte disturbances may trigger seizures, especially if the rate of change is rapid.
- Hyponatremia is commonest, which usually does not cause seizures until sodium falls below 115 millimoles per liter in blood.
- Others causes are hypernatremia, hypocalcemia, hypercalcemia, hypomagnasemia, hyperkalemia and hypokalemia.

Drug-Induced Seizures

- CNS-active drugs carry the greatest risk of drug-induced seizures (Table 13.2). Virtually all such drugs may cause this complication from time to time.
- Other drugs may also occasionally cause seizures.
- The mechanism of generating seizures may be a direct consequence of a drug's main mode of action. For example theophyllines act on adenosine that seems to have endogenous antiepileptic activity. Epileptogenicity may be a secondary effect, for example penicillins are highly effective convulsants when applied directly to the cerebral cortex, completely separate from their action on bacterial cell walls.
- Anti-epileptic drugs may sometimes have a paradoxical proconvulsant activity and the clinician must be alert to this possibility (Case 10, Chapter 9).

BIBLIOGRAPHY

Denison H, Berkowicz A, Wendestam C, Wallerstedt S. Ischemic heart disease and epilepsy: two major causes of out-hospital natural death in male alcoholics. Forensic Sci Int 1995;73:19–33.

Genton P. When antiepileptic drugs aggravate epilepsy. Brain Dev 2000;22:75–80.

Hart YM, Sander JWAS, Johnson AL, Shorvon SD. National general practice study of epilepsy: recurrence after a first seizure. Lancet 1990;336:1271–1274.

Ng KS, Brust JCM, Hauser WA, Susser M. Illicit drug use and the risk of new-onset seizures. Am J Epidemiol 1990;132:47–57.

Ng KS, Hauser WA, Brust JCM, Susser M. Alcohol consumption and withdrawal in new-onset seizures. N Engl J Med 1988;319:666–673.

Venna N, Sabin TD. Tonic focal seizures in nonketotic hyperglycemia of diabetes mellitus. Arch Neurol 1981;38:512–514.

Zaccara G, Muscas GC, Messori A. Clinical features, pathogenesis and management of drug-induced seizures. Drug Safety 1990;5:109–151.

14

Status Epilepticus

DEFINITIONS

- Status epilepticus is seizures occurring continuously or recurrently for at least 30 minutes without recovery. Most seizures stop within 5 minutes and there is a significant risk of evolving into status epilepticus if a seizure lasts longer than five minutes.
- Convulsive status epilepticus (CSE) is immediately life-threatening and non-convulsive status epilepticus is dangerous and may evolve into CSE.

PATHOPHYSIOLOGY

- Children are more susceptible to status than adults, pointing to a developmental influence.
- A positive feedback loop may stimulate a seizure circuit into status. In temporal lobe epilepsy (TLE), intimate connections with the adjacent entorhinal cortex may provide this re-entrant function. Status is more likely to occur in brain slices if the original animal had a previous history of epilepsy, suggesting some kind of conditioning process.

• As status proceeds, GABAergic mechanisms fail and the ability of benzodiazepines to terminate status through GABA also declines within hours. Later the ability of other anti-epileptic drugs (AEDs) to stop status is also affected and this may be due to failure of ion homeostasis – phenytoin acts through sodium channels. This causes excess glutamatergic activity which may result in secondary neurotoxicity.

EPIDEMIOLOGY OF STATUS EPILEPTICUS

• The population incidence of all status epilepticus is probably 441 to 646 per million and of convulsive status epilepticus of 180 to 280 per million (Table 14.1).
• Status epilepticus is the first presentation of epilepsy in 12 percent of patients.
• The age-related incidence of status epilepticus follows a U-shaped curve, reflecting the incidence of epilepsy as a whole.
• Status is commoner in males at all ages.
• Recurrence is common only in children under 5 years old. Most patients suffer status epilepticus only once.
• Children are more commonly affected by status epilepticus, 4 to 8 per 1,000 children may develop status before the age of 15. Status affects 5 to 10 percent of all patients with epilepsy and 16 to 24 percent of children with epilepsy under the age of 16. In a series of 239 children with status, 37 percent were under the age of 1 and 85 percent were under 5. In 76 percent of children with status, it is the first epileptic event. Approximately 70 percent of neonatal seizures and 5 percent of febrile seizures manifest as status.

ETIOLOGY OF STATUS EPILEPTICUS

• The age of the patient and their previous history determine the likely etiology of status epilepticus. Risk factors for status epilepticus include symptomatic seizures, especially lesions of the frontal lobes and mental handicap.
• First presentation of epilepsy with status often means a serious cause. Status in the context of pre-existing epilepsy is much less likely to have a new, serious cause and is commonly due to AED withdrawal.

Table 14.1. Epidemiology of Status Epilepticus

Diagnosis	Incidence Per 1, 000, 000 Persons
Newly diagnosed epilepsy with convulsive status	80
Established epilepsy with convulsive status	40–80
Febrile seizures with convulsive status	20–40
Acute symptomatic seizures	40–80
Non-convulsive status in mentally handicapped	100–200
Neonatal status	120
Other	41–46
Total	441–646

Adapted from Shorvon 1994, with permission.

- At all ages hypoxia, trauma, metabolic disturbances, tumors or cerebrovascular disease are common causes of status.
- Most cases of neonatal status are associated with a serious cause, for example infection, hypoxic-ischemic encephalopathy, cerebral malformations, or hypoglycemia.
- In older children, acute causes become less likely and chronic encephalopathies or status epilepticus secondary to previous epilepsy become more common. Approximately half of childhood cases are idiopathic and about half of these are due to febrile status epilepticus. Febrile seizures most commonly cause status between six months and three years of age. Fixed lesions, such as cerebral malformations, continue to cause status into later life.

Case History 1

An 82-year-old woman had suffered epilepsy since childhood that had been treated with methobarbital. When this drug was withdrawn from use her GP converted her to an equivalent dose of phenobarbital. The drug was dispensed as a liquid, which was too heavy for her to carry home, so she stopped her medication. She was admitted to hospital in a fugue-like state and with a convulsive seizure. She remained in absence status epilepticus, which did not respond to loading with valproate, but responded rapidly to intravenous phenobarbital.

This case illustrates an unusual cause of status epilepticus due to treatment withdrawal. It shows that status due to AED withdrawal tends to respond to reinstituting the missing AED rather than trying something else.

MORTALITY AND MORBIDITY OF STATUS EPILEPTICUS

- The overall mortality of status epilepticus in community-based studies is approximately 23 percent but is strongly age-dependent. Under age 15 it is less than 10 percent; from age 16 to 59 mortality is about 13 percent and over the age of 60 it is 38 percent.
- Convulsive status epilepticus carries a higher risk than other forms.
- The incidence of new neurological deficits after convulsive status is 9.1 percent of survivors in childhood.
- The cause of status epilepticus is the main determinant of outcome.
- The duration of status epilepticus is another major factor.

STAGES OF CONVULSIVE STATUS EPILEPTICUS

1. Prestatus is a phase of escalating seizures lasting hours to days, which precedes status epilepticus in many cases. Treatment at this stage may prevent status.
2. Early status is the first 30 minutes when there is continuous convulsive seizure activity paralleled by continuous electrographic seizure activity. The metabolic consequences of status are contained by homeostatic mechanisms (Figure 14.1, Table 14.5).
3. Established status occurs from 30 to 60 minutes when homeostatic mechanisms start to fail and there is unmet demand. From about 60 minutes decompensation occurs and there are major changes in vital parameters.

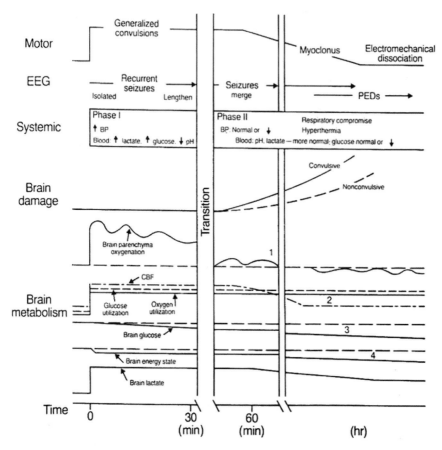

Figure 14.1. Systemic changes in status epilepticus. Reproduced with permission from Lothman 1990.

4. Refractory status lasts over 1 hour and persists despite first-line treatments There is a high risk of brain injury for example from hypoxic-ischemic damage or hypoglycemia.
5. Subtle status may emerge if the seizures are maintained for hours. Convulsive motor activity gradually declines in amplitude and extent. Coma deepens and the motor manifestations may become limited to just twitches around the eyes or mouth. The diagnosis is easily missed at this stage. This sequence is paralleled by changes in the EEG: the electrographic seizures merge and the EEG becomes flattened between discharges. Periodic lateralized epileptiform discharges appear in the later stages. Mortality of subtle status is 65 percent compared to 27 percent for overt status in adults, probably mediated via glutamatergic excitotoxic damage.

CHRONIC NEURONAL TOXICITY OF STATUS EPILEPTICUS

- Seizures induced acutely in animals may lead to later epilepsy. Whether the same occurs in humans is not yet clear. The animal models show that status epilepticus is associated with loss of cells in hippocampal regions CA1 and CA3 and alterations in the sensitivity of $GABA_A$ receptors that may themselves predispose to epilepsy.

- In humans, status epilepticus is associated with acute changes in hippocampal neurons in Sommer's sector This region is implicated in the etiology of mesial temporal epilepsy. In addition, prolonged febrile seizures of childhood are associated with later mesial temporal lobe epilepsy providing circumstantial evidence of the epileptogenicity of status epilepticus, especially in children.
- Status epilepticus may cause typical MRI changes of mesial temporal sclerosis (MTS). In an experiment of nature some individuals accidently ingested a glutamate agonist, domoic acid. This caused an encephalopathy with status epilepticus and some went on to suffer partial epilepsy associated with histological changes of hippocampal sclerosis, supporting excitotoxic mechanisms in the etiology of MTS.

DIAGNOSIS OF STATUS EPILEPTICUS

The clinical presentation, diagnosis and differential diagnosis of status epilepticus depend on the clinical form of the disorder (Table 14.2).

Table 14.2. Differential Diagnosis of Different Presentations of Status Epilepticus

Clinical Presentation	Alternative Differential Diagnoses
Prolonged convulsion	Psychogenic non-epileptic seizure (PNES), hypoglycemic agitation
Confusional state	Toxic or metabolic disorder, PNES
Coma*	Structural brain lesion, metabolic disorder, drug overdose, infection including CNS infection
Progressive aphasia (usually children)	Focal structural lesion
Prolonged focal motor activity	Movement disorder, PNES

*Status epilepticus, especially myoclonic status, is a common complication of coma due to other causes as well as a cause of coma itself.

CONVULSIVE STATUS EPILEPTICUS (CSE)

Clinical Presentation

Convulsive status epilepticus evolves through the stages of prestatus, early status, established status and subtle status (above).

Management of Convulsive Status Epilepticus

The principles of management are

1. Standard first aid
2. Diagnose the seizure disorder

3. Treating seizures
    (a) Prestatus
    (b) Stopping status
    (c) Keeping seizures away
    (d) Refractory status
4. Treat the complications of the seizures
5. Diagnose and treat the cause of the seizures

Standard First Aid

-   The patient should be nursed in the recovery position on the floor or on a bed with sides, to prevent falls and injury. Dangerous or sharp objects should be removed from near the patient.
-   Oxygen should be administered but interfering with the airway during the convulsive episode may cause broken teeth, bleeding and aspiration.
-   Intravenous access should be established to administer fluids and drugs.

Diagnosis of the Seizure Disorder

-   Epileptic seizures are difficult to differentiate from psychogenic non-epileptic seizures (PNES) and the two types may co-exist in the same patient.
-   About 80 percent of patients with convulsive status epilepticus respond to first-line treatment on arrival in hospital. Around half the remainder have PNES mimicking status epilepticus.
-   Ictal EEG is best way of differentiating PNES from epilepsy but in the UK EEG is rarely available at presentation. The following guidelines may helpful:

    1. Incongruous clinical signs point to PNES. A single clinical feature should not be taken in isolation, the whole clinical picture needs to be included to make a diagnosis (Table 14.3 and Case 2).
    2. Hypoxia is rare in attacks with a psychological cause.
    3. Serum prolactin is generally unhelpful.
    4. If in doubt treat as epilepsy and seek specialist advice.

Case History 2

A 48-year-old woman had a large left fronto-parietal arteriovenous malformation, causing monthly focal motor seizures affecting her right arm with speech disturbance. There had recently been increasing problems with her ability to perform her secretarial work. She was admitted to hospital in a state of agitation with bilateral motor activity. Careful examination revealed dystonic posturing and jerking of her right arm and flailing of her left limbs with facial flushing and agitation. This was followed by flailing of all four limbs. The motor activity ceased after intravenous phenobarbital 12 milligrams per kilogram and she went to sleep. Repeated admissions followed a similar pattern. Clinically it appeared that she was suffering her well-defined focal motor seizures but that these were triggering panic and widespread and prolonged, abnormal motor activity. The threat to her job seemed to be the trigger for this change. After psychiatric treatment for her anxiety, the flailing component ceased. She settled back into the previous pattern of self-limiting focal motor seizures and was able to resume her normal life.

Table 14.3. Differentiation of Status Epilepticus and Psychogenic Non-Epileptic Seizures

Clinical Signs	Epilepsy	Non-Epileptic Seizures
Seizure activity	Attacks initially continuous or well-defined	Continuously fluctuating motor activity
Seizure variability	Usually stereotyped	Often variable
Eye deviation	Where present, fixed to one side	Always looks away from examiner
Tongue biting	Major injuries to sides of the tongue	Minor injuries to the tip of tongue
Cyanosis	Common	Rare but patient may look purple from Valsalva maneuver
Self protection during convulsion	No attempts at self protection.	Patient may withdraw from noxious stimuli.
Pattern of motor activity	Tonic with limb jerking commonest	Truncal and pelvic movements commonest
Responsiveness of motor activity	Activity continues independent of external stimuli	Activity is altered by external stimuli, often more violent when attempts are made at restraint

A new seizure pattern merits full assessment. It may be due to evolution of the underlying pathology, a change in the response to treatment or a completely new problem. In this case PNES evolved from epileptic attacks. Ictal EEG and close observation may be needed to make an accurate diagnosis.

Investigation of Convulsive Status Epilepticus

- The urgency and pattern of investigation depend on the likelihood of a serious cause (see Figure 14.3).
- All cases should have blood for blood count, electrolytes, renal function, liver function, glucose, calcium, magnesium, and AED levels, arterial blood gases, and urine for toxicology. All *de novo* cases should have a brain scan and if normal, a CSF examination. Patients with known epilepsy should also be investigated as *de novo* cases unless they recover to normal with treatment within 2 hours.

Treatment of Status Epilepticus

- Treatment depends on the stage of the status epilepticus, on whether it is a first presentation of epilepsy, previous AEDs taken, including recent AED changes, and any other potential causes (Figure 14.2).
- AED withdrawal is generally best treated by re-instituting the missing drug (Case 1).
- The urgency of treatment often means the clinician does not know the patient's previous treatment when making therapeutic decisions.
- There may be only 30 to 60 minutes available to attempt simpler treatments before the patient should be anaesthetized.

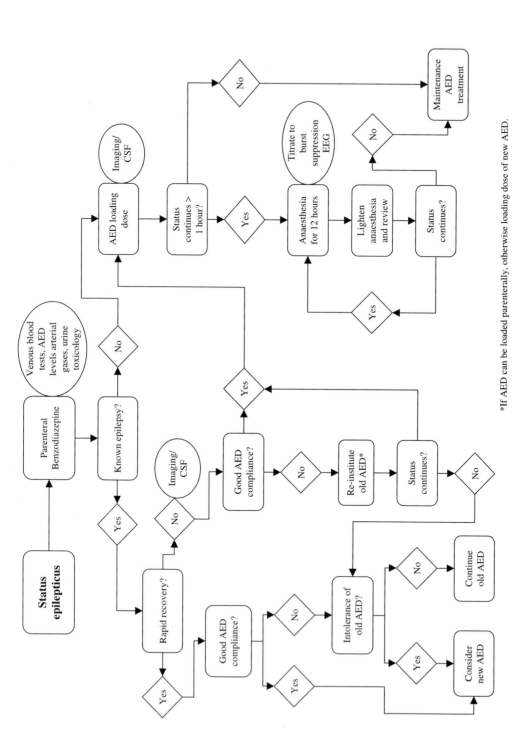

Figure 14.2. A scheme for the management of status epilepticus, illustrating the crucial differentiation of patients into *de novo* cases and those with known epilepsy.

*If AED can be loaded parenterally, otherwise loading dose of new AED.

Prestatus

- The recognition and aggressive treatment of prestatus may prevent status from ever occurring. This is easiest in those patients with a past history of epilepsy. in whom an escalation of seizures is readily recognizable. A benzodiazepine may stop a seizure cluster from evolving into status.
- If the patient is alert between seizures, oral clobazam 10 to 20 milligrams may stop the cluster of seizures and can be continued as 10 to 20 milligrams daily over a few days until the risk period is over or more permanent treatment is established.
- If the seizures are very close together or the patient is drowsy, an alternative route of benzodiazepine administration is safer (Table 14.4).
- Urgent measurement of AED blood levels may help decide whether the problem is due to treatment failure.

Stopping Status Epilepticus

- A benzodiazepine aborts status in about 80 percent of cases and the main risk is 10 percent of respiratory depression.
- Lorazepam is the drug of choice. It works as fast as diazepam but the rate of relapse of status is much lower: 55 percent at 24 hours, compared to 50 percent at two hours for diazepam. Additional therapy must be instituted promptly after a benzodiazepine.
- Phenobarbital has similar efficacy to lorazepam in adults but may cause more hypotension.
- Paraldehyde is an irritant drug and is difficult to use but has the advantage of rarely causing respiratory depression.

Keeping Seizures Away

- Once seizures have stopped, treatment needs to be given to prevent recurrence.
- AED should be reinstated if status is due to AED withdrawal and the relevant drug can be given as loading dose.
- IV phenytoin 15 to 18 milligrams per kilogram can be infused slowly with cardiac monitoring. Mild local reactions/phlebitis are common and severe local reactions (purple glove syndrome) or cardiac depression may occur. Fosphenytoin can be given IM or IV and is rapidly converted to phenytoin in the liver. Onset of effect is almost as fast as IV phenytoin and efficacy is equivalent. Local reactions are very rare and cardiac reactions are probably reduced with fosphenytoin.
- IV phenobarbital 15-20 milligrams per kilogram may also be given at this stage. Risk of respiratory depression is significant when combined with a benzodiazepine.
- Valproate may also be given at therapeutic doses but is less fully evaluated.

Case History 3

A 52-year-old man with a history of alcoholism and intravenous drug abuse was admitted with brief convulsive seizures, occurring serially. Repeated injections of benzodiazepines, including both diazepam and lorazepam with a loading dose of phenytoin had no effect. Between seizures he regained consciousness but clusters of seizures recurred several times over the next 24 hours. It was decided to try and

Table 14.4. Drugs Used in the Treatment of Status Epilepticus

Drug	Stage of Status	Mode of Administration	Adult Dose	Paediatric Dose	Comments
Clobazam	Prestatus	Oral	10–30 mg daily	Age 3–12 yrs, 5–15 mg daily	Useful in the prevention of escalation of seizures when the patient is able to take oral medication. May be given for a few days until high risk subsides
Diazepam	Prestatus, all stages of status	Oral, rectal Rectal or IV	IV 10–20 mg Rectal 10–30 mg	0.25–0.5 mg/kg	Given no faster than 5 mg/minute. Relapse of status is common but dose may be repeated. Respiratory depression is the main risk. Clonazepam 1 mg in adults, 0.25–0.5 mg in children is similar
Lorazepam	Prestatus, all stages of status	IV	4–8 mg can be repeated once	2 mg IV	Benzodiazepine of choice in first line treatment of status
Midazolam	Prestatus, all stages of status	IV, IM, intranasal, buccal	IV 5–10 mg, can be repeated once	IV 0.15–0.3 mg/kg	Midazolam is less fully evaluated than other benzo-diazepines but may compare favorably to diazepam. A wide variety of routes of administration may make it useful in the community
Paraldehyde	All stages of status	PR or IM	5–10 ml may be repeated once	0.07–0.35 ml/kg	Needs to be prepared and given straight away. May cause injection site abscess. Respiratory depression is rare and seizures rarely relapse once under control
Phenytoin	Prestatus, all stages of status	IV	15–18 mg/kg loading dose, then according to blood levels	15–18 mg/kg phenytoin equivalent loading then according to blood levels	Adverse effects include local ischemia (purple glove syndrome) hypotension and arrhythmia. Cardiac and respiratory monitoring are needed. For best effect lorazepam is given first
Fosphenytoin	Prestatus, all stages of status	IV or IM	15–18 mg/kg phenytoin equivalent loading then according to blood levels		A prodrug of phenytoin, it does not cause purple glove syndrome and cardiac adverse effects may be less common
Phenobarbital	Prestatus, all stages of status	IV	15–20 mg/kg loading dose then 3–4 mg/kg/day	IV 0.15–0.3 mg/kg loading dose then 3–4 mg/kg/day	Phenobarbital is as effective but slower than lorazepam and phenytoin together at aborting status epilepticus. Major side effects are respiratory and cardiac depression
Valproate	All stages of status	IV	5–10 mg/kg initial dose, then 20–30 mg/kg/day		Valproate is starting to be evaluated and may prove an effective alternative medication. Adverse effects are few.
Thiopental	Established status and subtle status	IV	Bolus 100–250 mg then 50 mg every 2–3 minutes followed by infusion 3–5 mg/kg/h		Dose calculated to maintain burst-suppression pattern on EEG withdrawal attempted 12 h after last seizure
Propofol	Established status and subtle status	IV	2 mg/kg bolus then 5–10 mg/kg/hr reducing to 1–3 mg/kg/h		Propofol works faster than thiopental, minutes rather than hours but thiopental may be effective in a greater number of cases. Contraindicated under age 16

avoid general anesthesia if possible. He received intravenous phenobarbital 15 milligrams per kilogram and seizures stopped immediately. Treatment was continued with phenobarbital 120 milligrams daily in the short term.

Although an old drug, with significant sedative effects in long-term use, phenobarbital remains a highly effective treatment for status epilepticus.

Refractory Status

If seizures persist for 1 hour despite appropriate intravenous therapy then they should be suppressed by general anesthetic in an intensive care unit.

- Barbiturate anesthesia with phenobarbital or thiopental is the standard. This is best guided by simultaneous EEG until the EEG evidence of seizures disappears or the EEG shows the pattern of "burst suppression."
- After 12 hours of seizure suppression, anesthesia can be lightened. The patient is monitored for the return of electrographic or clinical seizure activity that may necessitate repeat anesthesia. Usually a patient can be weaned to a standard AED. Even after several weeks of anesthesia patients may still have a good outcome from status.
- Propofol is also widely used although it is theoretically proconvulsant in low doses. It has a much shorter half-life, allowing more rapid weaning, although there may be some accumulation. It may cause acidosis and is contraindicated in children under 16.
- In one small trial, the incidence of severe hypotension and respiratory infection was similar with propofol and barbiturates. Propofol controlled seizures much more rapidly but was not always effective whereas phenobarbital achieved seizure control in all patients, including two for whom propofol had been unsuccessful.
- Regimes of intravenous sedatives such as benzodiazepines and chlormethiazole are not recommended. They may cause sudden respiratory depression and do not suppress seizures as fully as anesthesia.

Treating the Complications of Seizures (Table 14.5)

- Many complications reverse spontaneously on cessation of seizures if treatment is sufficiently early in the condition. If complications persist then they should be treated along conventional lines. The following points are worth emphasizing.

Table 14.5. Systemic Complications of Status Epilepticus

Metabolic	Hypoglycemia, hyperkalemia, myoglobulinemia, acute renal failure, respiratory and metabolic acidosis, dehydration, inappropriate antidiuretic hormone secretion
Autonomic	Pyrexia and hyperpyrexia, hypertension or hypotension, cardiac arrhythmia, urinary retention or incontinence
Hematological	Leukocytosis, disseminated intravascular coagulopathy
Others	Trauma including intracranial, aspiration pneumonia, venous thrombosis, pressure sores

1. Respiratory depression occurs in 10 to 17 percent and hypotension in 25 to 35 percent of cases and both are much more common in advanced status.
2. Pyrexia is common as epileptic motor activity raises body temperature like continuous shivering. This, combined with leukocytosis that often accompanies status epilepticus may lead to a presumptive diagnosis of infection. If in doubt, a full investigation should be carried out with blood cultures, neuroimaging and CSF examination to exclude infection.
3. Oliguric renal failure due to dehydration, seizure-induced myoglobinemia and hypotension can be avoided with adequate intravenous fluids.

Catches in Status Epilepticus

- Psychogenic non-epileptic seizure disorders mimicking status epilepticus
- Giving a benzodiazepine and failing to give another AED
- Inadequate AED loading doses
- Delay in anesthesia
- Missing subtle status epilepticus
- Failing to diagnose the cause of status epilepticus, including AED withdrawal
- Acute intermittent porphyria or ornithine transcarbamylase deficiency exacerbated by AEDs (rare)

NON-CONVULSIVE STATUS EPILEPTICUS

The following is a simple clinical classification of non-convulsive status epilepticus.

1. Focal motor status epilepticus
2. Status epilepticus causing confusional states
3. Rarer forms including
   (a) partial status causing sensory and other purely subjective symptoms
   (b) focal cognitive disturbances for example aphasia in adults
   (c) myoclonic status
4. Special forms of status epilepticus in children (Chapter 11)
   (a) status in neonates and infants
   (b) forms of status associated with mental retardation in children, including myoclonic status, atypical absences, and tonic status
   (c) syndromes of cognitive decline in young children such as Landau-Kleffner syndrome and epilepsy with continuous slow waves in sleep

Focal Motor Status Epilepticus FMSE (Epilepsia Partialis Continua)

FMSE is distinguished by the continuous jerking of one side of the body or part of one side of the body. The clinical manifestation may be very subtle with just twitching of the corner of the mouth or one eye. The patient is mostly fully conscious during the jerking although at times the seizures may spread to become more severe with alteration of awareness and even evolve into full tonic–clonic seizures. This is distinct from subtle status convulsive status in which similar motor manifestations may occur in a comatose patient (above).

Etiology

Commoner Causes

- In adults, episodes of FMSE lasting hours to days are usually due to cerebrovascular disease (Case 4) or metabolic disturbance, especially non-ketotic hyperglycemia. Other structural pathology may cause FMSE of much greater duration, including tumors, previous encephalitis, cerebral abscess, cysticercosis, trauma, vascular malformations, or cortical dysplasia.

Case History 4

A 55-year-old man suffered a swollen right hand when it became trapped in a gate. The swelling settled and 1 week after the injury, the hand began to jerk. The jerking continued for 2 weeks until he was admitted to hospital, where to his surprise, an MRI scan showed infarction (Figure 14.3). The jerking stopped without treatment but his hand remained weak and clumsy, recovering over several weeks.

FMSE may be the presentation of acute stroke. In this context FMSE is often prolonged, but eventually self-limiting and may not respond to treatment.

Rarer Causes

- Penicillin is a cortical irritant and may cause FMSE in the presence of a local break in the blood-brain barrier, for example after neurosurgery. Tick-borne encephalitis, is an endemic cause in Canada and Russia. Rasmussen's encephalitis is a rare but distinctive condition affecting mostly children and

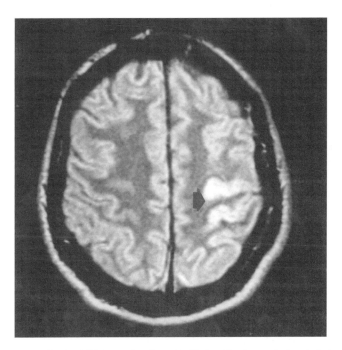

Figure 14.3. Proton density MRI scan showing a highly localized acute ischemic lesion associated with focal motor status epilepticus. Similar MRI changes can sometimes be seen in status epilepticus without a clear underlying lesion.

young adults and evolving over years. One whole cerebral hemisphere becomes progressively more affected by encephalitis and curiously the other hemisphere usually remains normal. The best clue to date to the etiology is the presence in many cases, of antibodies to a glutamate receptor (GluR3). The clinical presentation is with refractory focal seizures, most commonly focal motor seizures and FMSE, associated with a progressive decline in hemisphere function, with hemiparesis and cognitive deficits.

Case History 5
An 11-year-old boy developed focal motor seizures affecting his left arm and leg. These were very persistent but came under partial control with standard AEDs. Over the next four years he experienced a decline in motor function of his left side, until he became dependent on walking aids. His seizures deteriorated and he suffered several bouts of focal motor status, affecting his left arm and lasting hours to days. These required admission to hospital with alteration of his medication to bring them under control. At the age of 16, he again developed focal motor status epilepticus, but this time seizures sometimes spread to become tonic clonic seizures. All attempts to control his seizures with medication failed and he required barbiturate anesthesia and intensive care treatment. Attempts to wean him from barbiturates were unsuccessful. He underwent emergency left hemispherectomy. Following this all AEDs except phenytoin were withdrawn. One year later he was seizure-free and able to walk with a hemiparesis but without walking aids.

This case illustrates the course of Rasmussen's encephalitis. Hemispherectomy is the only definitive treatment and the response can be dramatic. It is usually undertaken electively. Corticosteroids or plasmaphoresis may also be beneficial.

Diagnosis

- Diagnosis of FMSE is clinical. The affected part is usually the hand or face, reflecting their greater representation in the motor cortex. There are rhythmical jerks often combined with a tonic contraction or a dystonic component. The seizures are occasionally painful. The affected part may be weak but it is often difficult to know in the acute phase whether this is a prolonged Todd's paresis or whether it is related to the underlying cause of the seizures.
- The EEG is unhelpful in 50 percent of cases. It may show focal slow activity from damage to the underlying cortex or spikes maximal in the frontoparietal region.
- Neuroimaging (see Figure 14.3) may show an obvious focal cause, such as a tumor or vascular abnormality. FMSE may be a manifestation of more diffuse disease such as double cortex. In Rasmussen's encephalitis, neuroimaging is usually normal in the early stages, followed by gradual unilateral, hemispheric atrophy, and sometimes an increased signal on T_2 weighted images.

Treatment

- FMSE is often self-limiting in the context of acute stroke or metabolic disturbance, although it may be protracted, lasting days or even 2 to 3 weeks (Case 4). Aggressive treatment may sometimes help to arrest seizures, improve outcome and prevent secondarily generalized seizures .

- Intravenous benzodiazepines may just induce sleep and respiratory depression, without stopping seizures. Oral clobazam may be helpful.
- Choice of anticonvulsant is between phenytoin, phenobarbital and sodium valproate, all of which can be given in therapeutic doses from the outset. Other agents such as carbamazepine are less practical as they require a titration period.
- Oral loading dose can be considered for patients at high risk of cardiotoxicity, as the urgency of treatment is less than in convulsive status epilepticus.
- General anesthesia is rarely indicated.
- More protracted FMSE should be treated as any other form of focal epilepsy but dose titration may need to be more rapid.

Status Epilepticus Causing Confusion (SECC)

Etiology

Confusional states are a rare first presentation of epilepsy and are less common than convulsive status epilepticus, except in the mentally handicapped, where they may affect up to 1 percent of epilepsy sufferers. Three main causes of SECC can be identified:

- Idiopathic generalised epilepsy; synonyms primary generalized absence status, typical absence status, petit mal status.
- Focal epilepsy causing SECC; synonym complex partial status, usually arising from temporal or frontal lobes.
- Secondarily generalized epilepsy such as Lennox-Gastaut syndrome; synonym atypical absence status (Chapter 11)

Diagnosis

1. Thinking of the diagnosis is crucial in any patient with altered mental state. SECC may manifest in different spheres (Table 14.6). There is often marked fluctuation with lucid intervals and in association with the mental changes there may be more obvious periods of absence, and motor manifestations, including myoclonus, automatisms or agitation.

Case History 6
A 56-year old man presented with seizures and bouts of confusion. When seizures were diagnosed 5 years earlier, he had to leave his previous, more demanding job.

Table 14.6. Clinical Features of Status Epilepticus Causing Confusion

Clinical Features of SECC	Clinical Presentations of SECC
Alteration of awareness	Declining school performance in children
Slowing of thought	Work failure and pseudo-dementia in adults
Behavioral change	Confused or psychotic behavior
Amnesia	Apathy or depression
Psychiatric disturbance	

His current employers found his work had declined over the previous year and were initiating redundancy proceedings. His wife described episodes when he appeared mildly confused and his eyelids flickered. During these times he was able to undertake some simple activities in the house but was unable to perform the more complex tasks demanded of him in his clerical work. At times these episodes terminated in tonic–clonic seizures and he was suffering convulsive episodes several times per month. His wife felt that his memory had generally deteriorated and she was concerned he was suffering from dementia. Treatment was with phenytoin 300 milligrams and lamotrigine 175 milligrams daily. An EEG showed bilateral, frontally predominant spike and wave activity and a CT scan was normal. A clinical diagnosis was made of idiopathic generalized epilepsy (IGE) absence status. Sodium valproate was started and built up to a dose of 1200 milligrams daily. Phenytoin was gradually withdrawn. Two months later he had had no further seizures but he developed headaches and gastrointestinal disturbance. Lamotrigine was reduced to 50 milligrams daily and he remained cognitively normal and seizure-free.

- Non-convulsive status may present with a pseudodementia but there are usually also overt seizures. Eyelid flickering and termination in convulsive seizures suggest IGE absence status. There is often less profound loss of contact than found in brief absence seizures. IGE status usually responds well to valproate.
- Changing concomitant therapy from an enzyme inducer (phenytoin) to an enzyme inhibitor (valproate) can cause lamotrigine levels to rise and side effects to emerge.

Table 14.7. Differentiation of Different Types of Status Epilepticus Causing Confusion

Clinical feature	IGE	Temporal Lobe SECC	Frontal Lobe SECC
Age of onset	a) 10–20 years, b) middle age to elderly	Usually adult	Usually adult
De novo status?	Rarer in children Commoner in late onset	Common	Common
Previous seizure patterns	Absence, myoclonus, TCS	Focal, TCS	Focal, absence, TCS
Myoclonus/ eyelid fluttering	**Common**	**Rare**	**Rare**
Mute	Common	Rare	Common
Fear, irritability	Rare	Common	Rare
Complex gestural automatisms	Rare	Common	Uncommon
EEG	Generalized	Focal or bitemporal	Frontal or generalized
Spontaneous termination in TCS	**Common**	**Uncommon**	**Uncommon**
Rapid response to IV diazepam	**Common**	**Variable**	**Variable**

The table shows features differentiating focal SECC from generalized SECC. Factors that are most diagnostically useful are in bold.

2. What type of SECC is it (Table 14.7)? It may be clear from the investigations and preceding seizure history into which category the epilepsy falls but it may be difficult to tell even after detailed evaluation. One study suggested that in focal SECC there is a previous history of epilepsy in only 70 percent of patients compared to 96 percent of patients with generalized SECC. In older patients generalized SECC may be a first presentation of epilepsy but is often due to identifiable factors such as psychotropic medication, intercurrent infection or benzodiazepine withdrawal.

Investigations

- Interictal EEG may be normal or abnormal.
- Ictal EEG is always abnormal in SECC. There is little correlation between the EEG change and the severity of the clinical changes, especially in generalized SECC.
- In generalized SECC, there is usually the classical frontally predominant spike-wave discharge. As status progresses, the frequency may slow, even to below 1 hertz and focal components may appear. Cessation of abnormal EEG activity is followed rapidly by clinical recovery.
- In focal SECC, the clinical state may be associated with two EEG patterns. The first is continuous epileptic activity. Spike-wave discharges may be frontally predominant and it may be difficult to tell the difference between frontopolar status with secondary bilateral synchrony and generalized SECC. The abnormalities may be restricted to the temporal lobes, in which case they are usually bilateral. The second pattern is of frequent focal seizures causing confusion, alternating with postictal confusion to cause a continuous, fluctuating confusional state.
- Neuroimaging is normal in generalized SECC and lesions causing focal SECC may be very subtle; all patients should undergo detailed MRI.

Treatment

- There are no formal trials of treatment for SECC.
- An IV benzodiazepine may abolish the seizures. This is best undertaken with simultaneous EEG monitoring and facilities for respiratory support to hand. In idiopathic generalized SECC there is often a dramatic clinical and EEG response, within one minute, but seizures may recur after a few minutes. In focal SECC, there may occasionally be as dramatic a response but it is less consistent. The patient may just fall asleep from the sedative affects of the drug, then seizure activity returns as the drug wears off.
- Clobazam 10 to 30 milligrams daily may help control status whilst more definitive therapy is established. This drug is also useful used intermittently in the prevention of status for patients who suffer recurrent bouts of SECC (Case 9, Chapter 9).
- First choice AED in IGE is sodium valproate. In focal SECC, loading doses of phenytoin or phenobarbital may be given. Medication can usually be given orally to avoid the toxicity of intravenous injection.
- General anesthesia may occasionally be justified to suppress refractory seizures.

Rarer Forms of Status Epilepticus

Sensory Partial Status Epilepticus (SPSE)

If a prolonged focal seizure remains restricted to the primary sensory cortex, then the result will be SPSE. As there are no objective changes, the only one aware of any abnormality is the patient themselves. These seizures are probably under-reported.

Diagnosis
- Persistent ictal hallucinations may affect vision (simple or formed), hearing, smell, somatosensory function, prolonged epigastric aura and rarely odd thoughts or memories. The diagnosis is easiest if the symptoms are the same as the aura to a patient's more obvious habitual seizures (Case 7). If a sensory symptom is the only manifestation of the patient's epilepsy then a definite diagnosis may be impossible. The differential diagnosis includes migraine aura, and psychological symptoms, including hyperventilation syndrome (Chapter 5).

Case History 7
A 23-year-old man developed complex partial seizures at the age of 6 that became regular after the age of 10. These were preceded by a butterfly sensation, usually felt in his abdomen. This sensation often lasted up to 2 days before overt seizures occurred and sometimes continued after a seizure. The seizures were characterized by a scream, abduction of his arms then rocking of his trunk and bicycling movements of his legs. They occurred in clusters, often terminating in a convulsive seizure. Continuous electrographic seizure activity occurred during a period of prolonged abdominal sensations after an overt seizure. He underwent right frontal resection and was seizure-free for 1 year, but seizures then recurred. The resected cortex was dysplastic.

- The EEG is often normal during epileptic auras.
- Abolition of the symptom with IV benzodiazepine may be a helpful diagnostic pointer and guide treatment of future episodes. However, it is neither specific nor reliable unless there are simultaneous concordant changes in the EEG. Failure of a response does not exclude epilepsy and anxiety states with somatic symptoms may respond to benzodiazepines.
- Neuroimaging may show an appropriately sited lesion.

Treatment

As there is no impairment of function, treatment is less urgent than in other forms of status. Nevertheless treatment should not be delayed.

- Clobazam 10 to 30 milligrams daily may be helpful, whilst long-term AEDs are titrated.

Status Epilepticus with Focal Cognitive Symptoms in Adults

- Focal status epilepticus may rarely present with focal cognitive symptoms, usually amnesia or aphasia, evolving over days to weeks but with no overt seizures.

A very fluctuating deficit is usual but the history may appear progressive. The patient may exhibit subtle signs of seizure activity such as twitching of the face or fingers. An EEG is often diagnostic, but may need to be repeated if the patient is in prestatus.
- Neuroimaging is mandatory to exclude a foreign tissue lesion.
- Treatment is as for status epilepticus causing confusion.

Case History 8 (from Manford *et al.* 1995, with permission)
A 74-year-old man developed a progressive disturbance of speech over several days. At this stage he was still ambulant and able to communicate his needs by pointing. After 2 weeks his family noticed some other errors such as holding his knife and fork in the wrong hands. On examination he would repeat the phrase: "I can't hear," and had a clear disturbance of receptive and expressive language, both spoken and written. A metabolic screen revealed hyperosmolar non-ketotic hyperglycemia (HONH) and his CT brain scan was normal. His EEG showed widespread but non-specific slow activity, which evolved into a clear seizure discharge over the left temporal region. Numerous anticonvulsants had no impact on his speech, just making him more sedated but his clinical state started to resolve 10 days after correcting his metabolic abnormalities. Six months later, antiepileptic drugs were withdrawn without seizure recurrence.

- Focal status epilepticus or frequently recurring focal seizures need to be considered in the differential diagnosis of any subacute progressive focal cortical deficit for which no structural cause is found. HONH is an under-recognized cause of focal status epilepticus, usually FMSE. Status epilepticus may persist for some time after correction of the metabolic cause and may respond poorly to medication.

Myoclonic Status Epilepticus (MSE) in Adults

Diagnosis

- A very sick brain may exhibit myoclonic status epilepticus, whatever the cause (Table 14.8). Commonest are metabolic coma and hypoxic-ischemic encephalopathy. In primary brain diseases such classical Creutzfeldt-Jakob disease or subacute sclerosing pan-encephalitis (a rare, fatal complication of early measles infection) the myoclonus is often stimulus-sensitive: a flurry of jerks may be triggered by a loud noise or by tapping a tendon reflex.

Table 14.8. Causes of Myoclonic Status Epilepticus

Acute diffuse hypoxic injury e.g. post cardiopulmonary resuscitation
Metabolic e.g. liver failure, renal failure, hyponatremia, hyperglycemia, Hashimoto's encephalopathy
Toxins e.g. lead
Drug overdose e.g. AEDs, tricyclics, sedatives
Degenerative disease e.g. CJD, Alzheimer's disease
Viral encephalopathy e.g. Herpes simplex encephalitis, subacute sclerosing panencephalitis, HIV, progressive multifocal leukoencephalopathy

- MSE may persist for days or weeks and may be punctuated by occasional convulsive seizures. Jerks are usually multifocal and typically affect the face and sometimes limbs. Epileptic nystagmus may be the only sign.
- Without an accurate history of previous convulsive seizures it may be difficult to tell the difference from advanced, subtle convulsive status epilepticus (above).
- The progressive myoclonus epilepsies are a group of metabolic and degenerative brain diseases in which myoclonus are prominent features (Chapter 3). They may be complicated by myoclonic status epilepticus.

EEG Changes in Myoclonic Status Epilepticus

- If coma is the cause, the EEG often shows non-specific diffuse slowing as a manifestation of a sick brain.
- More specific changes are periodic complexes in Creutzfeldt-Jakob disease and triphasic waves in hepatic encephalopathy.
- It may be difficult to identify specific EEG changes of the myoclonus itself. Sometimes there are paroxysmal sharp waves or spikes over the central regions. Combined EEG and EMG with back-averaging may show that the paroxysmal EEG changes are time-linked to the bursts of muscle activity, preceding them by a fixed interval.
- Giant somatosensory evoked potentials may be present, especially if the myoclonus is stimulus-sensitive.

Treatment

- Myoclonus is often sensitive to benzodiazepines, for example clonazepam or clobazam. Sodium valproate is the best established AED for myoclonus.
- Piracetam is a drug useful only in myoclonus. It is given in enormous doses of 15 to 25 grams per day but is very safe.
- Refractory myoclonus may respond to combination therapy of these agents, if a single agent is unsuccessful. Levetiracetam may be considered.
- Several drugs may make myoclonus worse – carbamazepine, phenytoin, gabapentin, vigabatrin, tiagabine.

Special Forms of Status Epilepticus in Children

- Status epilepticus in young children differs from that in older children and adults in several key respects (Chapter 11).
- The immature CNS of a newborn infant manifests status epilepticus in different ways from older children and adults. As a child with severe epilepsy matures the seizure patterns expressed go through recognizable age-dependent syndromes. Once the child reaches the age of 5, seizures become more like those of an adult.
- The etiology of status epilepticus changes as a child passes through various stages of development.
- Brain damage including MTS is more likely following severe seizures in children than in adults.

- Status epilepticus may cause specific syndromes of developmental delay, with few overt seizures for example Landau-Kleffner syndrome.

BIBLIOGRAPHY

Cendes F, Andermann F, Carpenter S, Zatorre RJ, Cashman NR. Temporal lobe epilepsy caused by domoic acid intoxication: evidence for glutamate receptor-mediated excitotoxicity in humans. Ann Neurol 1995;37:123–126.

DeLorenzo RJ, Hauser WA, Towne AR, Boggs JG, Pellock JM, Penberthy L, Garnett L, Fortner CA, Ko D. A prospective, population-based epidemiologic study of status epilepticus in Richmond, Virginia. Neurology 1996;46:1029–1035.

Gross DW, Li LM, Andermann F. Catastrophic deterioration and hippocampal atrophy after childhood status epilepticus [letter; comment]. Ann Neurol 1998;43:687.

Guberman A, Cantu-Reyna G, Stuss D, Broughton R. Nonconvulsive status epilepticus: clinical features, neuropsychological testing and long-term follow-up. Neurology 1986;36:1284–1291.

Hesdorffer DC, Hauser WA, Annegers JF, Rocca WA. Severe, uncontrolled hypertension and adult-onset seizures: a case-control study in Rochester, Minnesota. Epilepsia 1996;37:736–741.

Hesdorffer DC, Logroscino G, Cascino G, Annegers JF, Hauser WA. Incidence of status epilepticus in Rochester, Minnesota, 1965–1984. Neurology 1998;50:735–741.

Krishnamurthy KB, Drislane FW. Relapse and survival after barbiturate anesthetic treatment of refractory status epilepticus. Epilepsia 1996;37:863–837.

Leppik IE, Derivan AT, Homan RW, Walker J, Ramsay E, Patrick B. Double-blind study of lorazepam and diazepam in status epilepticus. JAMA 1999;249:1452–1454.

Manford M, Shorvon SD. Prolonged sensory or visceral symptoms: an under-diagnosed form of non-convulsive focal (simple partial) status epilepticus [published erratum appears in J Neurol Neurosurg Psychiatry 1992;55:1223]. J Neurol Neurosurg Psychiatry 1992;55:714–716.

Maytal J, Shinnar S, Moshe SL. Low morbidity and mortality of status epilepticus in children. Pediatrics 1989;83:323–331.

Rohr-Le FLoch J, Gauthier G, Beaumanoir A. Etats confusionnel d'origine epileptique interet de l'EEG fait en urgence. Revue Neurologique 1988;144:425–436.

Scholtes FB, Renier WO, Meinardi H. Non-convulsive status epilepticus: causes, treatment and outcome in 65 patients. J Neurol Neurosurg Psychiatry 1996;61:93–95.

Scholtes FB, Renier WO, Meinardi H. Simple partial status epilepticus: causes, treatment and outcome in 47 patients. J Neurol Neurosurg Psychiatry 1996;61:90–92.

Scott RC, Besag FM, Neville BG. Buccal midazolam and rectal diazepam for treatment of prolonged seizures in childhood and adolescence: a randomised trial [see comments.] Lancet 1999;353:623–626.

Stecker MM, Kramer TH, Raps EC, O'Meeghan R, Dulaney E, Skaar DJ. Treatment of refractory status epilepticus with propofol: clinical and pharmacokinetic findings. Epilepsia 1998;39:18–26.

Thomas P, Andermann F. Late-onset absence status epilepticus is most often situated-related. In: Malafosse A, Genton P, Hirsch E, Marescaux C, Broglin D, Bernasconi R (eds). Idiopathic Generalized Epilepsies: Clinical, Experimental and Genetic Aspects. London: John Libbey and Company Ltd. 1994;95–109.

Treiman DM. Generalized convulsive status epilepticus in the adult. Epilepsia 1993; 34(Suppl1):S2–S11.

Treiman DM, Meyers PD, Walton NY, Collins JF, Colling C, Rowan AJ, Handforth A, Faught E, Calabrese VP, Uthman BM, Ramsay RE, Mamdani MB (1998). A comparison of four treatments for generalized convulsive status epilepticus. Veterans Affairs Status Epilepticus Cooperative Study Group. N Engl J Med 1998;339:792–798.

Wakai S, Ito N, Sueoka H, Kawamoto Y, Tsutsumi H, Chiba S. Complex partial status epilepticus in childhood. Pediatric Neurology 1995;13:137–141.

REFERENCES

1. Lothman EW. The biochemical basis and pathophysiology of status epilepticus. Neurology 1990;40 (Suppl 2):13–23.
2. Manford M, Fuller GN, Wade JP (1995). "Silent diabetes": non-ketotic hyperglycemia presenting as aphasic status epilepticus. J Neurol Neurosurg Psychiatry 59:99–100.
3. Shorvon SD. Status Epilepticus: Its Clinical Features and Treatment in Children and Adults. Cambridge: Cambridge University Press; 1994.

15

Epilepsy Surgery

A BRIEF HISTORY

Hughlings-Jackson laid the foundations of the principles of clinical localization of focal epilepsy in the late 19th century and the first successful surgical treatment for focal motor epilepsy was in 1886. From the 1930s, EEG allowed more patterns of surgically treatable epilepsy to be identified especially temporal lobe epilepsy (TLE). In the 1960s mesial temporal sclerosis (MTS) was defined as the commonest pathological basis of TLE and subsequently most epilepsy surgery has been in the treatment of MTS. In these early stages the pathological basis of the epilepsy was rarely known prior to surgery. From the 1970s CT scanning allowed the presurgical identification of lesions underlying epilepsy in 10 to 20 percent of cases. It is only since the advent of MRI that it has usually become possible to identify the structural cause of refractory focal epilepsy prior to surgical resection and this has revolution-ized the approach to epilepsy surgery.

PRINCIPLES OF SURGICAL TREATMENT

- Surgery may be used to cure or palliate refractory focal epilepsy.
- The technical approaches include resection of brain tissue, interruption of seizure pathways or electrical stimulation techniques.
- Patient selection requires a multidisciplinary approach as each patient presents a unique profile.
- Only 1 percent of epilepsy is amenable to curative surgery at present. The pathway to surgery for each patient is long and complex and the final recom-mendation is always a balance of probabilities of risk *versus* benefit. In the most favourable TLE cases, the chance of seizure-freedom may approach 90 percent with about 2 percent risk of significant neurological consequences from surgery (Table 15.1).
- The patient embarking on presurgical evaluation must understand that the out-come of long and complex investigations may be that surgery is not feasible. This always comes as a severe blow.

RESECTIVE SURGERY – PATIENT SELECTION

What is Refractory Epilepsy?

- If three anti-epileptic drugs (AEDs) at therapeutic doses have proved unsuc-cessful then it is relatively unlikely that another drug will be able to render a patient seizure-free. It should take no longer than 2 years to decide that epilepsy is refractory to medical treatment.
- Delay of surgery whilst endless drugs are tried, may adversely affect education, employment or the patient's ability to form and maintain relationships.
- Non-specialists need to know whom to refer for further evaluation as the major-ity of patients will not benefit from surgery. A simple scheme is summarized in Figure 15.1.

The Principles of Epilepsy Surgery

- A preliminary assessment by a clinician is needed to decide whether there is a case for detailed presurgical evaluation on technical clinical criteria.

Table 15.1. The Standard Outcome Measures of Epilepsy Surgery

Seizure Outcome of Surgery	Adverse Effects of Surgery
1. Seizure-free or occasional auras only	A. None
2. Rare seizures	B. Minor or transient
3. Worthwhile improvement	C. Severe
4. No improvement	

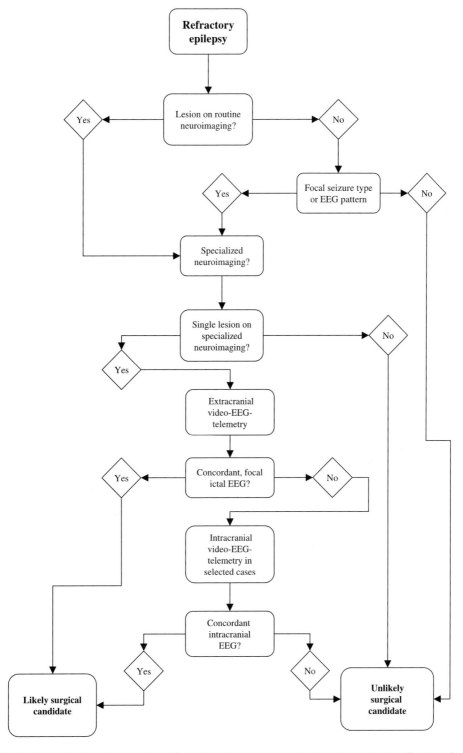

Figure 15.1. A scheme for the selection of candidates for epilepsy surgery relies heavily on the identification of a structural basis to the epilepsy with neuroimaging.

- The patient's key judgment is whether becoming seizure-free would sufficiently alter their lives to justify the risk of surgery.

Case History 1

A 37-year-old woman was referred for consideration of epilepsy surgery. She had suffered frequent focal seizures since her teens, which were refractory to medication. The seizures manifested with an epigastric aura followed by a brief period of absence. She was married with three children and worked as an administrator. Her colleagues were used to her minor seizures and her employment was secure. Investigations showed right hippocampal atrophy and interictal spiking in the right anterior temporal leads. Although there were features suggesting that her epilepsy could probably be cured by surgery, she was well adapted to her problem. There would have been relatively little psychosocial benefit from being rendered seizure-free and she declined further investigation.

- The clinician bases the final balance of risk and benefit of surgery on the results of three arms of investigation:

  1. Demonstrating that a single area of the brain is essential to seizure generation and that if it is removed seizures will stop. Sources of information for localizing epilepsy include: clinical pattern, EEG, neuroimaging and psychometric assessment. If all these sources are concordant in suggesting the same region is responsible for the epilepsy then there is a good chance of seizure remission after surgery
  2. Demonstrating that removal of that region will not result in unacceptable adverse effects, either physical or cognitive. Neuropsychometric testing is vital to judge the safety of epilepsy surgery. Routine testing may be by functional neuroimaging and by the Wada sodium amytal test (Chapters 8 and 16)
  3. Psychiatric evaluation to demonstrate that a patient's mental state is unlikely to be disturbed by the process of investigation, by surgery and by the life changes that may be triggered by becoming seizure-free.

- The outcome of surgery is conventionally assessed 2 years post-operatively. The majority of patients who become seizure-free do so immediately after surgery and stay seizure-free. A small number experience a winding down process with seizures declining before stopping. There is another small group in whom seizures stop after surgery but relapse months or years later (Figure 15.2).

The Central Role of Neuroimaging

- For most patients the criterion that predicts whether they are likely candidates for resective epilepsy surgery is whether there is an identifiable structural abnormality underlying their epilepsy.
- If there is a visible lesion, then the process of localizing epilepsy is geared to proving that the visible lesion is causing the epilepsy. If there is no lesion, then it is more difficult to guide subsequent investigations and surgery and the prognosis of surgery is less favorable.
- If there is a strong suspicion of a focal structural abnormality, for example very focal clinical seizure pattern or electrophysiological disturbance, standard MRI

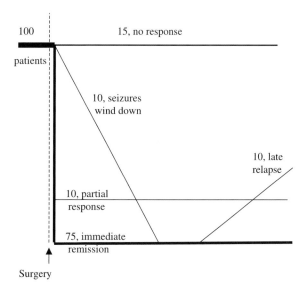

Figure 15.2. A graph illustrating potential outcomes after epilepsy surgery with approximate figures.

is insufficient to rule out a potential surgical target. Tailored neuroimaging needs to be undertaken at an epilepsy centre, often with specialized techniques (see Chapter 8).

- Patients with mesial temporal sclerosis or foreign tissue lesions stand out as having the best potential outcome from resective surgery.
- Patients with subtle lesions for example cortical dysplasia may also do well but are more difficult to identify.

The Role of the Etiology of the Epilepsy

- A history of complicated febrile seizures makes a diagnosis of MTS more likely, although only a minority of patients with MTS have had febrile seizures.
- A history of a diffuse or multifocal insult underlying the epilepsy, such as head injury or encephalitis makes multifocal onset of the epilepsy more likely and is generally an argument against surgical treatment. However, in some cases of multifocal disease, such as tuberose sclerosis, epilepsy may arise from a restricted part of the structural abnormality.
- An abnormal physical examination is often evidence against a sufficiently focal cause of epilepsy for resective surgery.

The Role of the Clinical Seizure Pattern

- A highly focal clinical seizure pattern makes an identifiable structural cause more likely. A non-focal seizure pattern such as tonic–clonic seizures is less likely to be treatable by resective surgery. However, frontal lobe epilepsy (FLE) may present with non-focal seizure patterns (Case 8, Chapter 6).

The Role of Interictal EEG

- Focal slow waves on the interictal EEG are often associated with underlying pathological changes and are supportive evidence for an underlying lesion.
- Focal interictal spikes are in favor of focal onset of epilepsy but the interictal abnormalities cannot be taken as proof of the electrophysiological region of onset of seizures.
- Multifocal or diffuse spikes are evidence against a single region of seizure onset but do not rule it out. For example some frontal lesions can cause the EEG pattern of secondary bilateral synchrony (Case 8, Chapter 6) and still be amenable to surgery. The proportion of spikes from one region is important: if abnormalities elsewhere are only occasional, then a focal seizure onset remains possible.

The Role of Ictal EEG

- The ictal EEG defines the region of onset of epilepsy. Although neuroimaging is important in establishing whether there is a resectable cause for the epilepsy, it is ictal EEG that confirms that the epilepsy arises in the region of the lesion.
- A highly focal EEG seizure onset provides strong evidence of a localized, resectable region underlying the epilepsy.
- A diffuse or multifocal EEG onset implies a poor prognosis for focal surgical resection.
- Some technical factors need to be considered in the interpretation of ictal EEG (Table 15.2).

The Role of Neuropsychometric Assessment

- Neuropsychometric assessment may show a focal pattern of cognitive dysfunction compatible with an observed lesion or an electroclinical seizure localization, supporting the suggested region of onset of seizures.

Table 15.2. Technical Considerations in Interpreting the Ictal EEG in Presurgical Evaluation

Factor	Interpretation
Have all the habitual seizure types been recorded?	If any has been missed, they may arise from a different part of the brain and may persist after resective surgery
Have enough seizures been recorded?	The same clinical seizure type may arise from different parts of the brain. The more seizures are recorded the less likely that independent sites of seizure onset have been missed
Was the EEG seizure onset before the first clinical seizure manifestation?	If the clinical manifestation came before any EEG changes then the EEG missed the crucial onset of the seizure
Do all the seizures have the same EEG pattern?	If attacks are highly stereotyped electrophysiologically and clinically then EEG localization is more reliable

- A more diffuse disturbance may be due to a number of factors (see Chapter 16) for example AED toxicity but raises the possibility of more widespread disease and therefore a worse post-operative prognosis of the epilepsy.
- A minor disturbance of cognitive function is generally a good prognostic sign.
- An unexpected focal pattern of disturbance raises concerns of non-concordance but may be due to plasticity changes after the development of epilepsy causing altered localization of function.

Resolving Discordant Investigations

- Discordance means that different investigations suggest different locations for the origin of epilepsy but does not always rule out resective surgery; discordance may be due to technical considerations. Not all investigations are equally important in epilepsy localization and different weighting is applied to different investigations (Table 15.3). For example, up to 20 percent of interictal EEG spikes may be contralateral to the origin of seizures without jeopardizing the outcome of temporal lobe surgery.
- Dual pathology is a major problem. One third of neocortical lesions are associated with MTS. One or both may trigger seizures.
- Discordance between EEG and imaging is common. It may be due to rapid spread of discharges so they are only detected distant to their site of origin. Occasionally a lesion may be coincidental, for example 75 percent of arachnoid cysts.
- Intracranial ictal EEG studies are the main way to resolve major discordance. For example if MRI points to left TLE but extracranial EEG points to right TLE, electrodes may be inserted into just the two temporal lobes.
- Functional neuroimaging may provide supportive evidence for seizure lateralization or localization and occasionally obviates the need for intracranial EEG.

Resective Surgery without a Lesion

- For patients with electroclinical evidence of TLE but no structural changes on sophisticated MRI, additional evidence may be found by other imaging techniques, for example magnetic resonance spectroscopy (MRS; Chapter 8). The chance of seizure freedom after surgery falls from over 80 percent with the clearest changes on structural imaging to around 50 to 60 percent if the abnormalities are only detectable by MRS.
- Extratemporal epilepsy surgery is even more difficult without imaging abnormalities. In some early series of surgery for frontal lobe epilepsy success rates

Table 15.3. Weighting of Different Investigations in Presurgical Epilepsy Localization

Strongest Weighting	Moderate Weighting	Weakest Weighting
MRI	Interictal EEG	Interictal SPECT/PET
Ictal EEG	Ictal SPECT	Neuropsychometry
	Clinical seizure pattern	

were only 20 percent. Neither the location nor the nature of the pathology is as consistent in extratemporal epilepsy as it is in TLE. Surgery has to be tailored to the individual patient's electroclinical syndrome and it is more difficult to resect the margins of an electrical disturbance than it is to remove an anatomically defined lesion. Intracranial EEG, including perioperative EEG, is needed more often.

Assessing the Safety of Resective Epilepsy Surgery

- There is approximately a 2 percent risk of serious or irreversible adverse events such as stroke after temporal lobectomy.
- Neuropsychometric tests are used to predict the consequences of technically successful surgery, which involves the resection of functioning brain tissue.
- For TLE surgery, the most important issues are the localization of speech and verbal memory. In nearly all right-handed people and in many left-handed people verbal memory is in the left temporal lobe. The Wada test (Chapter 16) is used to determine the lateralization of these functions in individual patients.
- The effects of extratemporal surgery on cortical function depend on the location of surgery. Some areas are relatively safe, for example the anterior frontal cortex. Others usually cause deficits, for example visual field deficits from occipital surgery.
- Plasticity of cortical function means that some functions may not be located exactly where expected and the function of the cortex to be resected may need to be established experimentally.
- Eloquent regions may be operable. For example there is bilateral motor cortex representation of the upper part of the face and resective surgery may be undertaken on one side of the upper but not lower face motor cortex, without compromising function.
- Electrophysiological localization of function can be undertaken with evoked potentials and cortical stimulation studies. Careful electrical stimulation can be used to map the precise location of crucial functions for example of the motor cortex. Electrodes inserted preoperatively to identify the region of onset of epilepsy can also be used to stimulate the cortex. Intra-operative stimulation can also be used but this means the patient has to be awake for part of their operation, when the brain is exposed.
- Functional imaging can be used to localize functions in eloquent cortical areas where a highly tailored resection may be possible (Chapter 8). The paradigm must be appropriate to the function being tested but in appropriately selected cases may obviate the need for intra-operative neurophysiological studies.

RESECTIVE EPILEPSY SURGERY TECHNIQUES

Lesional Epilepsy

- A lesion may be removed because it causes epilepsy or because of other reasons. For example, vascular malformations are removed to eliminate the risk of

Table 15.4. Reported Effects of Surgery on Epilepsy Due to Different Lesions (%)

Lesion	Percentage Seizure-Free After Surgery
Arteriovenous malformation	50–89 with complete resection
Cavernous hemangioma	84
Meningioma	80
Low grade glioma	>60 with complete resection
Ganglioglioma	>75
Dysembryoplastic neuroepithelioma	69

intracerebral hemorrhage, although the epilepsy often gets better at the same time (Table 15.4).

- Where there is discordance between the location of a foreign tissue lesion and the EEG localization of epilepsy, the best result usually comes from resection of the lesion rather than resecting the electrophysiological disturbance.
- Dual pathology may necessitate a second operation to remove the mesial temporal structures.
- Frameless stereotaxy is a technique that allows the surgeon to locate the position of his instruments in relation to three-dimensional coordinates defined pre-operatively. These coordinates are defined in the patient's head by reference to anatomical markers on a pre-operative MRI scan. Information from different investigations such as EEG is superimposed on the scan and related to these coordinates. The surgeon uses a mechanical arm with electronic sensors that tracks its own movement within three-dimensional space against the anatomical landmarks defined pre-operatively. The arm "knows" where it is in relation to the region that requires resection, and a lesion can be resected, which the surgeon may not easily see.

Mesial Temporal Sclerosis

- Anterior temporal lobectomy is the standard surgical treatment for TLE. Resection tends to be more extensive in the non-dominant than in the dominant temporal lobe.
- Selective amygdalohippocampectomy has been advocated by some authors as being less destructive and less likely to cause neuropsychological deficits.

Non-Surgical Ablation

- "Gamma knife" radiotherapy has been applied to lesions including cavernous hemangiomas with good results. Preliminary studies have also shown promise in the treatment of MTS. Seizures tend to run down after radiotherapy rather than stop abruptly as with surgery. Complications may prove to be fewer than with surgery, but it is nevertheless ablative treatment and requires the same rigorous "presurgical" assessment.

Cortical Developmental Abnormalities

- Cortical developmental abnormalities are the second commonest pathologies underlying refractory focal epilepsy.
- The location and extent of lesions is very variable and resections must be tailored to the individual. This often requires intraoperative neurophysiological evaluation.

Hemispherectomy

- Hemispherectomy is undertaken when a whole cerebral hemisphere is serving the patient little useful purpose but is triggering all their seizures.
- Hemimegelancephaly (Chapter 2) and Rasmussen's encephalitis (Chapter 14) are two commoner indications.
- Removal of a whole hemisphere often leaves the patient ambulant with some contralateral arm movement but with little contralateral hand function. If the cause arises under the age of about six years, there is a good chance that the remaining hemisphere will take over some higher cortical functions such as language.

Anti-Epileptic Drugs after Neurosurgery

- When a patient becomes seizure-free after epilepsy surgery, it is usually possible to start reducing AEDs to monotherapy very soon.
- Withdrawal of the last AED is often undertaken 1 to 2 years after surgery. Some patients may wish to remain on treatment for longer.

PALLIATIVE NEUROSURGERY

- The aim of palliative neurosurgery is to reduce the frequency or severity of seizures without the expectation of seizure-freedom.
- Lesion reduction is generally only helpful if at least 90 percent of the lesion is removed.
- Multiple subpial transection is a technique applied to epilepsy in eloquent cortex that cannot be resected. Multiple cuts are made through the thickness of the cortex at short intervals and with different orientations (Figure 15.3). The aim is to transect short intercortical fibres, interrupting local seizure spread but preserving the descending fibres and long intercortical fibres that are important in normal function. Its precise role remains uncertain but small series suggest that 50 to 60 percent of appropriately selected patients may gain more than a 50 percent seizure reduction.
- Corpus callosotomy is generally reserved for patients who suffer severe drop attacks due to focal epilepsy with rapid seizure spread. These patients are at risk of major head injury. Their seizures usually start in one frontal lobe and spread across the corpus callosum within milliseconds to produce a pseudogeneralized EEG pattern. Section of the corpus callosum may prevent this spread and the sudden and dangerous collapses associated with it. It is rarely used.

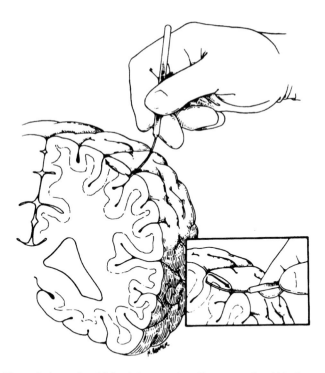

Figure 15.3. The technique of multiple pial transection. Cuts are made within the cortex to prevent local spread of discharges important in seizure propagation, whilst sparing deeper intercortical pathways more important in normal function. Reproduced with permission from Morrell (1989).

- Vagus nerve stimulation is undertaken for any form of refractory epilepsy. The technique involves inserting an electrode around the left vagus nerve, attached to an electronic stimulator that is implanted subcutaneously. Pulsed stimulation is given at regular intervals. It is thought that the afferent stimulation may desynchronize cerebral activity, reducing the chance of abnormal, synchronized seizure discharges. Some patients with auras may trigger the stimulator with an external device during the aura, to try to prevent more severe seizures. Adverse effects are a hoarse voice and throat irritation but cardiac effects are rarer than one might expect. The technique is helpful for about 25 percent of patients for whom it is tried but drug reduction is rarely possible.

BIBLIOGRAPHY

Aykut-Bingol C, Bronen RA, Kim JH, Spencer DD, Spencer SS. Surgical outcome in occipital lobe epilepsy: implications for pathophysiology. Ann Neurol 1998;44:60–69.

Britton JW, Cascino GD, Sharbrough FW, Kelly PJ. Low-grade glial neoplasms and intractable partial epilepsy: efficacy of surgical treatment. Epilepsia 1994;35:1130–1135.

Cendes F, Li LM, Andermann F, Watson C, Fish DR, Shorvon SD, Dubeau F, Arnold DL. Dual pathology and its clinical relevance. Adv Neurol 1999;81:153–164.

Dodick DW, Cascino GD, Meyer FB. Vascular malformations and intractable epilepsy: outcome after surgical treatment. Mayo Clin Proc 1994;69:741–745.

Ferrier CH, Engelsman J, Alarcon G, Binnie CD, Polkey CE. Prognostic factors in presurgical assessment of frontal lobe epilepsy. J Neurol Neurosurg Psychiatry 1999;66:350–356.

Fisher RS, Handforth A. Reassessment: vagus nerve stimulation for epilepsy. Neurology 1999;53:666–669.

Guerreiro MM, Andermann F, Andermann E, Palmini A, Hwang P, Hoffman HJ, Otsubo H, Bastos A, Dubeau F, Snipes GJ, Olivier A, Rasmussen T. Surgical treatment of epilepsy in tuberous sclerosis. Neurology 1998;51:1263–1269.

Hennessy MJ, Elwes RDC, Honovar M, Rabe-Hesketh S, Binnie CD, Polkey CE. Predictors of outcome and pathological considerations in the surgical treatment if intractable epilepsy associated with temporal lobe lesions. Journal Neurol. Neurosurg Neuropsychiatry 2001;70:450–458.

Jomin M, Lesoin F, Lozes G. Prognosis for arteriovenous malformations of the brain in adults based on 150 cases. Surg Neurol 1985;23:362–366.

Moran NF, Fish DR, Kitchen N, Shorvon S, Kendall BE, Stevens JM. Supratentorial cavernous haemangiomas and epilepsy: a review of the literature and case series. J Neurol Neurosurg Psychiatry 1999;66:561–568.

Morris HH, Matkovic Z, Estes ML, Prayson RA, Comair YG, Turnbull J, Najm I, Kotagal P, Wyllie E. Ganglioglioma and intractable epilepsy: clinical and neurophysiologic features and predictors of outcome after surgery. Epilepsia 1998;39:307–313.

Salanova V, Andermann F, Rasmussen T, Olivier A, Quesney L. The running down phenomenon in temporal lobe epilepsy. Brain 1996;119:989–996.

Smith DF, Hutton JL, Sandemann D, Foy PM, Shaw MD, Williams IR, Chadwick DW. The prognosis of primary intracerebral tumours presenting with epilepsy: the outcome of medical and surgical management. J Neurol Neurosurg Psychiatry 1991;54:915–920.

Smith MC. Multiple pial transection in patients with extratemporal epilepsy. Epilepsia 1998;38 (Suppl.4):S81–S89.

Wiebe S, Blume WT, Girvin JP, Eliasziw M. A randomized controlled trial of surgery for temporal lobe epilepsy. N Engl J Med 2001;345:311–318.

Wyllie E, Comair YG, Kotagal P, Bulacio J, Bingaman W, Ruggieri P. Seizure outcome after epilepsy surgery in children and adolescents. Ann Neurol 1998;44:740–748.

REFERENCE

1. Morrell F, Whisler WW, Bleck TB. Multiple pial transection: a new approach to the surgical treatment of focal epilepsy. J Neurosurg 1989;70:231–239.

SECTION 5
Psychosocial Issues

16

Cognitive Aspects of Epilepsy

Altered cognition is a common complaint amongst patients with epilepsy. The assessment of these disturbances may be difficult as there is often a poor correlation between the patient's subjective complaints and measures of cognitive disturbance on standard neuropsychological tests. Numerous factors may contribute to cognitive disturbance, including epilepsy etiology, epilepsy syndrome, seizure activity, interictal disturbances, medication and depression.

NEUROPSYCHOLOGICAL TESTING

Neuropsychometric testing involves applying a battery of tests of different cognitive processes to identify an individual's strengths and weaknesses. The tests include assessments of memory, speech, non-verbal skills, and tests of planning. This is related to an estimate of their previous level, which takes into account occupation and educational achievement. For an excellent explanation of these tests the reader is referred to Hodges 1994.

Purpose of Neuropsychometric Assessment

Identifying Problem Areas

- Patterns of neuropsychological deficits may help to determine whether any deterioration is more likely due to epilepsy, its cause, its treatment, or coincidental factors, for example depression.
- Serial testing may provide additional information in planning management.

Case History 1

A 35-year-old man had suffered typical temporal lobe epilepsy for eight years. After each seizure he was left dysphasic for a period of up to 30 minutes. His seizures were very infrequent and did not concern him. He noticed that he was finding it increasingly difficult to express himself. Serial neuropsychometric assessment confirmed a progressive, slow decline in language function. MRI showed a small temporal lesion, thought either to be a dysembryoplastic neuroepithelioma (DNET) or a low grade glioma. Serial MRI showed no evidence of progression of the lesion. Although his epilepsy was mild, he decided to consider surgery because of his speech disturbance. A DNET was removed and his epilepsy went into remission. There was no further speech deterioration over the next two years.

In this case the neuropyschometric assessment confirmed deteriorating function in the presence of mild epilepsy and an unchanging lesion. This formed the basis for a decision to excise the lesion, with a good outcome.

Presurgical Evaluation

- For presurgical localization of epilepsy (see Chapter 15) the pattern of cognitive deficits can be related to other measures of the region of epilepsy onset in order to assess concordance before surgical resection. In Case 1 the neuropsychometric abnormality was fully concordant with the known left temporal lesion. If there are deficits pointing to neurological dysfunction of brain regions, not shown up on MRI or EEG, then the prognosis for epilepsy surgery is poorer.
- Assessing safety of surgery is another crucial role of neuropsychometric assessment. HM is a celebrated case who underwent bilateral temporal lobectomy for epilepsy, resulting in a total amnesic syndrome: he has been totally unable to retain any new information since his surgery nearly half a century ago. Neuropsychometric testing now plays a central role in trying to predict the impact of surgery on cognition. An adverse assessment may mean that surgery is impossible or that the surgical approach has to be altered.

The Wada Test

- The risks of temporal lobe surgery can be assessed indirectly by the intracarotid amylobarbital or Wada test. The hippocampus is intimately involved in memory and hippocampal sclerosis is often associated with some memory disturbance. The dominant hemisphere hippocampus (left side in right-handers and variable in left-handers) is more involved with verbal memory and the non-dominant hippocampus more with non-verbal memory. Once it is determined that a patient's epilepsy is likely to respond to surgery, the Wada test is often undertaken as the final stage of investigation.

- The procedure involves an angiographic approach from the femoral artery. Amylobarbital, a very short-acting barbiturate anesthetic, is injected into each carotid artery in turn. This anesthetizes the ipsilateral half of the brain, leaving the other half functioning normally. The functional capacity of the awake hemisphere can then be assessed.
- The whole carotid territory is anesthetized, but the psychometric tests applied are more specific to the temporal lobes. If the patient performs well when the side to be operated is anesthetized, then surgery is unlikely to have a major adverse effect on memory. The test cannot detect altered functional localization within one hemisphere.

Case History 2

A 23-year-old left-handed woman gave a 12-year history of focal epilepsy. She had suffered two prolonged febrile convulsions as a child. Neuroimaging showed left mesial temporal sclerosis (MTS). Interictal and ictal EEGs confirmed epilepsy arising from the left temporal lobe. She underwent a Wada test. On injection of the left carotid artery there was minor impairment of memory for visually presented material but preserved memory for verbally presented material. On injection of the right carotid artery she became aphasic for 60 seconds. She was tested with verbal material, which she could not recall after a brief interval and had some milder impairment of memory for visually presented material.

The preservation of verbal memory with the left carotid injection suggests that this patient is right hemisphere dominant and that left temporal lobectomy should be safe. Some minor problem with visual memory may occur but there is bilateral representation of this function, suggesting it will not be a major problem.

Localization of Function in a Damaged Brain

- Children who suffer severe dominant hemisphere damage before the age of about six years are able to regain language function within the undamaged nondominant hemisphere. Plasticity is maximal in children, but there is increasing evidence that functions may redistribute in damaged adult brains. Brain functions in patients with epilepsy may be distributed in atypical brain regions. More anatomically selective procedures than the Wada test may be required to test the location of specific brain functions in planning for epilepsy surgery especially resections in other critical areas, for example the motor cortex.
- Functional neuroimaging is used increasingly with experimental paradigms designed to test specific brain functions (see Chapter 8).
- Intracranial recordings: brain activity may be recorded with intracranial electrodes during the performance of specific mental tasks. This may be undertaken with indwelling electrodes during the course of pre-surgical evaluation or during surgery itself. After a craniotomy has been performed, the patient is woken from the anesthetic and the activity is recorded at intracranial electrodes during specific tasks. The brain activity can be mapped against the grid of electrodes. Functional neuroimaging is gradually superseding these invasive and stressful techniques.
- Cortical activation studies: the brain is stimulated via the electrodes implanted for the purpose of seizure recording and the functional consequences are observed, enabling mapping of cortical function.

CAUSES OF COGNITIVE DEFICITS IN EPILEPSY

Epilepsy Etiology

- Focal epilepsies may be associated with focal cognitive disturbance referable to the region of onset of the epilepsy. For example many patients with left temporal lobe epilepsy (TLE) suffer memory disturbances or patients with frontal lobe epilepsy may suffer difficulties with organization and executive function. The structural lesion underlying the epilepsy is likely to be the major cause of the disturbance in these cases.
- Idiopathic generalized epilepsies (IGE) are not associated with major structural lesions and are not thought to cause major, persistent cognitive effects. Some subtle alterations in function have been suggested. For example frontal lobe dysfunction is postulated in juvenile myoclonic epilepsy. This may relate to subtle alterations that have been detected with structural and functional neuroimaging and the possible histopathological finding of mesial frontal microdysgenesis in this syndrome.
- Symptomatic generalized epilepsies such as West's or Lennox-Gastaut syndromes are commonly associated with major structural or metabolic brain disease. These epilepsies most commonly affect children with pre-existing cognitive deficits due to these etiologies (see Chapter 11) and cause further cognitive decline.

Epilepsy Activity

- Normal cognitive function is interrupted by most seizures. The more frequent the seizures, the greater their impact on cognition.
- Head injury is a common consequence of epileptic seizures and is probably under-recognized as a secondary cause of cognitive disturbance. Atonic and tonic seizures are particularly likely to cause severe head injury.
- Status epilepticus commonly causes brain damage and cognitive disturbance through hypoxic or excitotoxic mechanisms (see Chapter 14). The learning-disabled are more liable to status epilepticus and recurrent episodes may cause further cognitive decline and structural cortical change.
- Cognitive triggers may occasionally cause seizures, for example reading epilepsy or epilepsy caused by games or calculation. These problems often manifest in childhood or adolescence and may affect schooling and cognitive development.

Idiopathic Generalized Epilepsy

- Global loss of function with altered awareness is the rule during generalized epileptic seizures. Sometimes the seizures are so brief, for example myoclonic seizures, that it may be difficult to detect any change.
- Immediate recovery is usual after absences and myoclonic seizures but not convulsive seizures.
- Generalized absence status epilepticus causes a more persistent alteration of function that may be less dense than in brief absence seizures. For example patients may wander in a confused state with automatisms and partial responsiveness.

- Very frequent absences or absence status with no major motor phenomena may mean that the "brain is absent" for much of each day. Patients with this severity of disturbance often present with school failure or work failure, without a history of overt seizures.

Case History 3
A 17-year-old boy was referred after his employer had noticed episodes at work. Typically, he would appear blank and his head would move slightly backwards. There was no other movement and he returned rapidly to normal. In retrospect his parents realized these episodes had been occurring since the age of 3 or 4 but they had just thought he was daydreaming and this was never brought to medical attention. He had performed poorly at school leaving without any formal qualifications. During the consultation he had an episode in which he became staring and unresponsive for approximately five seconds, before recovering fully to normal. An EEG showed typical 3 hertz spike and wave of absence epilepsy.

Focal Epilepsy

- Most focal seizures cause altered awareness during the ictus.
- Postictal cognitive deficits often reflect the region of onset of the seizure. The commonest is dysphasia after a seizure arising in the dominant temporal lobe.
- An underlying lesion may be affected by ongoing epileptic activity. Animal models suggest that continuing epileptic activity may cause shrinkage of a damaged hippocampus. Whether this occurs in humans is not yet clear.
- Landau-Kleffner syndrome (LKS) is characterized by progressive speech disturbance in the context of electrographic seizure activity, sometimes without overt seizures. The abnormal activity may be interfering with the formation of normal connections during a critical period of speech development. Other severe childhood epilepsies may have a similar effect (see Chapter 11).
- Focal status epilepticus in adults may also present with a progressive disturbance of cognition, depending on the region of onset of the epilepsy (see Case 8, Chapter 14). Unlike in LKS, this disturbance largely reverses once seizures cease, although some excitotoxic damage may persist.

Interictal Electrographic Abnormalities

- Brief interictal electrographic discharges transiently affect cognitive function.
- Generalized discharges have the greatest effect.
- Focal discharges have an effect that relates to their region of onset. Patients can be assessed continuously with computerized tasks, which measure function of one or other hemisphere. Studies with these techniques show that during a lateralized discharge, there is a subtle alteration of function of the affected hemisphere.

Anti-Epileptic Drugs and Cognition

- Mental slowing is a common adverse effect of virtually all AEDs, which can be detected on reaction time tasks. Mental slowing underlies many of the

Table 16.1. A Guide to the Cognitive Adverse Effects of AEDs

Minor Cognitive Effects	Intermediate	Major Cognitive Effects Common
Gabapentin	Carbamazepine	Barbiturates
Lamotrigine	Oxcarbazepine	Benzodiazepines
Levetiracetam	Phenytoin	Topiramate
	Tiagabine	Zonisamide
	Valproate*	
	Vigabatrin	

*Rare encephalopathy in the context of urea cycle disturbances.

cognitive effects of AEDs. The problem is worst with rapid dose escalation or at high doses and tends to reduce as the patient gets used to the medication.

- Focal cognitive deficits occur occasionally with some drugs. For example topiramate occasionally causes dysphasia.
- Sleepiness has been shown to occur in patients with epilepsy whether or not they are taking AEDs. Disturbed nocturnal sleep may be a factor.
- All AEDs may cause cognitive adverse effects in susceptible patients at low doses but Table 16.1 gives a personal view of the major culprits supported by the limited evidence available. Of the older, commonly used drugs, the barbiturates stand out as being the worst. Patients may have been taking barbiturates so long that they don't realize the cognitive effects they have been suffering until the drug is stopped.
- Polytherapy is more likely to cause cognitive effects than monotherapy.
- Improvement of cognition may also occur as an AED brings seizures and interictal disturbances under control.

Depression and Cognition

- Depression is the commonest cause of memory disturbance in general neurological practice and affects one third of patients with epilepsy.
- The etiology of the depression may be multifactorial – the epilepsy itself, medication, and psychosocial factors (Chapter 17).
- Other clinical features of depression should be sought to support the diagnosis.

AN APPROACH TO A PATIENT COMPLAINING OF COGNITIVE DISTURBANCE

- A fluctuating cognitive disturbance with some periods much better than others is likely to be related to epilepsy activity, whether or not there are overt seizures. EEG studies, including ambulatory EEG may help to evaluate whether there is an increase in abnormal electrographic activity.
- A progressive cognitive disturbance is likely due to other factors, especially progression of the underlying cause. Neuroimaging is usually indicated (Figure 16.1).

Case History 4

A 34-year-old man developed epilepsy that was found to be due to a low grade glioma of the left temporal lobe. He remained well apart from refractory epilepsy. After several years he started treatment with topiramate. Within a few weeks his speech deteriorated. Neuroimaging showed massive enlargement of the left temporal glioma.

Although topiramate can cause speech disturbance, a progressive neurological deficit should lead to a search for a progressive neurological lesion.

- Recent drug changes should be re-evaluated and modification of treatment considered as indicated and evidence of depression should be sought.

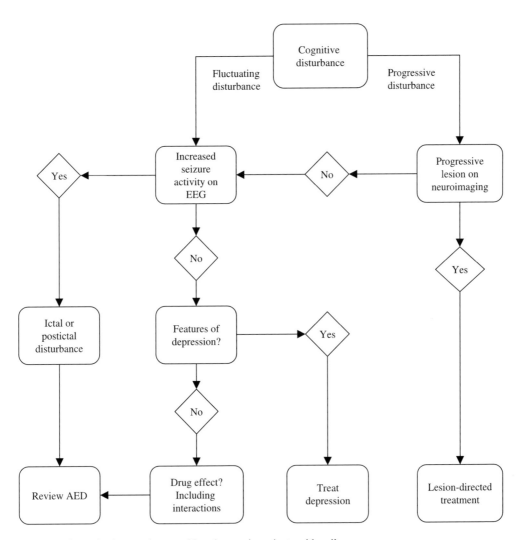

Figure 16.1. A scheme for interpreting cognitive changes in patients with epilepsy.

MEMORY DISTURBANCES IN EPILEPSY

- The hippocampus is crucial in memory formation and retrieval and MTS is the commonest cause of focal epilepsy. Fixed deficits of verbal and visuospatial memory commonly affect patients with TLE, especially when due to MTS. Other forms of amnesia are peculiar to patients with epilepsy.
- Patients have been described whose behavior appears normal during the seizure but who have no recollection of the event. This has been termed pure epileptic amnesia.
- Accelerated forgetting is a mechanism of amnesia, which has recently been recognized in patients with TLE, especially of the dominant hemisphere. These patients may recall information normally at the brief time interval of minutes to hours used in standard neuropsychological tests but cannot remember it normally weeks later. It is thought that the role of the hippocampus in consolidating memories is disrupted by MTS and associated seizures.
- Episodic memory disturbance is a curious phenomenon, which affects some patients with epilepsy.

Case History 5

A 64-year-old, retired school teacher was admitted to hospital as an emergency. His wife described an acute memory disturbance affecting him for the previous two weeks. Neuropsychometric testing confirmed severe anterograde amnesia and retrograde amnesia for recent events. Neuroimaging, EEG and CSF studies were normal including PCR for Herpes simplex virus. He had never abused alcohol. He was discharged without a clear diagnosis. Two weeks later he suffered a convulsive seizure and was admitted to another hospital. He started treatment with carbamazepine. Some weeks later he was reassessed and his anterograde and retrograde amnesia had resolved. However, he remained amnesic for the one month prior to starting AED therapy. In addition he seemed unable to remember important events in his life, such as holidays over the previous five years.

It is likely that the acute amnesic presentation was due to ongoing seizure activity, even though this was not detectable on scalp EEG. The selective loss of recall of major life events over the previous few years may be due to epilepsy interfering with the consolidation of memories.

Frontal Lobe Disturbances in Epilepsy

After TLE, frontal lobe epilepsy is the most frequent of focal epilepsy and is the commonest to be associated with neuropsychological and behavioral disturbances. Memory is less impaired than in TLE but patients suffer more problems with motor control, speed of executing tasks and maintaining or inhibiting responses. These are more subtle correlates of the more major symptoms of perseveration and reduced mental flexibility that affect patients with larger frontal lesions. It is difficult on the basis of neuropsychological tests to tell where in the frontal lobes the epilepsy is coming from or even to differentiate between left and right frontal lobes.

BIBLIOGRAPHY

Aldenkamp AP, Alpherts WC, Sandstedt P, Blennow G, Elmqvist D, Heijbel J, Nilsson HL, Tonnby B, Wahlander L, Wosse E. Antiepileptic drug-related cognitive complaints in seizure-free children with epilepsy before and after drug discontinuation. Epilepsia 1998;39:1070–1074.

Vermeulen J, Aldenkamp AP. Cognitive side-effects of chronic antiepileptic drug treatment: a review of 25 years of research. Epilepsy Res 1995;22:65–95.

Binnie CD. Cognitive performance, subtle seizures, and the EEG. Epilepsia 2001;42 (Suppl. 1):16–18.

Binnie CD, Kasteleijn-Nolst Trenite DG, Smit AM, Wilkins AJ. Interactions of epileptiform EEG discharges and cognition. Epilepsy Res 1987;1:239–245.

Blake RV, Wroe SJ, Breen EK, McCarthy RA. Accelerated forgetting in patients with epilepsy: evidence for an impairment in memory consolidation. Brain 2000;123:472–483.

Devinsky O, Gershengorn J, Brown E, Perrine K, Vazquez B, Luciano D. Frontal functions in juvenile myoclonic epilepsy. Neuropsychiatry Neuropsychol Behav Neurol 1997;10:243–246.

Elixhauser A, Leidy NK, Meador K, Means E, Willian MK. The relationship between memory performance, perceived cognitive function, and mood in patients with epilepsy. Epilepsy Res 1999;37:13–24.

Helmstaedter C, Gleissner U, Zentner J, Elger CE. Neuropsychological consequences of epilepsy surgery in frontal lobe epilepsy. Neuropsychologia 1998;36:681–689.

Jokeit H, Markowitsch HJ. Age limits plasticity of episodic memory functions in response to left temporal lobe damage in patients with epilepsy. Adv Neurol 1999;81:251–258.

Palmini A, Gloor P, Jones-Gotman M. Pure amnestic seizures in temporal lobe epilepsy. Definition, clinical symptomatology and functional anatomical observations. Brain 1992;115:749–770.

REFERENCES

1. Hodges JR. Cognitive Assessment for Clinicians. Oxford: Oxford Medical Publications, 1994.
2. Scoville WB, Milner B. Loss of recent memory after bilateral hippocampal lesions. J Neurol Neurosurg Psychiatr 1957;20:11–21.

17

Psychiatric Aspects of Epilepsy

Psychiatric illness and epilepsy morbidity have a complex relationship. Epilepsy is associated with an increased risk of affective and psychotic disorders through a variety of mechanisms. The medications used to treat psychiatric disorders may trigger seizures and anti-epileptic drugs (AEDs) commonly have psychotropic adverse effects.

Differentiating psychiatric illness presenting with psychogenic non-epileptic seizures (PNES) from epilepsy with associated psychopathology is a recurring diagnostic conundrum. Indeed, about 20 to 30 percent of patients with PNES also suffer epileptic seizures. The proportion of patients with epilepsy who also suffer PNES is much smaller.

PSYCHOGENIC NON-EPILEPTIC SEIZURES

- PNES can mimic virtually all types of epileptic seizures (see Chapter 5). The commonest kinds of attacks are swoons, tantrums and attacks with stiffening convulsion and often hyperventilation. The attack disorder must be diagnosed in its own right and not assumed to be PNES just because the patient has a psychiatric illness.
- A diagnosis can only be made for the seizures that have been observed. If this is the patient's only seizure type, one can make a confident diagnosis. If there are other seizure types, then the clinician must be cautious about unifying all the

seizures under one diagnostic label as some patients with PNES also have epilepsy.

- Neurological investigations, including interictal EEG, are more commonly abnormal in patients with PNES than in the general population.
- A positive psychiatric diagnosis is necessary in patients with PNES in order to target appropriate psychiatric treatment, (see Case 9, Chapter 5, and Figure 17.1).
- The psychiatric concept of dissociation applies to many forms of PNES (below). Although by definition a psychiatric disturbance, PNES may present as a mono-symptomatic dissociative disorder without the clinical features of commoner psychiatric disorders, which may lead clinicians into assuming an organic cause.
- Patients, carers and clinicians need to be taught to recognize and manage PNES differently from epileptic seizures when both coexist.

Hyperventilation Syndrome

- Hyperventilation syndrome (HVS) is common. It is commonest in young or middle-aged women but can occur in adolescents or adults of either sex and at any age. The presumed mechanism is anxiety triggering hyperventilation, causing alkalosis and hypocalcemia, which can cause a variety of neurological symptoms.
- Unexplained fluctuating neurological symptoms should lead to an evaluation for HVS. Common presentations are giddiness, paresthesiae and blackouts. The symptoms are almost continuous with major fluctuations in severity rather than truly paroxysmal. Often the hyperventilation is a persistent mild habit that at unpredictable intervals tips the patient into somatic symptoms, rather than occurring only when they feel under severe emotional stress.
- The patient may take deep sighs during the consultation, is often unable to hold their breath for more than five seconds and forced hyperventilation may reproduce their attacks within one minute.
- Epileptic seizures may occasionally be triggered by hyperventilation, most commonly idiopathic generalized epilepsy (IGE) absences. Hyperventilation may also occasionally be due to brainstem lesions, metabolic disturbance or drugs.
- Treatment is often easy as the physical basis can be demonstrated to the patient and there is less stigma than in a pure psychiatric diagnosis. Physiotherapy and breathing control techniques are useful.

Case History 1

Nine months earlier a 27-year-old traffic warden had been assaulted during the course of her work and suffered a head injury. She had been dazed but had not lost consciousness. Six weeks later she started to suffer attacks. At the onset her mouth felt dry with a strange taste. Then both hands started to tingle and she felt light headed and giddy. She fell to the ground and started to convulse. She developed opisthotonic posturing, carpopedal spasm and more generalized convulsive movements, which lasted 10 minutes. After the attack she was tearful. They only occurred during the day and were not associated with tongue-biting, incontinence or major injury. Because of these attacks she had been unable to return to work. On closer questioning she revealed poor sleep, flashbacks of the assault, reluctance to leave the house and a tendency to be tearful. Forced hyperventilation for 30 seconds caused

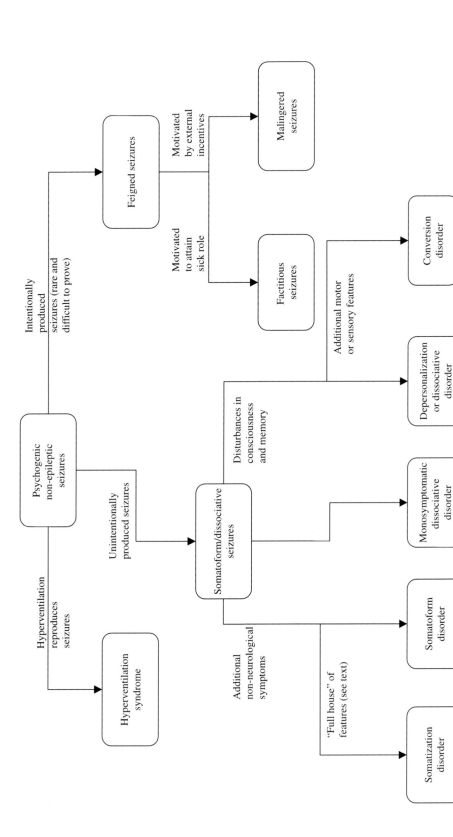

Adapted with permission from Martin R.L. and Gates J.R. Nosology, classification and differential diagnosis of non-epileptic seizures: an alternative proposal. In Gates J.R and Rowan A.J. Non-epileptic seizures 2nd edition. Butterworth-Heinemann, Boston. 2000. pp253-267.

Figure 17.1. A scheme for the differential diagnosis of non-epileptic seizures.

her right arm to start to shake. The shaking grew more violent and she was encouraged to cease overbreathing but was unable to stop, triggering a full-blown attack. A friend described this as typical of her habitual attacks.

Although a classical symptom of temporal lobe epilepsy, an odd taste can also be caused by HVS. The other features are typical of severe hyperventilation and the duration of the attack is unusually long for epilepsy. It is important to confirm that this is the patient's habitual attack with a witness or by video recording. Her psychological symptoms pointed to a post-traumatic stress disorder. There was a secondary gain from the attacks in that they kept her away from work, which was the source of her stress. Advice about breathing control techniques prevented the attacks and with counseling her mood improved and she was able to return to work.

Somatization Disorder

Somatization disorder has a lifetime prevalence of 0.5 percent and affects about five times as many women as men. The condition is commonest in women from a deprived background and they have often suffered physical or sexual abuse. There are usually co-existing psychiatric disorders, including affective disorders or drug abuse.

- Diagnostic criteria of The Diagnostic and Statistical Manual of Mental Disorders volume IV of the American Psychiatric Association (DSM IV) are complex:

    1. Onset of many physical complaints without physical cause before age 30. The symptoms are not due to malingering but cause significant psychosocial impairment
    2. Four pain symptoms
    3. Two gastrointestinal symptoms
    4. One sexual symptom
    5. One pseudo-neurologic symptom including seizures.

- Patients with fewer symptoms than this are sometimes termed as having a somatoform disorder.

A typical patient has a very thick set of hospital records and has attended many specialist clinics. They may have undergone repeated abdominal surgery for recurrent abdominal pain. If they had an appendectomy or cholecystectomy then often the removed tissue was histologically normal. The patient may be emotionally or culturally prevented from expressing psychological distress with mental symptoms, for example if psychiatric illness is stigmatized in the family.

Dissociation

- Dissociation is the breakdown of integration of memory, consciousness, identity and perception in response to an overwhelming stress. Dissociative disorders are triggered by anxiety. The patient develops dissociative symptoms, which cause them to separate themselves from the stress that has triggered them. Pseudo-unconsciousness or amnesia are archetypal dissociative mechanisms. Sometimes the symptom may be more obviously physical. Although attempts are made to separate conversion disorder from factitious disorders and malingering, they may represent a spectrum.

- Management of dissociative disorders involves a cognitive behavioral approach, addressing the idea of gain from attacks as the underlying cause and explaining the process of conversion of stress to physical symptoms. The clinician takes a history guiding the patient through the circumstances of their attacks. They are encouraged to record the events and sensations prior to the onset of future seizures. Once unpleasant feelings have been identified, the patient is helped to learn new strategies for dealing with these symptoms so that they do not evolve into seizures.

Conversion Disorder

Symptoms are exclusively neurological. Conversion disorder is commoner in young women but is seen in men who have been involved in severe trauma, for example in the military. First onset in individuals over the age of 30 is rare and the diagnosis should be questioned:

1. One or more symptoms affecting motor or sensory function or other neurological symptoms for example ataxia, amnesia, seizures, or dysphasia
2. Psychological factors judged to be the trigger
3. The process is unconscious
4. There is primary or secondary gain
5. The symptom is not due to a physical cause or a culturally sanctioned behavior
6. There is no other identifiable physical or psychiatric explanation.

- The neurological symptoms of conversion disorders are often characterized by marked fluctuations in severity and distractibility.
- Histrionic personality and previous conversion symptoms have commonly affected the patient or their relatives. The patient may appear indifferent to the severity of symptoms (belle indifference) and there may be a clear primary gain or secondary reinforcers of the abnormal behaviors but the gain may be difficult to identify when the behavior is very longstanding.

Case History 2

A 27-year-old man was brought to hospital as an emergency suffering from seizures. These proved difficult to control with diazepam but settled over the next few days. As he recovered it became clear that he had a left hemiparesis in a non-organic pattern and a bizarre form of dysphonia. Investigations confirmed no organic basis to these symptoms. He had recently suffered two close family bereavements and his admission occurred on the day he was due to attend a funeral.

This man suffered a conversion disorder with clear psychological triggers and a gain of avoiding the emotional stress of attending a funeral.

Other Forms of PNES

Factitious Disorder and Malingering

Factitious disorder is defined as the intentional production of symptoms and signs, usually in order to assume a sick role. Malingering is the intentional production of symptoms and signs with a clear incentive such as financial gain or avoiding some financial or legal responsibility. These diagnoses are difficult to make without the confession of the patient. Most clinicians will give a patient the benefit of the doubt unless there is overwhelming evidence to the contrary and clinicians' ability to detect malingering is poor.

Munchausen's Syndrome

- Males more commonly suffer Munchausen's syndrome. It is motivated by the need for medical attention and characterized by recurrent symptoms without physical basis, leading to medical intervention and patients may bear many surgical scars. Seizures are relatively uncommon. Patients present to numerous different hospitals. They may have antisocial personality disorders.

Case History 3
A 55-year-old male inpatient was referred with a history of collapse and loss of consciousness, lasting hours, followed by transient left hemiparesis, lasting one to two days. He had a distinctive appearance. Before I could see him, he discharged himself from the hospital. From his description, I recalled admitting him to another hospital, 200 miles away, 13 years earlier and seeing him in a third hospital 12 years earlier, each time with exactly the same story. Perusal of notes from each hospital confirmed it had been the same individual each time and showed he had given numerous addresses. He had undergone a brain scan and lumbar puncture at each presentation.

Munchausen's Syndrome by Proxy

- Women are more commonly involved in Munchausen's syndrome by proxy. A parent or carer induces illness in an infant or child with a significant mortality.
- Seizures are common and are usually secondary to induced asphyxia.
- A high index of suspicion is needed to make the diagnosis. Pointers are: recurrent and persistent unexplained illness, unusual or remarkable clinical features, signs or symptoms are only present when the caregiver is present, and the caregiver refuses to leave the hospital but is not unduly concerned about the child's prognosis.

Psychogenic Non-Epileptic Seizures Triggered by Epilepsy

- In a small proportion of patients, a distressing aura or focal seizure may trigger a psychological reaction, which manifests as a psychogenic non-epileptic seizure. Careful clinical evaluation and ideally video-EEG-telemetry is needed to make this diagnosis (see Case 2 Chapter 14).

Clinical Features of Psychogenic Non-Epileptic Seizure Patients

- There are some pointers that the psychiatric profile of patients with PNES differs from the profile of patients with epilepsy but one cannot assume that seizures occurring in the context of psychiatric disorder are necessarily PNES, as epilepsy is commonly complicated by psychiatric disorder.
- Features commoner in PNES are: dissociative tendencies assessed on questionnaires, escape-avoidance (akin to wishful thinking), histrionic personality, major life events and traumas, and other dissociative symptoms.

PSYCHIATRIC DISEASE ASSOCIATED WITH EPILEPSY

- Patients with epilepsy often suffer psychiatric illness, most commonly depression or anxiety but sometimes psychotic disorders (Table 17.1). Community-based studies of epilepsy show the lowest risk and hospital-based studies of highly refractory epilepsy show the highest risk.
- Of patients attempting suicide, 3 percent have had epilepsy, a six-fold increase compared to the non-epileptic population. In some groups such as postoperative patients and patients with temporal lobe epilepsy, the risk may be more than 25 times the population risk. Although many of these patients may be depressed, psychotic features are also very common.
- The timing of the psychiatric disturbance in relation to seizure occurrence is an important determinant of diagnosis and guides treatment strategy:

  1. Ictal disorders occur during the seizure and are a manifestation of the abnormal electrophysiological activity of the seizure itself.
  2. Peri-ictal disorders occur around the time of the seizures but not necessarily during the seizure.
  3. Interictal disorders happen independently of seizures and may affect patients who are seizure-free.

- As a general therapeutic strategy, the primary treatment of ictal and peri-ictal disorders is to improve control of seizures, whereas interictal disorders need independent treatment.

Table 17.1. Psychiatric Associations of Epilepsy (%)

Diagnosis	Approximate Lifetime Prevalence in Epilepsy Sufferers (Approximate Lifetime Prevalence in General Population)
Major depression	30 (15)
Anxiety disorder	15 (5–7)
Psychotic disorder	2–10 (1–2)
Obsessional compulsive disorder	5 (1–2.5)
Attempted suicide	3 (0.5)

Depression

Interictal Depression

Epidemiology and Etiology

- Interictal depression is the commonest psychiatric disorder to afflict patients with epilepsy. Depression is commoner in epilepsy than in many other chronic diseases, implying a more specific relationship than just a reaction to the patient's condition. All age groups including children and both sexes are affected.
- Risk factors for depression include epilepsy severity; focal epilepsy rather than IGE (some studies) and left hemisphere epilepsy rather than right (some studies).
- Most AEDs may trigger depressive reactions although some do so more frequently, including topiramate, vigabatrin, benzodiazepines, phenobarbital, tiagabine and zonisamide.
- Psychosocial factors are important in depression. In one study, three-quarters of patients with severe epilepsy were dissatisfied with their social lives and a similar number had moderate or severe employment difficulties. One-third of patients felt they never had any true friends and only one-sixth had a steady relationship. Epilepsy carries a significant social stigma. Even in the absence of overt discrimination, patients may feel ashamed of their condition and conceal it from others. In previous generations it was common for parents to concealed or deny the diagnosis, making it even more difficult for a child to come to terms with it.

Case History 4

A 55-year-old man had developed IGE at the age of 10. He had seen a physician and had received a prescription for medication. His father had denied the diagnosis and refused to allow him to take medication. When he was 17, he suffered a convulsive seizure and fell into a fire. He sustained severe burns to his face and lost one hand. He had never been able to work but had married and had a family despite these injuries.

Diagnosis

- Clinicians need a high index of suspicion for this common complication of epilepsy. Diagnostic criteria for depression complicating epilepsy are the same as in other patient groups but psychotic features such as paranoia, delusions or hallucinations are more common.

Treatment

- Support may be provided by specialist epilepsy nurses, and by patient support groups. More specialized therapy such as psychotherapy may sometimes be required.
- AEDs should be considered a potential cause of depression, especially if they have recently been changed. Readjustment may be necessary to establish if there is a diagnostic link and as treatment. The choice of AED may be

influenced by coexisting psychopathology. Carbamazepine, valproate, lamotrigine and gabapentin have been demonstrated to have some mood stabilizing effect. Carbamazepine has the most established history in this regard.

- Antidepressant medication is indicated in depressed epilepsy patients just as in non-epileptic patients.
- Electroconvulsive therapy (ECT) is not contraindicated by epilepsy and it may be beneficial, although AEDs may reduce the convulsive effect.

Use of Antidepressant Medication in Epilepsy

ANTIDEPRESSANTS AND SEIZURE RISK

- Antidepressants may trigger seizures in some patients with epilepsy and in up to 1 percent of patients without previous seizures. For patients without a previous history of seizures, antidepressants are more likely to trigger seizures if there is any evidence of neurological damage, such as dementia, learning disability, head injury, substance abuse or if there is a family history of seizures.
- Tricyclic antidepressants may trigger seizures in 0.5 to 4 percent of patients treated and there is a clear dose effect. Amitriptyline above 200 milligrams daily carries a risk above 5 percent and in overdose, may cause seizures in nearly 10 percent of patients.
- Newer antidepressants have also been reported to cause seizures, which comprise 1 to 4 percent of their reported adverse events.
- Lowest seizure rates are reported for moclobemide (reversible monoamine oxidase A inhibitor), nefazodone and citalopram (selective serotonin reuptake inhibitors, SSRI), but these drugs also have the fewest adverse reports of any kind implying less usage to date.
- Combinations of different psychotropic medications add to the risk of seizures.

PHARMACODYNAMIC INTERACTIONS OF AED AND ANTIDEPRESSANTS

- In theory monoamine oxidase inhibitors (MAOI) given with carbamazepine may trigger a hypertensive crisis. SSRIs may exacerbate carbamazepine-induced hyponatremia. The sedation caused by AEDs may be compounded by concurrent antidepressants.

PHARMACOKINETIC INTERACTIONS OF AED AND ANTIDEPRESSANTS

- Some SSRIs may influence cytochrome P450 and when given concurrently with phenytoin, it is wise to check phenytoin levels before and after starting treatment. Many antidepressants may be rendered less effective by an enzyme-inducing AED, unless given in higher dosage.

Ictal Depression

- Ictal depression may affect about 1 percent of epilepsy patients and is commoner in patients with focal epilepsy, especially temporal lobe epilepsy (TLE).
- It is characterized by sudden overwhelming feelings of depression and despair. These occur seconds to minutes prior to the onset of an overt seizure. Psychotic depression has rarely been reported as the main manifestation of

non-convulsive status epilepticus. Olfactory hallucinations are more common in ictal depression than in other causes of depression.

- Treatment is the prevention of seizures. If ictal depression is more prolonged, then a benzodiazepine may help to abort the ictus. In these circumstances it may be necessary to prove with ictal EEG recording that the depression is ictal rather than postictal, for which a benzodiazepine will have no beneficial effect.

Case History 5

An 18-year-old boy gave a long history of partial seizures of probable temporal lobe origin. In recent years his mood had become low. Just before the start of each seizure he would become profoundly depressed, expressing feelings of worthlessness. These feelings persisted for 30 minutes after each seizure and sometimes resulted in self-injurious behavior. He then settled back to his normal level of more moderate depression. Treatment with antidepressants had no effect. Attempts to control his seizures with AEDs were unsuccessful until he started vigabatrin. With this drug his episodes of severe depression improved, although the more persistent depression remained.

Exacerbations of this boy's depression were closely linked to his seizures. As a last resort a strategy of treatment with vigabatrin was attempted. This reduced his seizure frequency and helped the peri-ictal depression, even though this drug has been associated with exacerbations of interictal depression.

Psychosis

Epidemiology and Etiology

- Psychosis affects 2 to 10 percent of patients with epilepsy, depending on the patient group studied and is slightly more common in women.
- Psychoses usually occur in the context of longstanding epilepsy, established for many years, often with multiple seizure types and often a history of status epilepticus.
- Focal epilepsy is more frequently associated with psychosis, especially TLE.
- Patients with psychosis and epilepsy generally suffer less frequent seizures than patients with refractory epilepsy without psychosis.
- Schizophrenia and epilepsy may coexist as independent conditions and epilepsy is more common in patients with schizophrenia than in the general population. This kind of relationship is suggested if the psychosis precedes or arises very shortly after the development of epilepsy.
- Diagnosis depends on the timing of psychosis in relation to seizures (Figure 17.2).

Postictal Psychosis

Diagnosis

- Postictal psychosis is the commonest form of psychosis associated with epilepsy and may occur in 5 to 15 percent of patients with intractable epilepsy.
- A cluster of tonic–clonic seizures (sometimes partial seizures) usually precedes postictal psychosis.

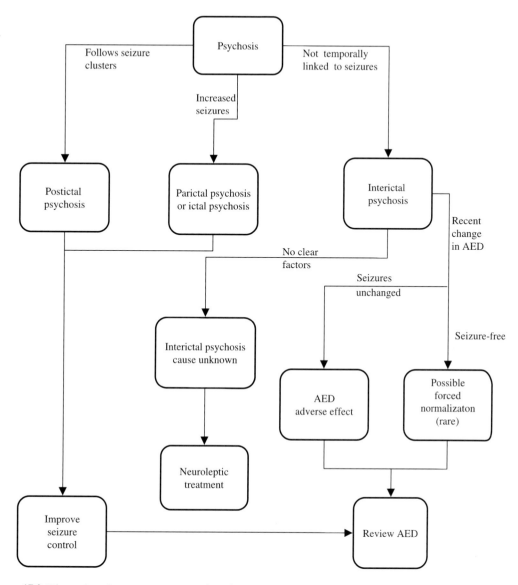

Figure 17.2. Diagnosis and management approach to the psychoses of epilepsy.

- A lucid interval usually follows the seizures before the onset of psychotic symptoms. The clinical features of the psychosis are indistinguishable from schizophrenic psychosis and agitation and paranoia are often prominent. The state persists for 1 to 6 days, then remits spontaneously unless further seizures perpetuate the process. The mechanism of postictal psychosis is unknown. Low-grade seizure activity has been suggested but not proven.

Case History 6

A 47-year-old woman had suffered temporal lobe epilepsy since her teens. In her forties the seizure pattern changed to clusters of nocturnal focal attacks. The day after each cluster she became agitated and believed that her husband was about to attack her with a knife. She became fearful and he was unable to approach her to reassure her. It was only with difficulty that he persuaded her to eat and drink. After two to three days the symptoms settled and she returned to her normal mental state until the next flurry of seizures. Her seizures had proved refractory to medication but use of rectal diazepam after the first seizure prevented the remaining seizures of the cluster and prevented the postictal psychosis.

Treatment

- Preventing seizure clusters prevents postictal psychosis. If regular AEDs are unsuccessful, intermittent benzodiazepines can abort flurries of seizures and reduce the chance of psychosis (Case 6). Neuroleptics given intermittently after each seizure cluster do not usually prevent the development of psychosis but may have a limited effect on its duration or severity. If the psychosis is severe and recurrent, continuous antipsychotic therapy may help reduce the severity of the bouts.

Interictal Psychosis

Diagnosis

- Interictal psychoses are independent of seizures and account for up to 30 percent of epilepsy-associated psychosis. Psychosis may arise *de novo* but recurrent bouts of postictal psychosis may evolve into persistent psychosis.
- AED-induced psychosis may be suggested by a recent change in AED. Psychotic reactions to AEDs are more common in those with a previous history of psychological disturbance. The clinical features may differ slightly from psychosis unrelated to drugs, with more visual or somatic hallucinations. Most drugs have been implicated, but vigabatrin, clobazam, topiramate and zonisamide have been implicated more frequently.
- The symptoms of interictal psychosis are very similar to those of schizophrenia. Delusions are common and auditory hallucinations occur in about a quarter of patients. Catatonia is rare. Interictal psychosis may be mild: some patients "coexist" long-term with their hallucinations and abnormal thoughts without major distress.

Treatment

- Review AEDs and consider simplifying treatment. Carbamazepine is used as a treatment for some psychiatric disorders and consequently is often favored for patients with epilepsy and psychiatric disturbances. However psychotic reactions have been reported very occasionally even with carbamazepine. Other drugs that may have separate AED and psychotropic functions are valproate, lamotrigine and gabapentin. Once interictal psychosis is established, improving seizure control has no effect on the psychosis. Even successful epilepsy surgery is unlikely to have an effect and psychotic reactions may even be triggered after epilepsy surgery.
- Psychological therapy may be indicated as for patients without epilepsy.
- Antipsychotic agents are usually required as for patients without epilepsy.

Neuroleptic Use in Epilepsy

- Seizure exacerbation occurs in 0.5 to 1 percent of patients taking neuroleptic drugs. Phenothiazines may carry a higher risk than butyrephenones and pimozide and sulpiride are favoured by some clinicians. Data are lacking that clearly differentiate between the drugs with the exception of chlorpromazine and clozapine, which carry a higher risk. The risk of seizures seems to increase with the speed of neuroleptic dose titration and the maximum dose achieved, for example higher doses of clozapine may cause seizures in 4 percent of patients.
- Interactions may occur between AEDs and antipsychotic agents. Haloperidol levels may be reduced by half when hepatic metabolism is induced by concomitant carbamazepine. Clozapine is not recommended in epilepsy and its levels are also reduced by carbamazepine. There is also a theoretical possibility of synergistic bone marrow suppression with these two drugs. The combination of carbamazepine and lithium may occasionally cause somnolence, ataxia and confusion, probably by a pharmacodynamic interaction, although it is a common treatment combination for mania.

Forced Normalization

- Forced normalization is a rare and somewhat contentious syndrome. It is characterized by the emergence of a psychotic state in parallel with normalization of a previously abnormal EEG. This usually occurs as the patient becomes seizure-free after a long history of recurrent seizures. For rare patients, the occasional seizure may be better than seizure-freedom, if it means their interictal mental state is normal.

Ictal Psychosis

- True ictal psychosis is very rare. Although hallucinations are common seizure symptoms, ictal auditory hallucinations are uncommon and very rarely have Schneiderian first rank features. There is almost invariably some clouding of consciousness, which excludes true psychosis.
- Ictal psychiatric features are probably most commonly seen as a complication of non-convulsive status epilepticus. A diagnostic clue may be other ictal features such as occasional limb or facial twitching. This diagnosis should be considered in any patient with epilepsy who develops abnormal psychiatric features and can only be excluded by EEG during the abnormal state. Treatment is to prevent seizures and sometimes the abnormal state can be terminated by intravenous benzodiazepines.

Parictal Psychosis

- Parictal psychosis is probably an intermediate form of psychosis between ictal, post-ictal and interictal psychoses. It is of gradual onset and is associated with a general increase in seizure frequency but its timing is not strictly linked to seizure occurrence. There may be an ictal component as alteration of awareness is more common than in other forms. Treatment is to improve seizure control.

Obsessive-Compulsive Disorder (OCD)

- Obsessions are recurrent intrusive thoughts and compulsions are recurrent urges to perform a particular action. In contrast to psychotic thoughts, the sufferer recognizes that the obsessions are senseless and that the compulsions are not due to external influences controlling their mind. The actions are purposeful and can be resisted, although this increases anxiety, in distinction to automatisms.
- Most OCD is idiopathic and not associated with structural pathology. Functional neuroimaging has consistently shown abnormalities in the anterior frontal regions in OCD.
- OCD may be secondary to structural lesions from a variety of causes in the frontal lobes or basal ganglia. These lesions may also cause seizures and obsessional traits are most frequent in patients with frontal lobe epilepsy.
- Obsessions or compulsive behavior are rare ictal manifestations of seizures arising in the pre-frontal cortex or cingulate gyrus. Obsessions need to be differentiated from ictal forced thoughts, for which there is no feeling of impulse.
- Hypergraphia and pathological hyper-religiosity are seen in non-dominant temporal lobe epilepsy.

Violent and Criminal Behavior in Epilepsy

- The terms "episodic dyscontrol" or "intermittent explosive disorder" are used to describe patients who are generally not pre-disposed to aggressive behavior but who suffer discrete episodes of failure to resist aggressive impulses that are out of proportion to the stimulus. The condition may be due to seizures or to organic brain damage without epilepsy, particularly affecting frontal or temporal lobes. Other causes include primary psychosis, drugs or alcohol.
- Ictal or post-ictal confusion and agitation are the commonest reason for epilepsy sufferers to express violent behavior. The agitation may evolve into violence if well-meaning observers try inappropriate measures to restrain the patient. Spontaneous undirected violence towards property or persons in the vicinity of the patient may also occur. Ictal violence may be a particular problem for patients who suffer bouts of non-convulsive status epilepticus with a twilight state.
- Ictal automatisms may occasionally be violent. Frontal lobe seizures may cause bizarre and agitated motor activity (Case 7). Temporal lobe seizures, usually secondary to encephalitis or tumors may cause an intense feeling of fear, which is associated with agitated and violent behavior. Sometimes ictal automatic activity can vary according to external stimuli, giving the appearance of directed behavior. This is most commonly seen in frontal lobe epilepsy but may occur in temporal lobe epilepsy with spread of discharges to the frontal lobes. Truly directed aggression is very rare in epilepsy.
- Post-ictal psychosis may cause paranoia and thought disturbance, which may lead to violence and aggression, which can be relatively directed. In these patients there is a history of seizure clusters and normal mental state at other times.

Case History 7

A 25-year-old man had suffered a very severe road traffic accident at the age of 17. There had been severe frontal injury with cerebral edema, requiring craniectomy to relieve intracranial pressure. He made a remarkable recovery with no physical deficit and only mild mental changes. About three years after his injury, he started to suffer tonic–clonic seizures, which responded to carbamazepine. After two years, carbamazepine was withdrawn, following which two different types of attack started. The first were absences lasting two to four minutes, with no specific features. Every few months he suffered a different type of attack at night. In these he would get out of bed, run round the room and sometimes down the stairs. He pulled over furniture and pulled down the curtains. He was unresponsive during these episodes that lasted about five minutes. If his mother tried to restrain him he would hit out and say he was trying to find his brother who was married and lived elsewhere. In the morning he had no recollection of these events and felt remorse over his actions.

Was this Violent Behavior Due to Epilepsy?

This question is often asked of clinicians involved with epilepsy, sometimes in relation to acts of criminal violence. A number of factors may help in making the decision:

- Is there definite evidence of epilepsy? A violent episode is highly unlikely to be a first presentation of epilepsy.
- Have previous seizures been associated with abnormal behavior such as ictal agitation or post-ictal psychosis? Presence of these features increases the probability that violent behavior may be seizure-associated.
- If the patient is not amnesic for the event an epileptic cause is highly improbable.
- Was there a witnessed overt seizure around the time of the abnormal behavior?
- Did the patient try to conceal the act of violence or seek help? Seeking help makes a seizure more likely and concealment makes it less likely.
- How structured or planned was the abnormal behavior? Picking up a nearby knife is possible in a confusional state, washing off the blood and burying it in the garden implies too much planning for a confused state.
- Was there an obvious build-up of behavior? A patient who becomes increasingly irritated over a period of minutes to hours, because of some external trigger, then lashes out, is unlikely to have had a seizure.
- Previous antisocial personality and non-epileptic violent behavior are in favor of an alternative cause.

BIBLIOGRAPHY

Hermann BP, Seidenberg M, Bell B. Psychiatric comorbidity in chronic epilepsy: identification, consequences, and treatment of major depression. Epilepsia 2000;41 (Suppl. 2):S31–S41.

Krishnamoorthy ES, Trimble MR. Forced normalization: clinical and therapeutic relevance. Epilepsia 1999;40 (Suppl. 10):S57–S64.

Lambert MV, Robertson MM. Depression in epilepsy: etiology, phenomenology and treatment. Epilepsia 1999;40:S21–S47.

Matsuura M. Epileptic psychoses and anticonvulsant drug treatment. J Neurol Neurosurg Psychiatry 1999;67:231–233.

Mellers JD, Toone BK, Lishman WA. A neuropsychological comparison of schizophrenia and schizophrenia-like psychosis of epilepsy. Psychol Med 2000;30:325–335.

Monaco F, Ciolin A. Interactions between anticonvulsant and psychoactive drugs. Epilepsia 1999;40:S71–S76.

Moore DP. Partial seizures and interictal disorders: the neuropsychiatric elements. Oxford: Butterworth-Heinemann 1997.

Schmitz EB, Robertson MM, Trimble MR. Depression and schizophrenia in epilepsy: social and biological risk factors. Epilepsy Res 1999;35:59–68.

Torta R, Keller R. Behavioral, psychotic, and anxiety disorders in epilepsy: etiology, clinical features, and therapeutic implications. Epilepsia 1999;40 (Suppl. 10):S2-S20.

18

Social Aspects of Epilepsy

Epilepsy is characterized by periods of loss of control that create some real risks for patients, which need to be anticipated and perceived; there can also be imagined risks. The clinician must try to allay the fears of patients and relatives. Carers may require training in the emergency management of a patient's seizures, sometimes including the administration of emergency medication. Many social spheres need to be addressed, including education, work, hobbies, relationships, sexuality, marriage, parenting and driving. The problems of altered family dynamics and stigmatization spread beyond the patient to family members, employers, schools, and the wider community. All may need to be involved in education about a patient's condition. Specialist nurses and active organizations can provide help, advice and contact with other patients (Table 18.1). Social under-functioning is more prevalent in patients with epilepsy than in patients with equivalent physical problems due to other chronic diseases such as asthma or diabetes.

SOCIAL EFFECTS OF EPILEPSY

Predictors of Psychosocial Underfunctioning

- Biological aspects of the epilepsy partly determine the quality of life measures in some but not all studies. Most studies show an effect of learning disability but

Table 18.1. Useful Organizations

National Society for Epilepsy, Chalfont St Peter, Gerrards Cross, Bucks, SL9 ORJ, UK
A source of information for patients, relatives, health care professionals and other interested
  parties
UK Epilepsy Helpline tel 01494 601 400.
http://www.epilepsynse.org.uk/

British Epilepsy Association
A source of information for patients, relatives, health care professionals and other interested
  parties

Freephone UK Helpline on 0808 800 5050
http://www.epilepsy.org.uk/index.html

American Epilepsy Society. Mostly a source of information for clinicians
http://www.aesnet.org/

Drivers Medical Unit, DVLA, Swansea, SA99 1TU, UK
http://www.dvla.gov.uk/drivers/drivers.htm

Epilepsy bereaved? PO Box 1777, Bournemouth BH5 1YR, UK
Patient support group for relatives of those bereaved through epilepsy
http://www.bodley.ox.ac.uk/external/epilepsy/

---

epilepsy severity is not consistently found to be a determinant of quality of life
(QOL).

- Supportive family dynamics are important in enabling patients to cope with
  their epilepsy in most studies (Table 18.2). Supported patients with severe
  epilepsy may lead remarkably normal lives, whilst others with relatively mild
  epilepsy may become over-protected and socially isolated. For children this may
  inhibit education and social development.

Education

- School failure may affect one-third of intellectually normal children with
  epilepsy, and one-third may require special educational support. Organic complications of epilepsy and its cause (Chapter 16), and social consequences,
  including the attitudes of teachers towards epilepsy are important.
- Psychiatric support may be needed by nearly a quarter of children with epilepsy
  during the education years.

Employment

- In a UK community-based study the number of patients who were unemployed
  or permanently sick correlated strongly with seizure-severity (Table 18.3).
- Cultural differences mean that for example in Holland, seizure-free patients are
  relatively less disadvantaged than in the UK, although they may have lower
  salaries than other employees with equivalent qualifications.
- Lower educational achievement than the non-epileptic population contributes to
  unemployment.

Table 18.2. Some Factors in Determining Social Outcome in Epilepsy

Factor	Effect
Learning disability	Affects employment and reduces the chance of having a partner in adult life
Seizure-frequency	Correlates inversely with QOL measures*, physical and social functioning and positively with perceived stigmatization
Multiple seizure types	More than one seizure type is associated with worse QOL measures* worse physical and social functioning and perceived stigmatization
Young onset and long duration of epilepsy	These are generally correlated with poorer social development, higher unemployment and less chance of marriage
Cultural background	Patients from different backgrounds may suffer different levels of under-functioning. Europeans may fare best
Family support	Good family support confers a higher chance of successful psychosocial outcome and improves self-esteem
Coping strategies	Favorable, active coping strategies are correlated with lower perceived epilepsy severity and less psychological complaints than more passive approaches

*QOL (quality of life) measures include family relationships, friendships, employment, feelings about self, plans and ambitions, standard of living, mental health, energy/vitality and pain.

Table 18.3. Unemployment among Patients with Epilepsy (%)

Seizure Severity	Percentage Unemployed or on Long-Term Sick
Seizure-free	19
<1 seizure per month	35
>1 seizure per month	52

Leisure Activities

- Individuals with epilepsy are less likely to pursue leisure activities than the unaffected population because of lack of self-esteem and fear of seizures in company. Epilepsy sufferers engage in less physical activity and are less physically fit than the rest of the population.

Stigma of Epilepsy

- Epilepsy is a highly stigmatizing condition and connotations of demonic possession remain in some cultures.
- Half of patients across Europe feel stigmatized by their epilepsy and one-fifth feel severely stigmatized.
- Cross cultural differences are marked. Around 30 percent of patients feel stigmatized in Spain or Poland and over 60 percent in France or Greece (UK 52%).
- Factors associated with stigma include worry, negative feelings, long-term health problems, injuries and adverse effects of anti-epileptic drugs (AEDs).
- Perceived stigma is much greater than clear evidence of having being subjected to stigmatizing behavior in most studies.

- Prejudice against epilepsy varies greatly between cultures. In one study in China, 57 percent of parents objected to their children playing with a child with epilepsy, compared with 7 percent in Denmark. Sixteen percent of Chinese thought that epilepsy is a form of insanity compared with only 1 percent in Denmark.

Marriage and Fertility in Epilepsy

- Marriage rates are inversely correlated and divorce rates are positively correlated with epilepsy severity in the UK. In Ireland, marriage rates amongst hospital outpatients with epilepsy are only half those in the general population.
- Fertility of married women with epilepsy is only 60 to 80 percent of fertility of married women without epilepsy. Reasons probably include reduced sexual arousal and satisfaction, altered gonadal function, effects of AEDs and concern about the effects of AEDs or the effects of epilepsy on the ability to care for children.
- Fertility of married men with epilepsy is also reduced and low marriage rate is probably the major factor. Other factors may include impotence, either psychogenic or AED-related and reduced spermatogenesis due to increased follicle-stimulating hormone, from enzyme-inducing AEDs.

EPILEPSY AND DRIVING

- Driving regulations vary between countries but epilepsy usually means a temporary ban from driving. The responsibility of reporting the onset of epilepsy to the driving authorities (DVLA in the UK) rests with the patient in the UK but in some countries it is with the clinician. This probably leads patients to withhold information from their clinicians. However, even in the UK the duty of a clinician to the community overrides their duty of confidentiality if a patient puts others at risk by continuing to drive. A strategy is first to inform the patient in writing, giving them an opportunity to contact the DVLA themselves, before reporting them.
- UK regulations are summarized in Table 18.4. They are regularly updated by the DVLA and are available on their website (Table 18.1).
- Vasovagal syncope is the only form of blackout for which there is no ban and which does not have to be reported.
- Group 2 licences (heavy goods or passenger-carrying vehicles) generally require the patient to be free of attacks for at least 10 years without medication.
- The etiology of the seizures may modify the ruling. For example if there is a malignant tumor underlying the epilepsy a 2-year ban usually operates for a normal driving licence and a group 2 licence will probably be revoked permanently, even if the patient is seizure-free.
- All seizures are the same to the DVLA, no matter whether consciousness is lost or preserved and no matter how brief. For example morning myoclonus is a bar to driving. The only exception is seizures purely from sleep.
- Insurance companies should be informed as well as the DVLA.

Table 18.4. Summary of DVLA Guidelines for Epilepsy

Situation	Regulation for an Ordinary Driving Licence
Newly diagnosed epilepsy	Driving ban until 1 year after seizures have ceased
Recurrent blackouts of uncertain cause	Driving ban until 1 year after blackouts have ceased
Single blackout of uncertain cause with epileptic features e.g. tongue-biting.	Driving ban for 1 year
Blackout of uncertain cause with no epileptic features	Driving ban for 6 months
Single provoked seizure or bout of status epilepticus	Driving ban is discretionary, sometimes until six months after the seizure providing the cause has been removed unless alcohol or illicit drugs were implicated
Single provoked seizure related to alcohol or illicit drugs	Driving ban until 1 year after seizures have ceased. A medical report and urine toxicology may be required to confirm current drug status before a licence is issued
Recurring seizures whilst awake	Driving ban until 1 year after seizures have ceased
Recurring seizures whilst asleep (case)	Even if seizures continue to occur, a patient may resume driving where it has been established for at least 3 years that they only occur in sleep
Withdrawal of all medication in a seizure-free patient	The clinician should advise the patient not to drive until 6 months after completion of drug withdrawal

Case History

A 47-year-old woman presented with a convulsive seizure in sleep. She had experienced a seizure in sleep 8 years previously, at which time she had surrendered her driving licence. She had resumed driving 2 years later. She re-informed the DVLA. The two episodes counted as purely sleep-related seizures consistent over more than 3 years and she was allowed to continue to drive.

SITUATIONS OF RISK – ADVICE TO PATIENTS AND CARERS

Each seizure carries a small risk. There is probably a gradient of risk according to seizure type: idiopathic generalized epilepsy (IGE) absences and focal seizures with preserved awareness carry the lowest risk, and tonic, tonic–clonic or atonic seizures the greatest risk. A patient's seizures can occasionally evolve unpredictably into a more serious seizure type and this needs to be taken into account in advising patients. A balance needs to be struck between alarmist over-protection and sensible precautions. This will depend on the frequency of seizures, whether they are nocturnal or diurnal and whether there is an aura, which allows the patient to take evasive action (Tables 18.5 and 18.6).

Sports

- Some sports pose unacceptable risks such as motor sports or aerial sports.
- Some sports are completely safe.

Table 18.5. Advice to Patients and Carers During a Seizure

Auras	Patient can try to make themselves safe, lying down away from sharp or dangerous objects
During the seizure	Bystanders should remove dangerous objects, place head on a cushion; do not interfere with airway; call for help after 5 minutes of convulsion
During postictal drowsiness	Bystanders should place the patient in the recovery position; remove ill-fitting dentures; allow recovery and observe for 20 minutes or until patient is guarding their airway
During postictal agitation	Bystanders should only interfere with the patient if at risk; gently guide the patient away from danger; lock doors if necessary; stay with the patient until no longer at risk
Criteria for calling for help	Convulsive seizures lasting more than 5 minutes
	Two convulsive seizures without recovery between
	More than two focal seizures without full recovery between
	Severe injury or burn
	Respiratory disturbance
	Failure to recover to normal neurological function within 2 hours of tonic–clonic seizure (TCS)

Table 18.6. Precautions against Injury from Epilepsy

Kitchen	Use cooker guards or microwave cooking
	Hot tap temperature control devices
	Tea or coffee-makers rather than kettles
Bathroom	Shower rather than bathe
	Fill a bath only to 5 cm
	Wash when others in the house and do not lock the door
	Bathroom doors, which open outwards rather than inwards
Bedroom	Use a firm pillow to avoid suffocation
	Sleep on a mattress on the floor if seizures are very violent
Elsewhere	Avoid sharp or glass objects/ornaments
	Avoid unguarded fires
	Reinforced glass for windows and door panels

- Many sports such as swimming are intermediate. Patients should not swim alone and they probably should not swim in open waters where first aid is more difficult.
- Many sports have regulatory authorities that can give advice.
- When engaging in sport, someone in a position of responsibility, such as a life-guard, should be aware of the problem.

Social Activities

- Individuals with epilepsy should be able to engage fully in social activities.
- Sleep deprivation and alcohol withdrawal may trigger seizures in susceptible individuals, most commonly those with juvenile myoclonic epilepsy (JME) but also other forms of IGE. It is reasonable to advise patients to avoid binge drinking.
- Photosensitivity affects only about 3 percent of patients with epilepsy. An EEG with photic stimulation can reassure the great majority that stroboscopic disco lights will not trigger seizures.

Employment

- Few jobs are closed to epilepsy sufferers. Examples involve flying, driving or working relatively unprotected at heights or close to dangerous machinery. An employer in the UK has a duty to try and accommodate an employee with a disability, where possible.
- Fear of seizures may make some jobs particularly stressful, for example where the individual is on show as a musician or as a barrister in court.
- Misunderstanding of epilepsy in the workplace may be helped by education of colleagues.

Applying for Work

- In the intensity of competition for employment, epilepsy sufferers find it particularly difficult find to work. One line of advice is to recommend to patients not to mention their epilepsy on a job application form as it may prejudice their application. At interview the epilepsy should be mentioned. If an individual conceals their epilepsy then their rights are reduced and their employer may fire them after their first seizure at work.

Travel

- There is no restriction on travel for patients with epilepsy but it is advisable for them to be accompanied.
- Medication should be to hand at all times and it is useful to have a spare supply. It is sensible to check whether medication is available at the destination, especially if traveling for a long period.
- A doctor's letter may help clarify the problems if the patient requires medical advice abroad.
- Long-haul flights and jet lag may cause sleep deprivation and trigger seizures. A benzodiazepine may ensure good sleep and act as an AED for the journey. If this strategy is used, the patient should first try the drug at home on a "dummy run" to ensure there are no untoward effects.

BIBLIOGRAPHY

Baker GA, Brooks J, Buck D, Jacoby A. The stigma of epilepsy: a European perspective. Epilepsia 1999;41:98–104.

Baker GA, Jacoby A, Buck D, Stalgis C, Monnet D. Quality of life of people with epilepsy: a European study. Epilepsia 1997;38:353–362.

Bjørholt PG, Nakken KO, Røhme K, Hansen H. Leisure time habits and physical fitness in adults with epilepsy. Epilepsia 1990;31:83–87.

Carlton FS, Miller R, Nealeigh N, Sanchez N. The effects of perceived stigma and psychological over-control on the behavioural problems of children with epilepsy. Seizure 1997; 6:383–391.

Chi-Wan Lai, Xishung Huang, Yen-Huei C, Zhiquang Zhang, Goujon Liu, Meng-Zhang Yang. Survey of public awareness, understanding and attitudes to towards epilepsy in Henan province, China. Epilepsia 1990;31:182–187.

Collings JA, Chappel B. Correlates of employment history and employability in a British epilepsy sample. Seizure 1994;3:255–262.

Jacoby A, Baker GA, Steen N, Potts P, Chadwick DW. The clinical course of epilepsy and its psychosocial correlates: findings from a UK Community study. Epilepsia 1996;37:148–161.

Jensen R, Dam M. Public attitudes towards epilepsy in Denmark. Epilepsia 1992;33:459–463.

Lassouw G, Leffers P, De KM, Troost J. Epilepsy in a Dutch working population: are employees diagnosed with epilepsy disadvantaged? Seizure 1997;6:95–98.

Swinkels WAM, Shackleton, Kasteleijn-Nolst Trenit. Psychosocial impact of epileptic seizures in a Dutch epilepsy population: a comparative Washington Psychosocial Seizure Inventory study. Epilepsia 2000;41:1335–1341.

Index

Notes:

Case histories are indicated by references followed by (CH)

To save space in the index abbreviations have been used as on pages ix–xi

WITHDRAWN